The Art and Science of Brief Psychotherapies

A Practitioner's Guide

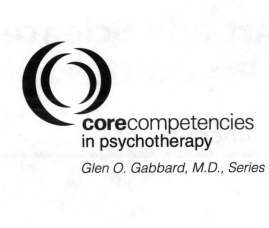

corecompetencies
in psychotherapy

Glen O. Gabbard, M.D., Series Editor

The Art and Science of Brief Psychotherapies

A Practitioner's Guide

Edited by

Mantosh J. Dewan, M.D.

Brett N. Steenbarger, Ph.D.

Roger P. Greenberg, Ph.D.

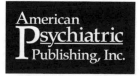

American Psychiatric Publishing, Inc.

Washington, DC
London, England

Note: The authors have worked to ensure that all information in this book is accurate at the time of publication and consistent with general psychiatric and medical standards, and that information concerning drug dosages, schedules, and routes of administration is accurate at the time of publication and consistent with standards set by the U.S. Food and Drug Administration and the general medical community. As medical research and practice continue to advance, however, therapeutic standards may change. Moreover, specific situations may require a specific therapeutic response not included in this book. For these reasons and because human and mechanical errors sometimes occur, we recommend that readers follow the advice of physicians directly involved in their care or the care of a member of their family.

Books published by American Psychiatric Publishing, Inc., represent the views and opinions of the individual authors and do not necessarily represent the policies and opinions of APPI or the American Psychiatric Association.

Copyright © 2004 American Psychiatric Publishing, Inc.
ALL RIGHTS RESERVED

Manufactured in the United States of America on acid-free paper
08 07 06 05 04   5 4 3 2 1
First Edition

Typeset in Adobe's Berling Roman and Frutiger 55 Roman

American Psychiatric Publishing, Inc.
1000 Wilson Boulevard
Arlington, VA 22209-3901
www.appi.org

Library of Congress Cataloging-in-Publication Data
The art and science of brief psychotherapies : a practitioner's guide / [edited by]
   Mantosh J. Dewan, Brett N. Steenbarger, Roger P. Greenberg.
     p. ; cm.
   Includes bibliographical references and index.
   ISBN 1-58562-067-X (pbk. : alk. paper)
     1. Brief psychotherapy. I. Dewan, Mantosh J. II. Steenbarger, Brett N.
   III. Greenberg, Roger P.
     [DNLM: 1. Psychotherapy, Brief—methods.   WM 420.5.P5 A784 2004]
   RC480.55.A78 2004
   616.89′14—dc22

                                                        2003065593

British Library Cataloguing in Publication Data
A CIP record is available from the British Library.

*With many thanks to our
patients, students, mentors, and families
for all they have taught us.*

*Mantosh J. Dewan, M.D.
Brett N. Steenbarger, Ph.D.
Roger P. Greenberg, Ph.D.*

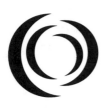

Contents

Part I
Six Key Brief Psychotherapies

Part II
Special Topics

Part III
Overview and Synthesis

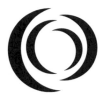

Contributors

Donald H. Baucom, Ph.D.
Professor and Director, Department of Psychology, University of North Carolina, Chapel Hill, North Carolina

Judith S. Beck, Ph.D.
Clinical Associate Professor of Psychology in Psychiatry, University of Pennsylvania; and Director, Beck Institute for Cognitive Therapy and Research, Philadelphia, Pennsylvania

Bernard Deitman, M.D.
Professor and Chair, Department of Psychiatry and Neurology, University of Missouri, Columbia, Missouri

Peter J. Bieling, Ph.D.
Assistant Professor, Department of Psychiatry and Behavioral Neurosciences, McMaster University, Hamilton, Ontario, Canada

Donald A. Bux Jr., Ph.D.
Research Associate, National Center on Addiction and Substance Abuse, Columbia University, New York, New York

Mantosh J. Dewan, M.D.

Professor and Chair, Department of Psychiatry and Behavioral Sciences, State University of New York, Upstate Medical University, Syracuse, New York

Rubén J. Echemendía, Ph.D.

Director, The Psychological Clinic, Department of Psychology, Pennsylvania State University, University Park, Pennsylvania

Norman B. Epstein, Ph.D.

Professor, Department of Family Studies, University of Maryland, College Park, Maryland

Edna B. Foa, Ph.D.

Professor and Director, Center for the Treatment and Study of Anxiety, Department of Psychiatry, University of Pennsylvania, Philadelphia, Pennsylvania

Roger P. Greenberg, Ph.D.

Professor and Head, Psychology Division, Department of Psychiatry and Behavioral Sciences, State University of New York, Upstate Medical University, Syracuse, New York

Elizabeth A. Hembree, Ph.D.

Assistant Professor, Center for the Treatment and Study of Anxiety, Department of Psychiatry, University of Pennsylvania, Philadelphia, Pennsylvania

Hanna Levenson, Ph.D.

Director, Levenson Institute for Training; and Director, Brief Psychotherapy Program, Department of Psychiatry, California Pacific Medical Center, San Francisco, California

John Manring, M.D.

Associate Professor and Director, Residency Training Program, Department of Psychiatry and Behavioral Sciences, State University of New York, Upstate Medical University, Syracuse, New York

Joël Núñez, Ph.D.

Graduate student, Department of Psychology, Pennsylvania State University, University Park, Pennsylvania

Deborah Roth, Ph.D.

Assistant Professor, Center for the Treatment and Study of Anxiety, Department of Psychiatry, University of Pennsylvania, Philadelphia, Pennsylvania

Brett N. Steenbarger, Ph.D.

Associate Professor, Department of Psychiatry and Behavioral Sciences, State University of New York, Upstate Medical University, Syracuse, New York

Scott Stuart, M.D.

Associate Professor and Co-Director, Iowa Depression and Clinical Research Center, Department of Psychiatry, University of Iowa, Iowa City, Iowa

Laura J. Sullivan, M.A.

Graduate student, Department of Psychology, University of North Carolina, Chapel Hill, North Carolina

Introduction to the Core Competencies in Psychotherapy Series

With the extraordinary progress in the neurosciences and psychopharmacology in recent years, some psychiatric training programs have deemphasized psychotherapy education. Many residents and educators have decried the loss of the "mind" in the increasing emphasis on the biological basis of mental illness and the shift toward somatic treatments as the central therapeutic strategy in psychiatry. This shift in emphasis has been compounded by the common practice in our managed care era of "split treatment," meaning that psychiatrists are often relegated to seeing the patient for a brief medication management session, while the psychotherapy is conducted by a mental health professional from another discipline. This shift in emphasis has created considerable concern among both psychiatric educators and the consumers of psychiatric education—the residents themselves.

The importance of psychotherapy in the training of psychiatrists has recently been reaffirmed, however, as a result of the widespread movement toward the establishment of core competencies throughout all medical specialties. In 1999 both the Accreditation Council for Graduate Medical Education (ACGME) and the American Board of Medical Specialties (ABMS) recognized that a set of organizing principles was necessary to measure competence in medical education. These six principles—patient care, medical knowledge, interpersonal and communication skills, practice-based learning and improvement, professionalism, and systems-based practice—are now collectively referred to as the *core competencies* in medical education.

This movement within medical education was a direct consequence of a broader movement launched by the U.S. Department of Education approximately 20 years ago. All educational projects, including those involving accreditation, had to develop outcome measures. Those entrusted with the training of physicians were no exception.

Like all medical specialties, psychiatry has risen to the occasion by making attempts to translate the notion of core competencies into meaningful psychiatric terms. The inherent ambiguity of a term like "competence" has sparked much discussion among psychiatric educators. Does the term mean that practitioners are sufficiently skilled that one would refer a family member to them for treatment without hesitation? Or does the term imply rudimentary knowledge and practice that would ensure a reasonable degree of safety? These questions are not yet fully resolved. The basic understanding of what is meant by core competencies will be evolving over the next few years as various groups within medicine and psychiatry strive to articulate reasonable standards for educators.

As of July 2002, the Psychiatry Residency Review Committee (RRC) mandated that all psychiatric residency training programs must begin implementing the six core competencies in clinical and didactic curricula. Those programs that fail to do so may receive citations when they undergo accreditation surveys. This mandate also requires training directors to develop more sophisticated means of evaluating the progress and learning of residents in their programs.

As part of the process of adapting the core competencies to psychiatry, the Psychiatry RRC felt that reasonable competence in five different forms of psychotherapy—long-term psychodynamic psychotherapy, supportive psychotherapy, cognitive behavioral psychotherapy, brief psychotherapy, and psychotherapy combined with psychopharmacology—should be an outcome of a good psychiatric education for all psychiatric residents.

Many training programs have had to scramble to find faculty who are well trained in these modalities and teaching materials to facilitate the learning process. American Psychiatric Publishing, Inc., felt that the publication of basic texts in each of the five mandated areas would be of great value to training programs. So in 2002 Dr. Robert Hales, editor-in-chief at American Psychiatric Publishing, appointed me to be the series editor of a new line of five books. This series is titled Core Competencies in Psychotherapy and features five brief texts by leading experts in each of the psychotherapies. Each volume covers the key principles of practice in the treatment and also suggests ways to evaluate whether residents have been trained to a level of competence in each of the therapies. (For more information about the books in this series and their availability, please visit www.appi.org.)

True expertise in psychotherapy requires many years of experience with skilled supervision and consultation. However, the basic tools can be learned during residency training so that freshly minted psychiatrists are prepared to deliver necessary treatments to the broad range of patients they encounter.

These books will be valuable adjuncts to the traditional methods of psychotherapy education: supervision, classroom teaching, and clinical experience with a variety of patients. We feel confident that mastery of the material in these five volumes will constitute a major step in the acquisition of competency in psychotherapy and, ultimately, the compassionate care of patients who come to us for help.

Glen O. Gabbard, M.D., Series Editor
Brown Foundation Chair of Psychoanalysis
Professor of Psychiatry
Director of Psychotherapy Education
Director, Baylor Psychiatry Clinic
Baylor College of Medicine
Houston, Texas

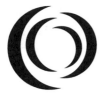

Introduction

Brett N. Steenbarger, Ph.D.
Roger P. Greenberg, Ph.D.
Mantosh J. Dewan, M.D.

For more than a decade, we have taught and supervised psychiatry residents and predoctoral interns in clinical psychology in the practice of the brief psychotherapies. Throughout that time, we lamented the absence of a single book that could guide the developing practitioner in learning the core concepts and skills of short-term work. Necessity spurring invention, we decided to pool our efforts and bridge this gap. In this book, you will learn about six eminently teachable and learnable models of brief psychotherapy and issues pertinent to their application. Our goal goes beyond a mere compilation of approaches. We hope that the following chapters provide you with a working sense of brief therapy as a whole: its science and its artistry.

How many times have we heard trainees in the mental health professions assert that they knew the theory but wanted guidance about what to *do* in the therapy room? In soliciting contributions from our authors, we challenged them to provide such practical guidance. We wanted to provide not only a book *about* brief therapy but also a guide to *doing* brief work. This means that our goal differs from that of many texts. We are not attempting to review all literature pertinent to short-term work, nor are we making any effort to cover all of the many schools of brief therapy in current use. Rather, we have selected a set of authors who are intimately involved in the teaching and training of brief therapy and who are uniquely qualified to supply readers with hands-on information about the practice of their chosen approaches. In making this selection, we sought to cover a variety of short-term models, emphasizing those that have found empirical support in the research literature and that can be readily learned. We present these models in the order that we have taught the brief therapies in the Department of Psychiatry and Behavioral Sciences at Upstate Medical University, Syracuse, New York, for more than a decade: cognitive, behavior, solution-focused, interpersonal, time-limited dynamic, and couple therapies. It has been our experience as educators that beginning with highly structured therapies is useful and reassuring to new therapists. Once they have internalized these structures, they feel more prepared to deviate from the manuals and make the improvisations that are necessary in the more fluid psychodynamic and couple therapies. Together, these modalities provide invaluable tools for handling the most common presenting concerns in private practice, clinic, and hospital settings.

We believe the authors have admirably shown that the practice of brief therapy is much more than the application of intuitively applied guidelines. Our task as editors has been to supplement their how-to expertise by highlighting the common themes behind the various chapters, providing readers with overarching principles and techniques to draw on in their own practice. Whether you are a beginning therapist wishing to learn more about brief therapy or an experienced clinician looking to expand your repertoire, we think you will find the chapters in this book to be excellent starting points.

Why Brief Therapy?

Never before in the history of psychotherapy have therapists been asked to do so much, so quickly. Tight economic conditions in community clinics, counseling centers, and hospitals—and especially among insurers—have guaranteed that most psychotherapy is swift and targeted. Indeed, surveys suggest that more than three-quarters of all therapists are conducting planned brief therapy and that such short-term work accounts for 40% of their clinical hours (Levenson 1995). Limited time and financial resources among patients also help to ensure that much therapy is brief. Indeed, even when the number of sessions is not limited by clinic policies or insurance constraints, the average number of sessions per client[1] tends to fall within parameters recognized as brief (Steenbarger and Budman 1998). If your clinical practice will include psychotherapy, it almost certainly will include brief therapy.

There are other reasons for developing knowledge and skills in brief work, however. One of the most important is that short-term therapies are proven effective in treating a wide range of emotional disorders (Barlow 2001; Dewan and Pies 2001; Koss and Shiang 1994; Steenbarger 1992). Furthermore, brief therapies not only treat symptoms and dysfunction as effectively as medications but also change brain function in a comparable manner. This has been shown in studies of behavior therapy for obsessive-compulsive disorder and with interpersonal therapy for depression (Baxter et al. 1992; Brody et al. 2001). Although the trajectory for change over time hinges on a variety of variables—including the outcome measures used, the patient population, and the points at which outcomes are assessed—it nonetheless seems clear that many adjustment, anxiety, mood, and relationship problems can be successfully treated with brief therapy (Steenbarger 1994). As several authors have observed, the vast majority of outcome studies in psychotherapy have been conducted with short-term interventions, making most of the literature a literature on brief therapy outcomes.

A third, and more personal, reason for learning brief therapy is that it opens the door to creative, as well as efficacious, ways of assisting individuals and couples. A common refrain in the practice literature is the role of therapist activity in short-term work. As time frames for intervention narrow, the therapist assumes a more hands-on, active stance in catalyzing change. This frequently entails reframing presenting issues, creating therapeutic experiences within sessions, assigning homework tasks, and teaching coping skills. Many trainees tell us that they find such work particularly rewarding because it challenges them to make the most of each session and draw on novel strategies for dislodging problem patterns and instilling promising new ones. It is not unusual for a brief therapist to integrate interventions drawn from many approaches, including cognitive, behavioral, interpersonal, and strategic. This variety lends spice to the daily challenge of helping people change their lives.

---

[1]In deference to the fact that people seeking therapeutic assistance do so in both medical and nonmedical settings, the terms *patient* and *client* will be used interchangeably in this chapter.

What Is Brief Therapy?

Defining *brief therapy* is every bit as difficult as conducting it. The brevity of behavior therapy—often concluding in fewer than 10 sessions—is not the brevity of cognitive restructuring work, which frequently extends from 10 to 20 sessions. Adding to the confusion, we commonly find short-term psychodynamic therapies lasting 20 sessions or more and solution-focused treatments lasting 3 or fewer sessions. Health maintenance organization plans typically limit the mental health benefit to 20 outpatient sessions annually, which, by some definitions, would make all therapy brief!

A further dilemma occurs when sessions are distributed intermittently, allowing for extended time between sessions to rehearse skills and consolidate changes. It is not unusual for brief therapists to hold fewer than 10 sessions with a patient spaced out over a 12-month period. Is such work brief or long-term?

For all of these reasons, it may make greater sense to define *brevity* by clinician intent rather than by an absolute number of sessions. Some elements in this intent include

- *Planning*—Short-term work is brief by design rather than by default (Budman and Gurman 1988), with planned strategies for accelerating change.
- *Efficiency*—The goal of the brief therapist is time-effectiveness: efficiency in achieving a particular set of objectives (Budman 1994). A 20-session course of treatment for a client with a personality disorder may be more time-effective than a 10-session course of therapy for an adjustment concern.
- *Focus*—The clinician and client seek focused changes in short-term work rather than broad personality change. The therapist takes responsibility for actively maintaining this focus and ensuring that it is a mutual one.
- *Patient selection*—As we will see later in this chapter, brief therapy is not appropriate for all patients and disorders, placing the responsibility on the therapist to screen individuals before initiating short-term work.

In short, we can think of interventions falling within the broad designation of brief therapy when time is an explicit consideration in treatment planning (Steenbarger 2002), placing the therapist in the role of actively stimulating and encouraging change. The intent and orientation of the therapist, rather than adherence to a session limit, characterize brevity.

When Is It Appropriate to Conduct Brief Therapy?

A review of the practice of, as well as research on, short-term work indicates several potential indications and contraindications (Steenbarger 1994, 2002; Steenbarger and Budman 1998). Some of these include

1. *Duration of the presenting problem*—When a problem pattern is chronic, it has been overlearned and often will require more extensive intervention than a pattern that is recent and situational.
2. *Interpersonal history*—For therapy to proceed time-effectively, a rapid alliance between therapist and patient is a necessity. If the client's interpersonal history includes significant incidents of abuse, neglect, or violence, it may take many sessions before adequate trust and disclosure can develop.
3. *Severity of the presenting problem*—A severe disorder is one that interferes with many aspects of the client's life. Such severity often also interferes with the individual's ability to actively use therapeutic strategies between sessions, a key element in accelerating change.
4. *Complexity*—A highly complex presenting concern, one that has many symptomatic manifestations, often requires more extensive intervention than highly focal problem patterns. For instance, a client who presents with an eating disorder may be abusing drugs and alcohol and experiencing symptoms of depression. Often, such complex presentations require a combination of helping approaches—psychotherapeutic and psychopharmacological—to address each of the problem components, extending the duration of treatment.
5. *Understanding*—Brief therapy tends to be most helpful for patients who have a clear understanding of their problems and a strong motivation to address these. In situations in which people's readiness to change is low (Prochaska et al. 1994), they enter therapy denying the need for change, being unclear about the changes they need to make, or having ambivalence over the need for change. As a result, they may require many weeks of exploratory therapy and self-discovery before they are ready to make a commitment to more action-oriented, short-term approaches.
6. *Social support*—Many clients enter therapy not only to make changes in their personal and interpersonal lives but also to obtain ongoing social support. This is particularly true of individuals who are socially isolated because of a lack of social skills and/or fears of rejection and abandonment. Although social support is a necessary and legitimate

end of psychotherapy, situations requiring extensive support will necessarily preclude highly abbreviated courses of treatment. Indeed, clients who are particularly sensitive to interpersonal loss may find it impossible to tolerate a therapy in which a working bond is quickly dissolved.

These six criteria, which form the acronym *DISCUS*, represent a useful heuristic for trainees first learning the brief psychotherapies. Whereas the presence of any single factor may not preclude short-term work, such presence often will require longer-term intervention within the range of treatments normally associated with brevity. The presence of multiple DISCUS criteria at client intake is almost certain to identify a situation in which highly abbreviated treatment will raise the odds of future relapse (Steenbarger 1994).

That having been said, we note that brief therapeutic strategies are finding wide application to chronically ill populations, even as part of longer-term intervention. Thanks to pioneering work on cognitive-behavioral therapy with borderline patients (Linehan et al. 2001), there is increased interest in treating chronic, complex, and severe disorders with a series of targeted brief therapies rather than single, ongoing long-term treatments. In Linehan's work, for instance, skills training for reducing suicidal behaviors and behaviors that interfere with therapy and quality of life may be followed by exposure-based strategies for reducing posttraumatic stress and cognitive work for resolving life problems and increasing self-respect. By stringing together brief therapies with specific targets, each of which addresses a particular facet of a syndrome, short-term work becomes useful with even the most challenging patient populations.

Because the brief therapies require a high degree of activity for both parties, it is generally helpful to assess the ability and willingness of the patient to engage in such hands-on efforts at change. Many brief modalities require individuals to reexperience their problems, even as they rehearse coping strategies. This may be more than some can or wish to tolerate. An initial set of experiential exercises and/or homework assignments is often an effective way of determining a client's appropriateness for active, short-term work. Successful and enthusiastic completion of an initial in-session or homework task is an excellent prognostic sign for compliance with the demands of short-term work.

The briefest of the brief therapies—solution-focused and behavioral approaches—are often used for focal problems of adjustment, anxiety, grief, and relationship conflicts. Longer-standing and more pervasive concerns—depression and eating disorders, for example—are frequently addressed by the lengthier of the brief schools, such as cognitive restructuring and short-term dynamic therapy. When brief methods are brought to bear on the most chronic and severe problems—including personality disorders—they are generally components of longer-term treatment or modules within overarching treatment and rehabilitation plans. Although not all problems can be solved briefly, it is difficult to find disorders for which short-term methods do not have value.

What Makes Brief Therapies Brief?

A major theme in this book, which we elaborate in Chapter 12, is that brief therapies owe their brevity to an intensification of the elements that facilitate change in *all* psychotherapies (Steenbarger 1992; Steenbarger and Budman 1998). In other words, brief therapy is not wholly different from time-unlimited treatment, just as lightning chess is closely allied to its traditional counterpart. For the therapist, however, doing brief work can *feel* quite different from undertaking longer-term therapy, much as the experience of driving laps in a race car differs from the experience of regular open-highway driving.

Perhaps the greatest shift of mind-set that helps to abbreviate the change process is the therapist's assumption of responsibility for making things happen in brief therapy. Shorn of the luxury of time to work through client resistances and historical antecedents of current problems, the short-term clinician actively avoids resistance by maximizing the alliance, framing treatment approaches and goals in ways that can be readily assimilated by the client. Moreover, once an agreement is reached as to the means and ends of therapy, the brief therapist takes an active role in both evoking client patterns and introducing ways of interrupting and modifying these. In a very important sense, nondirective brief therapy is an oxymoron. At its best, short-term work is a copiloting, with both client and clinician taking active roles in navigating change.

If brief therapy truly is an intensification of change processes found in all of the empirically supported therapies,[2] then our first question becomes "How do people change in *any* therapy?"

We have found a schematic of the change process, grounded in the process and outcome literatures of psychotherapy, to be especially helpful for trainees learning short-term work (Steenbarger 1992; Steenbarger

---

[2]We would further submit that therapy itself is an intensification of the change processes encountered in everyday life.

and Budman 1998). This schematic emphasizes three phases of therapeutic change:

1. *Engagement*—This opening phase of therapy features a development
   of a favorable working alliance between therapist and patient, a ven-
   tilation of client concerns and gathering of information by the clinician, a search for patterns among the presenting concerns, and a
   creation of a treatment plan to address these patterns.
2. *Discrepancy*—In therapy, as in chess, the opening moves tend to be
   highly circumscribed, giving way to a more freely flowing mid-game.
   In the middle phase of therapy, maladaptive client patterns that appear in their daily lives and/or in their therapy sessions become a focus
   for change. The therapist aids in the discovery of new, constructive
   ways of thinking and behaving that are discrepant from these maladaptive patterns and encourages their exploration and possible adoption.
3. *Consolidation*—Once the client recognizes his or her maladaptive patterns and identifies promising new, discrepant modes of thinking,
   feeling, and interacting, the goal of therapy becomes a consolidation
   of these new patterns. This can entail repeated application of the new
   insights, skills, and experiences to daily-life situations, including situations encountered in the therapy office. In "working through" past
   patterns and finding constructive replacements, the patient is able to
   internalize and maintain a new behavioral, interpersonal, and emotional repertoire.

As we shall see in Chapter 12, what makes the different approaches to
therapy unique is their implementation of these three phases. Some focus
more on the present, whereas others focus on the past and present. Some
emphasize interactions with the therapist as a primary locus of change
efforts; others stress out-of-session experiences. Some tend to define
broader treatment goals; others use more targeted, focal ones.

Identifying this common process underlying all therapies helps us understand what brief therapists do to help abbreviate treatment. Brief
therapy, it appears, takes advantage of the fact that learning under emotional circumstances is more enduring than learning tackled in ordinary
states of experiencing (Greenberg et al. 1993). By actively evoking problem patterns, brief therapists afflict the comfort of their clients, heightening their emotional experience. Once in this heightened state, individuals are more open to processing new ways of thinking, feeling, behaving,
and relating to others. Indeed, we submit that the various schools of
short-term work simply represent different means to the same end: accelerated learning in nonordinary states of awareness (Steenbarger 2002).

This formulation helps to explain why brief work is not appropriate for some clients. Individuals at risk for regression and decompensation in the face of stress may not tolerate the elicitation of symptoms that is key to brevity. They may require supportive interventions that build defenses, not challenges to those already present. A careful history at the outset of therapy is essential to discriminate between those clients who can benefit from an afflicting of their comfort and those who require comfort from their afflictions. Trial interventions under carefully controlled, in-session conditions, such as guided imagery exercises in which a patient must evoke a recent troubling event, can be useful in ascertaining the degree to which brief work is likely to be helpful or harmful.

Finally, we would be remiss if we did not point out that brief therapy is often brief precisely because of patient selection criteria that are typically used. Outcomes in any kind of therapy are most likely to be rapid and favorable if clients are motivated for change, actively engaged with their therapists, and free from chronic and severe symptoms that would interfere with the ability to sustain change efforts. Prudent adherence to the indications and contraindications of brief work will ensure the best outcomes for all patients.

How Can Brief Therapy Be Learned?

A classic prescription for medical education is "see one, do one, teach one." In the case of acquiring competence in brief therapy, we might modify the formulation to "read one, see one, do one." In the chapters that follow, practitioners with considerable experience in training mental health professionals in brief work will take you through their favored approaches step by step. You will be able to read about the therapies and why particular interventions are used. You will also be able to see how those approaches are implemented through illustrative case material. The idea is to describe not only what to do but also why to do it, so that you can start thinking like a brief therapist in your own work.

Although individual chapters may not always provide enough read-one, see-one experience to jump in and do one, our hope is that they will provide a solid foundation for further training efforts: workshops, direct supervision, and specialized readings and videotapes. In an important sense, the change process for therapists is no different from that among patients. We, too, come to our profession with patterns, and sometimes these prove limiting. A good book on therapy—like good supervision— needs to provide elements of discrepancy and consolidation, challenging those old patterns and juxtaposing them with promising alternatives. As you read through the various case histories and examples, try to think through how you would normally tackle such cases. Then examine how the authors proceeded and how their work differs from your own. The discrepancy may prove jarring at first, but it also may open the door to new ways of thinking about and responding to your clients.

With enough exposure—book reading, observation, supervision—you will start to think differently about your clinical work. Formerly foreign thoughts will creep into your mind, such as "How can I make this happen?" To be sure, therapy will always be a joint enterprise, requiring the consistent efforts of both parties. To date, however, practitioners have relied perhaps too much on talking as a sole source of cure. People change by *doing* things differently and by internalizing those experiences. Recognition of the ways in which we can catalyze change has the potential to invigorate our work and extend our repertoire. Brief treatment is not less of the same; it is a distillation and an intensification of what has worked all along. There is an art to working briefly, and there is a science. We hope that these chapters are a useful starting point in learning both.

References

Barlow DH: Clinical Handbook of Psychological Disorders: A Step-by-Step Treatment Manual, 3rd Edition. New York, Guilford, 2001

Baxter LR, Schwartz JM, Bergman KS, et al: Caudate glucose metabolic rate changes with both drug and behavior therapy for obsessive-compulsive disorder. Arch Gen Psychiatry 49:681–689, 1992

Brody AL, Saxena S, Stoessel P, et al: Regional brain metabolic changes in patients with major depression treated with either paroxetine or interpersonal therapy: preliminary findings. Arch Gen Psychiatry 58:631–640, 2001

Budman SH: Treating Time Effectively. New York, Guilford, 1994

Budman SH, Gurman AS: Theory and Practice of Brief Therapy. New York, Guilford, 1988

Dewan MJ, Pies RW (eds): The Difficult-to-Treat Psychiatric Patient. Washington, DC, American Psychiatric Press, 2001

Greenberg LS, Rice LN, Elliott R: Facilitating Emotional Change: The Moment-by-Moment Process. New York, Guilford, 1993

Koss MP, Shiang J: Research on brief psychotherapy, in Handbook of Psychotherapy and Behavior Change, 4th Edition. Edited by Bergin AE, Garfield SL. New York, Wiley, 1994, pp 664–700

Levenson H: Time-Limited Dynamic Psychotherapy: A Guide to Clinical Practice. New York, Basic Books, 1995

Linehan MM, Cochran BN, Kehrer CA: Dialectical behavior therapy for borderline personality disorder, in Clinical Handbook of Psychological Disorders, 3rd Edition. Edited by Barlow DH. New York, Guilford, 2001, pp 470–522

Prochaska JO, Norcross JC, DiClemente CC: Changing for Good. New York, Avon, 1994

Steenbarger BN: Toward science-practice integration in brief counseling and therapy. The Counseling Psychologist 20:403–450, 1992

Steenbarger BN: Duration and outcome in psychotherapy: an integrative review. Prof Psychol Res Pr 25:111–119, 1994

Steenbarger BN: Brief therapy, in Encyclopedia of Psychotherapy. Edited by Hersen M, Sledge W. New York, Elsevier, 2002, pp 349–358

Steenbarger BN, Budman SH: Principles of brief and time-effective therapies, in Psychologists' Desk Reference. Edited by Koocher GP, Norcross JC, Hill SS. New York, Oxford University Press, 1998, pp 283–287

Part I

Six Key Brief Psychotherapies

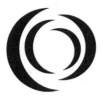

2

Cognitive Therapy

Introduction to Theory and Practice

Judith S. Beck, Ph.D.
Peter J. Bieling, Ph.D.

Cognitive therapy is an empirically validated form of brief psychotherapy that has been shown to be effective in more than 350 outcome studies for a myriad of psychiatric disorders, including depression, generalized anxiety disorder, panic, social phobia, obsessive-compulsive disorder, posttraumatic stress disorder, bulimia, and substance abuse. It is currently being tested for personality disorders as well. Several studies have documented its effectiveness as an adjunctive treatment to medication for serious mental disorders such as bipolar disorder and schizophrenia. It has been extended to and studied for adolescents and children, couples, and families (A. T. Beck and Weishaar 2000). It also has been applied and found effective in the treatment of medical disorders such as chronic fatigue syndrome, hypertension, fibromyalgia, post–myocardial infarction depression, noncardiac chest pain, cancer, diabetes, migraine, and other chronic pain conditions (White and Freeman 2000).

Aaron T. Beck, M.D., developed cognitive therapy in the mid-1960s. The first cognitive therapy outcome study of unipolar depression was published in 1977. Since that time, cognitive therapy has seen tremendous interest and growth. As of 2001, psychiatric residents in the United States are required to show competence in cognitive therapy. Several cognitive therapy training centers have been established around the world, and the Academy of Cognitive Therapy has been formed to certify individuals as cognitive therapists.

Cognitive therapy is a comprehensive system of psychotherapy, with an operationalized treatment based on an elaborate and empirically supported theory of psychopathology. In this chapter, we examine the roots of cognitive therapy, describing its origin and its theory of psychiatric disturbance. The cognitive model of psychological functioning and psychopathology is described to provide the reader with a theoretical foundation for understanding principles of therapy, case formulation, conceptualization of individual patients, treatment planning, general strategies, and common techniques. Depression and anxiety disorders are emphasized, and a case example, used throughout the chapter, is elaborated on at the end of the chapter.

Origins of Cognitive Therapy

Cognitive therapy is a short-term structured therapy that uses an information-processing model as the key to understanding and ameliorating psychopathological conditions. According to A. T. Beck and Weishaar (2000), the theory is based, in part, on a phenomenological approach to psychology, as espoused by Epictetus and other Greek Stoic philosophers and more contemporary theorists, including Adler, Alexander, Horney, and Sullivan. This approach emphasizes the role of individuals' views of themselves and their personal worlds as being central to their behavioral reactions. Kelly's description of individuals' personal constructs and beliefs helped shape cognitive theory, as did Arnold's and Lazarus's cognitive theories of emotion.

The identification of *cognition* as the critical element in psychopathology was a revolutionary view in the 1960s because psychoanalytic theory and therapy dominated the treatment of psychopathology at the time. In fact, Beck had trained in and practiced psychoanalysis. In the late 1950s and early 1960s, he conducted a series of experimental studies that he predicted would support psychoanalytic constructs but found the opposite to be true. He failed, for example, to find empirical support for the theory that depression resulted from inner-directed or retroflected anger.

Through further experimentation and a great deal of clinical observation, he began to conclude that a key element in depression was the negatively biased judgments patients had of themselves, particularly their negative thoughts about themselves, their worlds, and their futures.

Beck drew on the work of many other influential theorists, including Ellis, whose rational-emotive therapy posited that irrational beliefs were the basis of psychological dysfunction. Beck also was influenced by the other prevailing school of psychology at the time: behaviorism. Theorists such as Bandura, Lewinsohn, Mahoney, and Meichenbaum were influential, as were the burgeoning behavioral and cognitive-behavioral approaches: social learning, stress inoculation training, problem-solving training, and self-control therapy.

Cognitive Theory of Psychopathology

At the most superficial level, the *cognitive model* states that people's perceptions or spontaneous thoughts about situations influence their emotional and behavioral (and often physiological) reactions. When individuals are distressed, many of their perceptions are incorrect and dysfunctional to some degree. By learning to identify and evaluate their spontaneously occurring thoughts, they can correct their thinking so that it more closely resembles reality. When patients do so, they generally feel better and behave more functionally. Especially in patients with anxiety, physiological arousal is also decreased.

Ms. A, a depressed woman, will be used throughout this chapter as a case example. She had numerous distorted thoughts that led to sad, hopeless feelings and dysfunctional behavior. The following vignette illustrates the cognitive model:

> Almost every day when Ms. A returned to her apartment after work, opened the door, and noticed the disarray [situation], she thought, "I'm a total basket case. I'll never get my act together" [automatic thoughts]. She felt very sad [emotion] and heavy in her body [physiological reaction]. Then she lay down on the sofa, without even taking off her coat [behavior] (Figure 2–1).

According to A. T. Beck (1963), individuals show characteristic patterns or themes in their thinking. The idea of helplessness and inadequacy was prominent in Ms. A's perceptions. When she arrived late at work one day (an infrequent occurrence), she thought, "I can't do anything right." When she discovered a bill she had forgotten to pay, she thought, "I'm so stupid. I can't believe I did that." When her kitchen sink

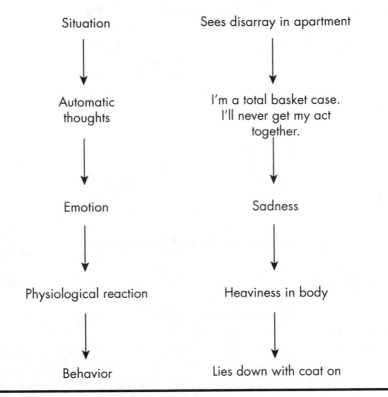

Figure 2–1. The cognitive model.

leaked, she thought, "I don't know what to do." It was apparent that Ms. A had a basic or core belief: "I am helpless and inadequate." This belief shaped her perception of her experience. She distorted reality by processing information in light of this belief, interpreting even neutral situations negatively and ignoring or discounting (positive) evidence to the contrary.

In a psychopathological state, individuals typically hold negative *core beliefs* about themselves that fall into one of two broad categories: those related to helplessness and those related to unlovability (J.S. Beck 1995; see Table 2–1). Helpless beliefs are expressed in various ways, each with a somewhat different nuance. Patients may believe that they are powerless, vulnerable, out of control, ineffective, weak, or inferior in achievement. Patients with a belief that they are unlovable may state that they are defective, bad, unworthy, or likely to be rejected and abandoned. Some patients hold beliefs in both categories.

Patients with straightforward depression and anxiety disorders, who were psychologically healthy before the onset of their disorder, may have

Table 2–1. Categories of core beliefs

Helpless	Unlovable
I am incompetent.	I am unlikable.
I am a failure.	I am ugly.
I am powerless.	I am bad.
I am weak.	I am evil.
I am vulnerable.	I will be rejected.
I am trapped.	I will be abandoned.
I am out of control.	I am different.
I am inferior.	I am worthless (so I won't be loved).
I am worthless (because I don't produce).	There is something wrong with me (so I won't be loved).
I am defective. (I don't measure up.)	I am defective (so I won't be loved).
I'm not good enough. (I don't measure up.)	I'm not good enough (so I won't be loved).

Source. Adapted from J.S. Beck 1995.

had relatively positive or benign beliefs about themselves throughout their lives (e.g., "I am reasonably adequate"; "I am reasonably lovable.") Their negative beliefs may be activated only during the course of their disorder. Patients with personality disorders, in contrast, may have had negative beliefs activated more or less continuously throughout their lives. Negative beliefs about the self in Axis II patients usually originated in developmental experiences in which the child negatively construed events relevant to himself or herself (J.S. Beck 1997).

As she was growing up as a young adolescent and adult, Ms. A had significant traits of dependence. She was often expected to perform tasks that were beyond her developmental capability. She began to view herself as inadequate (not recognizing, of course, that she was generally an adequate child who was being told she had to accomplish unreasonably difficult tasks). A series of experiences such as these at home, as well as a slight learning disability that hindered her achievement at school, led to the development of her negative belief. Soon she became hypervigilant for perceived signs of inadequacy and began, at times, to see herself as inadequate, even when she clearly was not. Because Ms. A believed so strongly that she was inadequate, she began to act inadequately at times.

Patients' dysfunctional reactions to situations make sense given how they perceive themselves, others, and their worlds. Whenever her belief of incapability was activated, Ms. A had a series of automatic thoughts with that theme. These thoughts affected her not only emotionally and physiologically but also behaviorally. Because Ms. A believed that she was incapable, she avoided tasks she found challenging, avoided making decisions for fear she would inevitably make mistakes with serious consequences, and gave up easily when a task proved to be difficult.

Many dysfunctional behaviors of patients have consistent patterns. Depressed patients show avoidance and isolation; anxious patients are hypervigilant for threat (A.T. Beck 1967). If these patients have a good premorbid history, they may show dysfunctional patterns of behavior primarily during an acute episode. Axis II patients, in contrast, have lifelong patterns of dysfunction. To compensate for or cope with a very rigid, global, negative self-view, these patients often overdevelop a small set of behaviors, or *compensatory strategies*, to get along in the world. And they fail to develop a full repertoire of behaviors that are adaptive in many situations (J.S. Beck 1998).

Ms. A, like many patients with strong Axis II features, developed over time some assumptions to guide her behavior and protect her from the activation of her core beliefs, such as "If I avoid challenges, I won't fail" and "If I rely on others, I'll be okay." She also developed the opposite for each belief: "If I take on a challenge, my inadequacy will show" and "If I rely on myself, I'll make terrible mistakes and have a bad life."

Thus, the cognitive model explains individuals' emotional, physiological, and behavioral responses as mediated by their automatic thoughts. Perceptions of experience, which are influenced by core beliefs, play a central role in one's characteristic ways of interacting with the world.

According to cognitive theory, core beliefs are stored in mental structures called *schemas*. Cognitive theory posits that the processing of information is crucial for the survival of any organism. Given that the number of external stimuli in the environment is practically infinite, organisms need to be able to filter out the most relevant information if they are to survive and thrive. Schemas are responsible for processing, storing, and retrieving information, such as people's perceptions of themselves and others, their goals and expectations, memories, fantasies, and previous learning (A.T. Beck 1964).

Schemas vary in their density, breadth, permeability, and salience (A.T. Beck et al. 1990). They have specific content in the form of beliefs, assumptions, and rules. Because schemas are flexible to some degree, they may be altered by experience, particularly by carefully designed learning experiences in therapy (Clark et al. 1999).

Two kinds of schemas operate within the individual's information-processing system. *Constructive schemas*, which are under conscious control, consist of personal goals and guiding principles of society. These guide productive, goal-oriented activity. They are relatively flexible, accessible, and elaborated and facilitate problem solving, rational thought, and creativity. *Primal schemas*, in contrast, are rigid, absolute, unelaborated, and evolutionarily linked to survival. Processing tends to occur at an automatic, or preconscious, level. Because they are associated with ensuring basic organismic needs (preservation, dominance, sociability, and reproduction), they tend to dominate the information-processing system when they are activated (Clark et al. 1999).

When a primal schema is activated, the individual tends to process information in a distorted way. When Ms. A was depressed, she saw evidence of what she believed was her fundamental inadequacy everywhere. She continually noted tasks at work that were more difficult for her. She blamed herself for not keeping her apartment in order. She was self-critical of her procrastination in buying food and returning telephone calls. Rather than understanding that her behavior reflected a psychiatric illness, she instead construed her actions as a reflection of her incompetence.

At the same time, when primal schemas are activated, the individual tends to process positive information in a different way, discounting or ignoring it. Ms. A began to focus on only the tasks at work that she did not complete, or did not complete well enough, in her estimation. She failed to recognize the tasks that she did well. Even when they were called to her attention, she discounted her successes: "Those things were easy to do. Anyone could have done them." While Ms. A exaggerated the importance of her perceived weaknesses, she minimized her accomplishments ("So what if I finally got my taxes done. It took me long enough."). Initially, Ms. A was not aware of her tendency to interpret information in this biased way. Once her therapist pointed it out, however, she understood the concept and was able to learn to correct her thinking.

Schemas are cognitive, behavioral, affective, motivational, and physiological in nature. Clusters of schemas activated together are called *modes* (A. T. Beck 1996). The cognitive underpinnings of psychopathology are rooted at a primal level at which information processing is dominated by primary modes. In an anxiety mode, for example, themes of threat are hypervalent. Patients view themselves or others as vulnerable to harm, perhaps weak. They feel anxious and fearful. Their systems become physiologically aroused to deal with perceived threat. They are motivated to act in a way to reduce threat, and if the threat is perceived as sufficiently severe, they may run, escape, freeze, or fight.

In a depressive mode, on the other hand, individuals see themselves, their worlds, and their future in a very negative light. They are dominated by ideas of loss or deprivation. They feel sad, empty, hopeless, and guilty. Their motivation for productive activity decreases significantly. They feel weighed down, heavy, and slow. Their behavior becomes markedly impaired as they isolate themselves and avoid (Clark et al. 1999).

How do modes become activated? Triggers of psychiatric symptoms involve individuals' interpretations of their experiences. The *diathesis–stress* model posits that not all negative events lead to depression, even in vulnerable individuals. Instead, the depressive mode is activated when the type of negative stressor that has occurred matches the person's underlying vulnerability. A person with a latent schema of unlovability may become depressed following the breakup of a relationship. An individual with a schema of inferiority may become depressed following a demotion at work. A recent comprehensive review found considerable empirical support for the diathesis stress model of depression (Clark et al. 1999).

Ms. A, for example, experienced several serious losses when her husband left her for another woman. She had lost her partner of 20 years, one who had provided financial, emotional, and practical support. She experienced this as a severe blow to her self-esteem. She began to view herself as even more incapable than usual (and, to a lesser degree, as unlovable), even though from a rational viewpoint, there was evidence to the contrary. Her motivation to act productively declined. She developed physiological signs of depression; she began to have difficulty sleeping, felt weighed down, and experienced a loss of energy. She interpreted her lack of motivation, her changed behavior, and her lack of energy in a negative light—as evidence that she was lazy, irresponsible, and inadequate. Soon she began to lose interest and pleasure in everyday activities and events. She began to isolate socially and was thus deprived of social support. Her depressive mode was fully activated, and she developed a full-blown major depression.

Principles of Cognitive Therapy

The overall aim of cognitive therapy is to help patients achieve a remission of their disorder by solving problems and reducing symptoms. This is achieved through a collaborative, empirical approach, which teaches patients to view reality more clearly through an examination of their central, distorted cognitions. Correcting their faulty ideas leads to improvement in mood and functioning. A summary of the basic principles of cognitive therapy is provided below.

During initial assessment, the practice of cognitive therapy involves a cognitive formulation of patients' disorders and an ongoing individualized *cognitive conceptualization* of patients and their difficulties. An accurate conceptualization helps the therapist to organize the multitude of data presented by the patient to identify the patient's most central dysfunctional cognitions and behaviors. It allows the therapist to select key thoughts, beliefs, and behaviors to target for change. The concepts described earlier concerning the general cognitive model are applied to patients' idiosyncratic presenting problems. J.S. Beck (1995) described different time frames for this formulation process. The first is the patient's thinking, emotional reactions, and problematic behaviors at the current time. The second involves the precipitating factors, the unique stressors or events that triggered the current episode. The third is particularly important in the treatment of personality disorders; a developmental framework is used to understand how early life events and experiences led to the development of core beliefs, underlying assumptions, and compensatory behaviors.

Figure 2–2 depicts how therapists organize data derived from the patient to complete a *cognitive conceptualization diagram*. The case of Ms. A is used as an example; the bottom half of the diagram illustrates the basic cognitive model: in specific situations, the patient's automatic thoughts influence her emotional, behavioral, and physiological reactions. The top half of the diagram shows how Ms. A's early experience influenced her self-concept and led to the development of conditional assumptions and compensatory strategies.

Clinicians start collecting data from their first contact with a patient. When they recognize consistent patterns in patients' thoughts, beliefs, and reactions, clinicians start to fill in the cognitive conceptualization diagram; question marks are used to note any hypothesis not yet checked out with the patient. Clinicians assume, until proven otherwise, that most patients are able to assess the validity of their clinicians' hypotheses. When Ms. A's therapist suggested to her that perhaps she had a belief that she had to please other people to gain their assistance, she offered confirmation. When her therapist made an incorrect hypothesis, that her expectations for herself were unreasonably perfectionistic, Ms. A validly corrected him, offering specific data and an alternative view.

Cognitive therapy requires a *strong therapeutic alliance*. The interpersonal factors—empathy, concern, and unconditional positive regard—that are important in any form of counseling are also essential in cognitive therapy. Cognitive therapy emphasizes providing rationales for interventions and eliciting and responding to patients' feedback, which not only strengthens the alliance but also allows the clinician to plan treatment more effectively. Clinicians aim to create a collaborative relationship in which they function as a team with patients, mutually deciding on problems to be discussed, homework assignments, frequency of visits, and so forth.

This teamwork is evident, too, as clinician and patient engage in a process of *collaborative empiricism* to investigate the validity of the patient's thoughts and beliefs. Clinicians do not know a priori whether any given

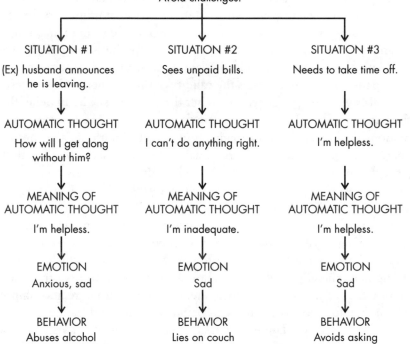

RELEVANT CHILDHOOD DATA

Mother had mood swings, was unreliable.
Parents expected patient to take on age-appropriate responsibilities.
She had a slight learning disability, did only "fair" at school.

↓

CORE BELIEF(S)

I am helpless/inadequate.

↓

CONDITIONAL ASSUMPTIONS/BELIEFS/RULES

Positive assumption(s): If I rely on others, I'll be okay.

Negative assumption(s): If I have to rely on myself, I'll fail.

↓

COMPENSATORY STRATEGIES

Rely on others.
Defer to others' wishes.
Avoid challenges.

SITUATION #1	SITUATION #2	SITUATION #3
(Ex) husband announces he is leaving.	Sees unpaid bills.	Needs to take time off.
↓	↓	↓
AUTOMATIC THOUGHT	AUTOMATIC THOUGHT	AUTOMATIC THOUGHT
How will I get along without him?	I can't do anything right.	I'm helpless.
↓	↓	↓
MEANING OF AUTOMATIC THOUGHT	MEANING OF AUTOMATIC THOUGHT	MEANING OF AUTOMATIC THOUGHT
I'm helpless.	I'm inadequate.	I'm helpless.
↓	↓	↓
EMOTION	EMOTION	EMOTION
Anxious, sad	Sad	Sad
↓	↓	↓
BEHAVIOR	BEHAVIOR	BEHAVIOR
Abuses alcohol	Lies on couch	Avoids asking

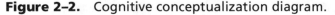

Figure 2–2. Cognitive conceptualization diagram.

Source. Copyright J.S. Beck, Ph.D., 1993.

cognition a patient reports is wholly true, wholly false, or partly true and partly false. Together, they test thoughts through an examination of the evidence or by setting up "experiments" for the patient to perform between sessions. By weighing the evidence, Ms. A was able to see that her thought "I can't do anything right" was patently false. She found that her thought "My boss won't give me any time off" was also untrue when she tested it by asking him (after role-playing how to do so with her therapist).

Cognitive therapy is *educative* in nature. The therapist's stated goal is to teach patients to become their own therapists. As with evaluating automatic thoughts, clinicians teach patients skills that they practice for homework, ultimately integrating them so that they become more automatic. Research shows that cognitive therapy reduces the frequency and severity of relapse (Strunk and DeRubeis 2001). The chance of relapse is reduced in several ways. Patients' core beliefs are modified (so that they are less vulnerable to an activation of negative schema under stress). They also develop cognitive and behavioral skills to use when they encounter stressors and note early warning signs of a recurrence.

Because of its educative nature and its emphasis on acquisition of skills, cognitive therapy aims to be *time limited*. Axis I conditions such as anxiety disorders and unipolar depression usually respond to 6–12 sessions of cognitive therapy. Sessions are usually scheduled weekly (unless distress is severe), then spaced out to every second, third, and fourth week as patients use their skills independently and start to achieve a remission of symptoms. Longer courses of treatment (6 months to 1 year or more) are often required for patients with Axis II disorders, with comorbid diagnoses, or with chronic or treatment-resistant symptoms.

Cognitive therapy is also *goal oriented*. During initial sessions, clinicians help patients specify their goals of treatment in behavioral terms (e.g., "How would you like to be different by the end of therapy? What would you like to see yourself doing?"). Clinicians share their treatment plan and general strategies with patients so that patients can visualize more clearly how they will be able to reach their goals. Treatment begins by discussing current problems of greatest distress to the patient.

Structure of the Therapeutic Interview

The structure of the standard 45-minute interview generally follows a set format to maximize efficiency, learning, and therapeutic change. Key elements include

- Mood evaluation and initial setting of the agenda
- Bridge between sessions

- Prioritization of the agenda
- Discussion of agenda topics and teaching of skills
- Homework
- Summary
- Feedback

Each structural element is briefly described below.

Patients are usually asked to complete objective, self-administered symptom scales before each session. Scales such as the Beck Depression Inventory (A.T. Beck et al. 1996), Beck Anxiety Inventory (A.T. Beck and Steer 1990), and Beck Hopelessness Scale (A.T. Beck and Steer 1989) or the Beck Youth Inventories (J.S. Beck and Beck 2001) are invaluable in providing the clinician with important data to guide the planning of the session and in helping the clinician and patient track progress. During the *mood evaluation*, the clinician reviews patients' total scores and individual symptoms, in addition to requesting a verbal comparison of how patients have been feeling that week compared with other weeks. If clinicians find that patients are suicidal, they focus the session on alleviating their hopelessness and developing safety plans.

The mood evaluation often suggests important topics for the agenda (e.g., "It looks as if your sleep has deteriorated. Can we put that on the agenda?"; "In a few minutes, I'd like to talk about why you think you're feeling worse, if that's okay."; "So, you're getting a lot more pleasure out of your activities. I'm glad to see that. Maybe we should take a few minutes to talk about that later.").

Concurrent with or subsequent to the mood evaluation, clinicians ask patients what problem(s) they want to put on the *agenda*. Usually, there is time to discuss only one or two problems in depth. Then therapists make a connection, or *bridge*, between the previous session and the current one by asking patients what important events (positive and negative) have occurred. They also ask patients to recall the important skills they learned in the previous session and the important conclusions they reached, so they can build from one session to the next. They also review *homework* patients have completed during the week, discussing what they learned and deciding whether to continue the assignment in the coming week.

Next, the clinician and patient collaboratively *prioritize the agenda*, with both contributing important topics. During the *discussion of agenda topics*, the clinician does a combination of data collection, conceptualization, presenting hypotheses, and eliciting key cognitions, affects, and behavior. The clinician and patient then may perform a combination of problem solving, evaluating and responding to dysfunctional thoughts and beliefs, and behavioral skills training. *Homework* assignments are a natural outgrowth of the discussion, and many include identifying and responding to distressing thoughts, doing experiments to test their thoughts, rehearsing new viewpoints, practicing skills learned in sessions, and taking steps to solve problems.

Throughout the session, the clinician makes *capsule summaries.* For example, the clinician may summarize the patient's narrative in the form of the cognitive model ("I want to make sure I've got it right. The situation was that your car broke down. You thought, 'This is the last straw. I can't handle life anymore.' These thoughts made you feel hopelessly sad, and you sat in the car and cried. Did I get that right?").

The purpose of another kind of capsule summary is to help clinicians assess the degree to which patients understand, and agree with, what they have discussed:

> Therapist: Can you summarize what we just talked about?
> Patient: Well, I see how I let my thoughts run away with me again. I just bought into the idea that there was nothing I could do to fix the situation, and I gave up. Next time, I should use that hopeless feeling as a cue to figure out what I was thinking and remind myself that my thoughts may or may not be completely true, especially because I am depressed.

Several minutes before their time is up, clinicians or patients *summarize* the session. Because most patients forget most of what was said during a given therapy session, the clinician ensures that the most important points and the homework assignments are recorded in some way. Throughout the session, the clinician continually thinks, "What do I wish [this patient] would remember this week?" This question prompts the therapist to guide the patient in writing important points, responses to common automatic thoughts, coping skills, and so on in a therapy notebook or on index cards. If the patient prefers, the clinician can do the writing. Or the two of them can make a 2-minute audiotape with the same information.

The clinician also elicits *feedback:* "What did you think of today's session? Was there anything you thought I misunderstood or anything that bothered you? Anything you want to make sure we do differently next time?" If clinicians believe that patients are distressed during the session, they do not wait until the end to ask for feedback. Rather, noting the patient's negative verbal and nonverbal responses, body language, facial expressions, and tone of voice, the clinician elicits the patient's automatic thoughts right on the spot. Many Axis II patients benefit greatly from evaluating their cognitions about the therapist, correcting their thinking, and learning to apply what they learned from the therapeutic relationship to specific relationships outside of therapy.

Specific Applications

Depression

Cognitive therapy was initially developed for working with depressed patients, and a voluminous literature supports the efficacy of cognitive therapy for this disorder, including more than 75 outcome trials (Butler and Beck 2000). In a recent meta-analysis, cognitive therapy was shown to be as efficacious as pharmacotherapy for even severe depression (Strunk and DeRubeis 2001). In addition, depressed patients who have been treated with cognitive therapy have half the relapse rate of patients treated with medication (DeRubeis et al. 1999).

The cognitive formulation of depression was introduced by A.T. Beck and colleagues in 1979. Initial treatment strategies usually include an emphasis on problem solving and behavioral activation. This has the simultaneous effect of raising the patient's energy level, directly countering some of his or her distorted thinking, providing a sense of pleasure and mastery, and reducing his or her sense of hopelessness. Behavioral activation also can provide the necessary energy and concentration to help the patient record and examine his or her thoughts. Although cognitive strategies are also used from the beginning, patients with severe depression often have difficulty modifying their extremely negative, rigid views at first and respond more positively to behavioral strategies. When patients are suicidal, clinicians explore the reasons behind their hopelessness and help them appraise their situations more realistically.

The cognitions of depressed patients center on negative appraisals of themselves, their personal world, and their future, termed the *cognitive triad of depression* (A.T. Beck et al. 1979). The content of their thoughts is pervasively pessimistic and negative. These patients overly attend to negative events and data, while minimizing or failing to register positive events and data. Overall, patients are helped to change their depressed way of processing information and to engage in more functional behaviors. When these goals are achieved, symptomatic reduction is usually complete.

Anxiety

The cognitive model of anxiety states that when individuals perceive significant risk and assess their ability to cope with the threat as low, they feel anxious. Features of anxiety disorders can be seen as excessive functioning of normal survival mechanisms. The evolution-based strategy for coping with threat is a physiological response that facilitates escape or self-defense. The same physiological reaction occurs in response to *perceived* threats from usually benign everyday stimuli (a crowd, an airplane, an audience). Therapy generally involves having patients learn skills to assess risk more realistically, to judge their resources more realistically, and to increase their internal and external resources to deal with the threat (A.T. Beck and Emery 1985). Because anxiety has several forms, the particular formulation and strategies vary somewhat from disorder to disorder. Several anxiety disorders are described in this section.

Generalized Anxiety Disorder

The effect of cognitive therapy on generalized anxiety disorder has been addressed in several outcome studies. A total of 11 clinical trials, whose control groups included a variety of conditions ranging from wait list to nondirective therapy to pill placebo, were reviewed by DeRubeis and Crits-Christoph (1998). In 10 of the 11 studies, cognitive therapy outperformed the control condition, and in one study, cognitive therapy was equivalent to nondirective therapy.

Patients with generalized anxiety disorder have patterns of negative predictions and excessive worry in several areas. In addition, they find their anxiety difficult to control, have physical manifestations of fear, and experience a reduction in functioning. The cognitive hallmark of generalized anxiety disorder is that almost anything can be a source of worry, from minor details (e.g., an automobile repair, a missed dental appointment) to larger issues (e.g., deciding whether to take a new job or worrying about the illness of a family member).

The critical cognitive distortion is related to catastrophizing. The individual sees problems as leading inevitably to disaster. The cognitions of the individual with generalized anxiety disorder represent a kind of worry tree, with spreading branches of doom that become wider and wider (e.g., "What if I don't get home in time to greet my son after school? What if he can't get in the house himself? What if no neighbors are home to let him in? What if he wanders in the street? What if he gets hit by a car?"). In addition to worrisome thoughts, patients often have scary images of the moment of catastrophe.

The automatic, rapid branching of worries results in considerable exaggeration of the odds of negative outcomes—that is, the patient is not likely to be evaluating all the different ways that things can turn out less drastically or even positively. Patients with generalized anxiety disorder also vastly underestimate their ability to cope with and handle problems that do come up. Even if they do know what should be done, they tend to perceive themselves as unable to implement the solution properly. This sense of inadequacy needs to be combated directly by having the patient engage in active problem solving, learning new skills when necessary, and practicing them. Thus, patients are taught to assess risk more accurately and to enhance self-efficacy by expanding their resources.

Many patients with generalized anxiety disorder need to modify dysfunctional assumptions and beliefs. Some assumptions involve a negative assessment of their abilities and stem from a core belief of helplessness ("If I try to solve problems myself, I'll fail," "If I make a mistake, something terrible will happen," or "If I make a decision, I'll make the wrong one"). Other beliefs involve a theme of vulnerability about themselves or others: "If the situation I'm in is not completely safe, then I'm in danger" or "If someone has an unexplained symptom, his or her health is in great jeopardy." Other assumptions are about the benefits of worry itself, such as "If I worry about something, maybe it won't happen" or "If I'm alert to danger, I'll be able to protect myself."

Patients with generalized anxiety disorder may benefit considerably from strategies designed to reduce physiological arousal. Thus, relaxation training can be very helpful in the early stages of treatment. Also, once the patient has the cognitive tools to defuse worry, behavioral strategies such as exposure exercises to anxiety-provoking situations can be useful to test the patient's coping and worry-control skills.

Panic Disorder

A review of 11 outcome studies examining cognitive therapy for panic disorder and panic disorder with agoraphobic avoidance concluded that cognitive therapy was an efficacious treatment for these disorders (DeRubeis and Crits-Christoph 1998).

Panic patients misinterpret a particular unexplained symptom or sensation (or a small set of related sensations) as a sign of an immediate mental or bodily catastrophe. Therapy focuses on helping patients see alternative (benign) explanations for their catastrophic misinterpretations. Common misinterpretations include the following: "My rapid heartbeat and chest pain mean I'm having a heart attack," "This feeling of unreality in my head means I'm going crazy," and "This feeling of dizziness means I'm going to pass out."

In treatment, panic patients are educated about the particular panic cycle in which they notice a bodily or mental change, make a negative attribution, feel anxious, experience an intensification of their symptoms, and, finally, catastrophically misinterpret their symptoms. The aim of treatment is to have patients prove to themselves that their symptoms, although extremely uncomfortable, are not dangerous. To do so, clinicians perform panic inductions with patients (often by having them hyperventilate) to show patients that they brought on their symptoms and were then able to reduce them through their own behavior and change in thinking. Patients learn that their feared sensations can be produced in a variety of ways and do not lead to the feared consequence. Clinicians ask patients to monitor their safety behaviors, or actions to avoid or reduce symptoms (such as distracting themselves, stopping an activity, leaving the situation, asking others for reassurance, or taking benzodiazepines). As long as patients engage in these safety behaviors, they reinforce the idea that panic attacks are dangerous and must be averted.

For patients who also have agoraphobia, it is critical to deal with anticipatory fears of being in a variety of situations. In some cases, a single panic attack in one location (e.g., a bookstore) can lead to avoidance of an entire class of stimuli (e.g., all stores and malls). Clinicians and patients construct a fear hierarchy, in which the least fear-provoking situations to those that are most fear provoking are listed. Patients are encouraged to practice entering these situations on a daily basis; recording their thoughts, feelings, and sensations for discussion in session; and using anxiety management techniques they have learned in therapy. Patients learn that the physical setting itself is not dangerous and gain confidence in their ability to manage their anxiety.

Specific Phobia

For the specific phobias, a particular stimulus (e.g., an animal, an insect, heights, closed spaces, blood or injury) provokes both anticipatory anxiety and a physiological fear response. As in panic disorder and agoraphobia, benign stimuli (such as a spider) are seen by the patient as having dangerous properties. A host of studies (e.g., Craske et al. 1995) have shown that cognitive-behavioral strategies are efficacious for the treatment of specific phobias. Reviewers of this literature suggest that effective treatment includes exposure to feared stimuli, enabling patients to disconfirm their cognitions about harm (Antony and Swinson 2000). As in the treatment of panic disorder, a fear hierarchy may be established. For patients with animal phobias, for example, therapy may begin with patients viewing pictures, imagining having contact with the animal, seeing the animal in a cage or another room, followed by closer and closer contact. Throughout these exposures, patients' predictions are recorded and evaluated to help them gain a more realistic sense of actual danger.

Social Phobia

Several studies have been carried out to examine the efficacy of cognitive therapy for social phobia. In all of these studies, cognitive therapy outperformed the control condition. A meta-analysis of outcome studies also suggested that cognitive therapy (combined with exposure) was the approach that most consistently led to improvement (Taylor 1996). In social phobia, the critical cognitive factor usually involves a bias concerning what other people are thinking. Patients are excessively preoccupied with thoughts that others do not like them or are evaluating them negatively. They engage in considerable mind reading and experience increased physiological arousal in response to actual or anticipated social interactions. Many of these patients also believe that their anxiety is visible to others and that *any* visible signs of anxiety will be interpreted as weakness if detected by others. In addition, many patients with social phobia are poor at taking in external data; they assume that others are reacting to them negatively. At the belief level, patients with social phobia tend to see themselves as unlikable, inferior, or socially defective in some manner. These patients also may believe that others are harsh, critical, and demanding. As a result, they may believe that they are constantly falling short of others' expectations.

Cognitive therapy for social phobia combines both cognitive and behavioral strategies to reduce levels of anxiety and to combat concerns about negative evaluation. Many patients with social phobia avoid or endure with dread a whole host of social situations, some of which they may not reveal in a brief assessment. An initial goal is usually to construct a list of feared and avoided situations, as in specific phobia or agoraphobia; patients then expose themselves to each of the situations in order of difficulty.

Exposure to anxiety-provoking social situations also may uncover *safety behaviors* that patients use to reduce their anxiety. For example, at parties or social gatherings, they may assiduously avoid making eye contact with others, consume alcohol or other substances, stay rooted to a specific spot in a room (often a corner), or discuss only certain safe topics in conversation. Such behaviors are only short-term solutions, of course, and reinforce the notion that negative consequences would ensue if they were to behave differently. The clinician points out the self-defeating cycle of patients with social phobia (avoidance of socializing and engagement reinforces their negative beliefs about themselves and others, making it more difficult to socialize and engage, and so on) and encourages patients to practice new strategies learned in therapy. Finally, patients' negative beliefs about themselves are modified.

Other Conditions

In addition to the examples presented here of cognitive therapy's applications in depression and anxiety, cognitive therapy also has been shown to be efficacious in a variety of other disorders, including obsessive-compulsive disorder (e.g., Emmelkamp et al. 1988), posttraumatic stress disorder (Tarrier et al. 1999), substance abuse (Woody et al. 1983), eating disorders (e.g., Fairburn et al. 1991), and marital problems (Baucom et al. 1990). Most recently, cognitive therapy has been found to be an effective adjunct to medication in patients with schizophrenia (A.T. Beck and Rector 2000).

Cognitive Therapy Techniques

In order to select which technique to pursue at any given point in a session, clinicians consider many variables, including the nature of the problem under discussion, their overall plan for the session, the stage of therapy, skills previously taught, patients' and therapists' goals, patients' current degree of distress, and the strength of the therapeutic relationship. Clinicians continually ask themselves, "How can I help this patient feel better by the end of the session, and how can I help the patient have a better week?" These questions also guide clinicians in planning strategy. We discuss common techniques in this section.

Problem Solving

Problem solving is a central part of cognitive therapy treatment. Every patient brings real-life problems to therapy, some of which are exacerbated by their faulty interpretations. At times, clinicians engage in straightforward problem solving with patients. Often, though, they need to help patients identify and respond to their distorted thinking before patients are ready to brainstorm options, examine their choices, and select a course of action. Ms. A, for example, needed to evaluate her cognition "I shouldn't inconvenience others" before she was ready to consider certain solutions, such as asking for reasonable, and needed, help from a friend and a co-worker. Clinicians assess the degree to which they need to teach patients problem-solving skills directly.

Graded Task Assignments

Graded task assignments are especially important for depressed patients. Clinicians help patients break down seemingly insurmountable problems into component parts they can work on step-by-step. Ms. A's apartment was in general disarray. She and her therapist discussed working on one room at a time, whichever seemed easiest, for 10–20 minutes at a time. Feeling much less overwhelmed by the task, Ms. A found that she could actually continue working for much longer periods.

Activity Monitoring

Activity monitoring is often used with depressed patients. They keep a log of what they are doing each hour and rate either their mood during each activity or their sense of pleasure or mastery. This log can be invaluable in identifying activities that patients are engaging in too much or too little. When Ms. A and her therapist examined her log, they discovered that she was spending far too much time in the evenings and on weekends lying on the couch, watching television, and feeling very sad. They recognized that she was not spending much time at all, if any, calling friends, managing the household, exercising, reading magazines, or gardening (her hobby).

Activity Scheduling

Behavioral activation and activity scheduling are particularly important for patients who, like Ms. A, are relatively inactive or whose lives are disorganized. Depressed patients often believe that they should wait until they are feeling better before they attempt to engage in activities that can give them a sense of mastery or pleasure. However, these patients invariably find that their mood improves when they push themselves to engage in formerly pleasurable activities and to perform tasks from which they can derive a sense of accomplishment. Such efforts are especially important when patients simultaneously experience interfering negative thoughts.

Psychoeducation

Psychoeducation is a key element in cognitive therapy. Clinicians educate their patients about many aspects of therapy, including the symptoms of their disorder, how cognitive therapy proceeds, their mutual responsibilities as patient and therapist, the structure of the session, the importance of setting agendas, the need for honest feedback, and the cognitive model. Clinicians often encourage patients to read cognitively oriented pamphlets and chapters of self-help books to reinforce what they learned in therapy.

Giving Credit

Many patients benefit from learning how to give themselves credit. Especially when patients are depressed, they focus unduly on the negative and fail to register the positive things they are doing. They tend to see their difficulties as being caused by an inherent character flaw instead of their illness. One way to help them see the broader picture is for them to note (preferably in writing) whatever they do that is even a little difficult for them but that they do anyway. Getting out of bed, performing their usual hygiene activities, getting to work on time, calling a friend, and paying a bill are all activities that merit credit, if they were difficult for the patient to accomplish.

Functional Comparisons of the Self

Functional comparisons of the self are an important skill for many depressed patients. Learning to compare themselves with how they were at their worst point reduces the hopelessness and self-blame they experience when they (automatically) compare themselves with others who are not depressed, with how they were before they became depressed, or with how they wish they would be.

Guided Discovery

A major part of cognitive therapy is, of course, to modify patients' dysfunctional cognitions. To aid patients in evaluating their automatic thoughts and beliefs, identify the distortions in their thinking, and develop more objective and adaptive viewpoints, clinicians use guided discovery, a gentle, Socratic questioning process. Therapists not only help patients respond to their dysfunctional thinking but also teach patients how to do so. Providing them with a list of questions (Table 2–2) allows patients to practice evaluating and responding to their thoughts between sessions. The questions guide patients in evaluating the validity of their thoughts, seeking alternative explanations or perspectives, decatastrophizing, examining the utility of their thinking, getting distance from their thoughts through reflecting on advice they would give to others, and planning a course of action.

Because patients show characteristic errors in their thinking (Table 2–3), learning to label these cognitive distortions also helps them gain some perspective on their thoughts. Ms. A, for example, engaged in considerable all-or-nothing thinking: "Either I do everything well and I'm a good employee or I don't, and I'm not." She also made personalization errors: "Since my accountant was short with me, he must be mad at me." She often catastrophized or engaged in fortune-telling: "[My friend] won't want to get together with me."

Table 2–2. Questioning automatic thoughts

---

1. What is the evidence that supports this idea?
   What is the evidence against this idea?

2. Is there an alternative explanation?

3. What is the *worst* that could happen?
   How could I cope if it did?
   What is the *best* that could happen?
   What is the most realistic outcome?

4. What is the effect of my believing the automatic thought?
   What could be the effect of changing my thinking?

5. If [friend's name] was in this situation and had this thought, what would I tell him or her?

6. What should I do now?

Source. Adapted from J.S. Beck 1995.

Table 2–3. Cognitive distortions

All-or-nothing thinking	Also called *black-and-white, polarized,* or *dichotomous thinking.* You view a situation in only two categories instead of on a continuum. *Example:* "If I'm not a total success, I'm a failure."
Catastrophizing	Also called *fortune-telling.* You predict the future negatively without considering other, more likely outcomes. *Example:* "I'll be so upset, I won't be able to function at all."
Disqualifying or discounting the positive	You unreasonably tell yourself that positive experiences, deeds, or qualities do not count. *Example:* "I did that project well, but that doesn't mean I'm competent; I just got lucky."
Emotional reasoning	You think something must be true because you "feel" (actually believe) it so strongly, ignoring or discounting evidence to the contrary." *Example:* "I know I do a lot of things OK at work, but I still feel like I'm a failure."
Labeling	You put a fixed, global label on yourself or others without considering that the evidence might more reasonably lead to a less disastrous conclusion. *Examples:* "I'm a loser." "He's no good."

Table 2–3. Cognitive distortions *(continued)*

Magnification/ minimization	When you evaluate yourself, another person, or a situation, you unreasonably magnify the negative and/ or minimize the positive. *Example:* "Getting a mediocre evaluation proves how inadequate I am. Getting high marks doesn't mean I'm smart."
Mental filter	Also called *selective abstraction.* You pay undue attention to one negative detail instead of seeing the whole picture. *Example:* "Because I got one low rating on my evaluation [which also contained several high ratings], it means I'm doing a lousy job."
Mind reading	You believe you know what others are thinking, failing to consider other, more likely possibilities. *Example:* "He's thinking that I don't know the first thing about this project."
Overgeneralization	You make a sweeping negative conclusion that goes far beyond the current situation. *Example:* "Because I felt uncomfortable at the meeting, I don't have what it takes to make friends."
Personalization	You believe others are behaving negatively because of you, without considering more plausible explanations for their behavior. *Example:* "The repairman was curt to me because I did something wrong."
"Should" and "must" statements	Also called *imperatives.* You have a precise, fixed idea of how you or others should behave, and you overestimate how bad it is that these expectations are not met. *Example:* "It's terrible that I made a mistake. I should always do my best."
Tunnel vision	You only see the negative aspects of a situation. *Example:* "My son's teacher can't do anything right. He's critical and insensitive and lousy at teaching."

Source.　Reprinted from Beck JS: *Cognitive Therapy: Basics and Beyond.* New York, Guilford, 1995. Used with permission.

Dysfunctional Thought Record

A tool that is useful for most patients (although sometimes in a simplified form) is the dysfunctional thought record (Table 2–4). This worksheet allows patients to record and respond to their thoughts in an organized way. Many patients use this worksheet not only during therapy but also for months and years after therapy is over, when they find that they are overreacting to situations or developing early warning signs of their disorder.

On the dysfunctional thought record, the first three columns after the date parallel the cognitive model: patients record their thoughts and emotions in specific situations. Patients are also instructed to note their degree of belief in each thought and the intensity of their emotion. The questions listed in Table 2–2 are printed at the bottom of the record so that patients can refer to them in formulating an adaptive response (which they write in the next column). Finally, patients re-rate how much they still believe their automatic thought. They also re-rate their degree of emotion in the outcome column, to determine whether further intervention with the distressing thought is needed. Patients are told that the efforts are worthwhile if they achieve even a 10% reduction in their distress, although frequently they gain much more relief if they have been able to complete the worksheet appropriately. Correctly identifying and differentiating among the initial elements (situation, automatic thoughts, emotion) requires practice. Clinicians do not ask patients to complete dysfunctional thought records at home until patients show facility with these tools in session.

Behavioral Experiments

Behavioral experiments help patients test their automatic thoughts that are in the form of predictions. Predictions such as "I won't get any enjoyment from having lunch with my friend," "If I try to sort out my medical records, I'll make serious mistakes," "My mother won't listen to me at all if I try to explain why I can't come home next week," and "My friend will get mad if I suggest that we do something else" can be empirically tested. The clinician helps set up the experiment carefully, to increase the odds of success, and may help the patient compose a useful response to read in case the experiment does not go well.

Responding to Patients' Valid Thoughts

Sometimes patients' thoughts are valid. When patients' thoughts are valid, clinicians usually do one or more of the following: problem solving, evaluating the patient's conclusion, or examining the utility of the thought. For example, Ms. A's thought "I can't concentrate well enough to do my work" appeared to be substantially true. Ms. A and the clinician talked about improving her sleep, taking brief walks outside during her work breaks, and reading her therapy notes at work when she was dis-

Table 2–4. Dysfunctional thought record

Directions: When you notice your mood getting worse, ask yourself, "What's going through my mind right now?" and as soon as possible, jot down the thought or mental image in the "Automatic thought(s)" column.

Date/ time	Situation	Automatic thought(s)	Emotion(s)	Alternative response	Outcome
	1. What actual event or stream of thoughts, or daydreams, or recollection led to the unpleasant emotion? 2. What (if any) distressing physical sensations did you have?	1. What thoughts and/or image(s) went through your mind? 2. How much did you believe each one at the time?	1. What emotion(s) (e.g., sad, anxious, angry) did you feel at the time? 2. How intense (0%–100%) was the emotion?	1. (optional) What cognitive distortion did you make? (e.g., all-or-nothing thinking, mind reading, catastrophizing) 2. Use questions at bottom to compose a response to the automatic thought(s). 3. How much do you believe each response?	1. How much do you now believe each automatic thought? 2. What emotion(s) do you feel now? How intense (0%–100%) is the emotion? 3. What will you do (or did you do)?
6/15	Seeing how messy the apartment is	I'm a total basket case. (100%)	Sad (85%)	Labeling error 1. My house is messy; I'm behind at work; I cry all the time. But I am still going to work every day and getting some things done. 2. I'm struggling with depression and still functioning even if I'm not doing as well as when I'm not depressed.	1. 70% 2. Sad (70%)

Table 2–4. Dysfunctional thought record (continued)

Date/ time	Situation	Automatic thought(s)	Emotion(s)	Alternative response	Outcome
				3. *Worst outcome: I'll stay depressed.* *Best outcome: I'll start feeling great today.* *Most realistic outcome: Maybe this therapy will continue to help.*	3. *I cleaned the kitchen.*
				4. *Thinking this way makes me feel worse. If I change my thinking, I'll function better.*	
				5. *I would tell Ms. G that she has an illness caused by depression and that doing something about the messiness will make her feel better.*	5. 80%
				6. *I should start cleaning the kitchen for 10 minutes.*	

Note. Questions to help compose an alternative response: 1) What is the evidence that the automatic thought is true? Not true? 2) Is there an alternative explanation? 3) What is the worst that could happen? Could I live through it? What is the best that could happen? What is the most realistic outcome? 4) What is the effect of my believing the automatic thought? What could be the effect of changing my thinking? 5) If [friend's name] were in this situation and had this thought, what would I tell him or her? 6) What should I do now?

Source. Copyright J.S. Beck, Ph.D., 1993.

tracted by her usual automatic thoughts. Ms. A had also reached a distorted conclusion from her valid thought "Since I can't concentrate well enough on my work, it means I am an utter failure." Evaluating and responding to this conclusion reduced Ms. A's distress. She and her therapist also examined the usefulness of the thought. Eventually, Ms. A was able to see that continually saying to herself, "I can't concentrate, I can't concentrate," just served to prolong her distress.

Weighing Advantages and Disadvantages

Another common technique when patients must make decisions is helping them identify, record, and perhaps weigh advantages and disadvantages. Ms. A's therapist used this technique to help her decide whether to talk to her boss about her depression, whether to take medication, and whether it would be worthwhile to take social risks to enlarge her network of friends. She and her therapist also discussed advantages and disadvantages of her belief "I should avoid conflict at any cost."

Coping Cards

Coping cards (Figure 2–3) are really just therapy notes on index cards that patients can carry with them and read several times a day. Usually they contain responses to patients' key, recurrent automatic thoughts or behavioral instructions. As Table 2–4 illustrates, Ms. A needed a robust response to her distressing automatic thought "If I don't do well at work, it means I'm a failure." Her therapist used several of the cognitive techniques discussed earlier to help Ms. A modify her thinking and then asked Ms. A to record her response on a card to read on her way to work, at lunchtime, and at break time. Ms. A also benefited from a card designed to get her up and going on weekends; again, this card was collaboratively composed.

Imagery Work

Imagery work is quite important for many patients, especially those who experience automatic thoughts in an imaginal form. In addition to verbal automatic thoughts, Ms. A had images of her boss yelling at her, images of an acquaintance rejecting her, and memories of difficult times in a previous job. Ms. A's clinician taught her some imaginal techniques to reduce her distress: checking the reality of an image, following an image through to completion, and changing a key element of the image.

> **Automatic thought:** I'm a failure.
>
> **Response:** I'm having problems because I'm depressed. And even though I'm depressed, I'm still going to work every day, getting some things done, and doing essentials such as going to the store and doing laundry. A real failure is someone who is not depressed but still makes no effort at all to do anything. That's not me.

Figure 2–3.   Sample coping card.

Relaxation Training

Many patients, especially patients with anxiety, find relaxation training (e.g., imaginal exposure, muscle relaxation, meditation) or controlled breathing (especially those who tend to hyperventilate) useful.

Graded Exposure

Graded exposure is often used with anxious patients, who create a fear hierarchy and gradually expose themselves to feared situations, using cognitive and behavioral skills they learned in therapy to decrease their anxiety and obtain a sense of mastery.

Response Prevention

Response prevention is used with obsessive-compulsive disorder patients to decrease their compulsive behavior, increase their anxiety tolerance, and test their predictions. Likewise, other patients with anxiety are encouraged to eliminate their use of safety behaviors (e.g., avoiding situations, trying to keep their emotions in check) that perpetuate their dysfunctional beliefs.

Modification of Underlying Beliefs

Modification of underlying beliefs entails many of the techniques listed in this section. Rigid, long-standing beliefs usually require a variety of interventions over time, a full description of which is beyond the scope of this chapter. Some techniques include examining advantages and disadvantages of holding a particular belief; creating cognitive continua; developing more realistic, more functional beliefs; explaining faulty information processing; monitoring the operation of the schema; identifying alternative explanations for patients' experiences when the belief has been activated; learning to recognize evidence that disconfirms the dysfunctional belief; using metaphors and analogies to help patients develop new perspectives; using rational–emotional role-plays; and examining the developmental origin of beliefs (see A.T. Beck et al. 1990 and J.S. Beck 1995 for a thorough presentation of these interventions).

Other Techniques

Many other techniques have cognitive and behavioral aspects but may be classified differently:

- *Emotional techniques* may include teaching patients to regulate affect through behavioral activities: distraction, controlled breathing, self-soothing activities, seeking support, and reading therapy notes. Clinicians also help patients tolerate negative affect and modify dysfunctional beliefs about emotions: "If I start to feel distressed, I'll get completely overwhelmed and will not be able to cope with it."
- *Interpersonal techniques* include correcting faulty beliefs about others; solving interpersonal problems; and learning communication, assertiveness, and other social skills. Clinician and patient may collaboratively decide to bring significant others into one or more sessions.
- *Supportive techniques* include empathy, showing an accurate understanding of the patient's experience, and providing positive reinforcement.
- *Experiential techniques* include role-playing, inducing positive imagery, responding to distressing imagery in imaginal form, and modifying beliefs through imaginal reexperiencing of previous trauma.
- *Biological interventions* might include use of medication (if indicated), reduction of caffeine or other drugs, exercise, and learning to focus externally instead of on internal sensations.
- *Environmental interventions* might include helping patients make changes in living or work environments.
- *Transference techniques* framed in a cognitive manner may be needed for Axis II disorders, as clinicians note patients' verbal and nonverbal signs of distress, elicit their automatic thoughts about the therapist and therapy, and help them evaluate and respond to their cognitions and generalize what they have learned to other relationships.

Summary Case Illustration: Ms. A

Ms. A was a 52-year-old divorced woman with three grown children living in other cities. She had worked full-time as a nurse's aide in a community clinic for the past 10 years. She was given a diagnosis of major depression, recurrent, moderate (score of 33 on the Beck Depression Inventory II at intake), and she also showed strong dependent features on Axis II. Her most severe episode of depression, which lasted for more than a year, had occurred nearly 20 years before, when her first husband announced that he was in love with another woman. Feelings of rejection were bad enough, but Ms. A was even more despondent over her loss of a partner for financial security, emotional support, and day-to-day activities of living, such as paying bills and making major and minor decisions. During the subsequent separation and divorce, she drank heavily and continued to do so for many years until she completed an inpatient substance abuse program 6 years ago.

Ms. A's current episode of depression was triggered 5 months ago when a relationship with a boyfriend ended. Although it had been a casual relationship that had ended by mutual agreement, she began to have thoughts such as "I'll never find anyone else" and "If I am alone, I will be lost." Although she had not taken a drink, she feared a potential relapse.

Early in treatment, Ms. A and her therapist focused on several problems: responding to her mild suicidal thoughts, dealing with urges to drink, and getting her behaviorally activated. She had withdrawn from friends and spent most of her nonwork hours watching television. Through activity scheduling, reading coping cards reminding her of the advantages of being active, graded task assignments to guide her in straightening up her apartment, and posing assignments as experiments to test her thoughts that she could not do things, Ms. A started functioning much better. Her mood improved, and she became willing to reach out to friends.

During the first part of treatment, Ms. A's therapist taught her cognitive skills as well. These included identifying her automatic thoughts when she was distressed or noticed herself avoiding situations and then evaluating and responding to them. In the following example, the therapist loosely follows the list of questions in Table 2–2. Ms. A reported that she had felt terrible earlier that day. She had been in a computer class mandated by her workplace. The specific situation was that the instructor had told the class to switch on their computers. Not knowing which of several switches was the right one, Ms. A had a series of thoughts that led her to feel sad (80%) and anxious (60%). Ms. A and the therapist initially agreed to work on the thought "I'm a complete idiot [because I can't even turn the computer on]," which she believed 100%. Initially, they discussed the validity of the thought:

> Therapist: Okay, so you couldn't find the "on" button. Any other evidence that you're an idiot?
> Ms. A: I always have trouble with machines. Always.

After Ms. A notes a few other things, the therapist helps her focus on positive data that she has not been taking into consideration.

Therapist: Any evidence on the other side? That maybe you're not an idiot?

Ms. A: I don't know.

Therapist: How about the fact that you recently got a bonus at work? Doesn't that indicate that your boss feels you're doing a good job?

Ms. A: Well, maybe, but not with computers.

Therapist: So, are you saying that at worst, you're an idiot with computers and maybe other machines but not a complete idiot?

Ms. A: I guess so.

After eliciting more data that contradict Ms. A's thought that she is an idiot, the therapist helps her recognize an alternative explanation for her difficulty.

Therapist: [pauses] Can you think of any other explanation for why you didn't know where the right switch was? Was there more than one switch? Was it marked?

Ms. A: There were lots of buttons and stuff. I didn't know what any of them meant. Not until the instructor had to come over and show me.

Therapist: [collecting data] Have you ever worked on a computer before?

Ms. A: No, I've been afraid of them. I've avoided them totally.

Therapist: Let me ask you this. [providing an analogy] Let's imagine I take someone who has had no experience with cars at all, has never even been in a car, and I put that person in my car and I say, "Start it up." Would they know what to do?

Ms. A: Well, you wouldn't expect so if they had not seen one before.

Therapist: I think you're right; they probably would be a little lost. Is that a reflection on their intelligence?

Ms. A: Not necessarily. You'd have to teach the person first, then see if they learned once they had been shown.

Therapist: Absolutely. Does that tell you anything about your computer class experience?

Ms. A: I suppose it does; I guess there's no way I would know which button to push.

Therapist: That seems more fair to me, and so what does that say about whether you're really "an idiot"?

Ms. A: You know, when you say it now, it sounds extreme to me.

Therapist: Yeah, I'd call that more than unfair. [providing psychoeducation] This is an example of what happens when we are depressed and anxious; we tend to zero in on negative information about ourselves and don't really consider all of the facts before we reach a conclusion.

Next, the therapist decatastrophizes the situation.

Therapist: Ms. A, what's the worst that could happen if you don't learn the computer?

Ms. A: I guess I'd be fired.

Therapist: Or might they move you to some job that didn't require computers?

Ms. A: Maybe.

Therapist: If you did get fired, what would you do?

Ms. A: Wow, it's been a while since I looked for a job.

Therapist: Well, what did you do last time?

Ms. A: I looked in the newspaper.

Therapist: If worse came to worst, would you do that again? Would you find another job?

Ms. A: I suppose so.

Therapist: Ms. A, what's the best thing that could happen in this situation?

Ms. A: I guess I'd be able to learn to do the computer. That I'd keep my job. I do know how to type. It's the other stuff I don't know.

Therapist: What do you think is the most likely outcome? Did you learn something from that first class? Will you have more classes?

Ms. A: The instructor went over a lot of things. I don't remember most of it.

Therapist: Were other people doing everything easily?

Ms. A: No, everyone was complaining afterward.

Therapist: So, maybe rather than your being an idiot, the instructor wasn't that good—if he was going too fast for other people, too. *[pauses, then does problem solving]* Do you think if you and the others went to him and asked him to slow down that you'd be more likely to catch on?

Ms. A: Yeah, I think so.

Therapist: Could you talk to other people or to him?

Ms. A: Yeah.

Therapist: Assuming you do so, would the most likely outcome be that it might take time and a lot of practice but that you would catch on?

Ms. A: Yeah, probably.

Next, they discuss the effect of Ms. A's telling herself that she is an idiot and the benefits of seeing this situation from the new perspective. Then the therapist asks Ms. A what she would tell her friend Ms. G if Ms. G were ever in this situation. Finally, the therapist has Ms. A re-rate how much she still believes she is "a complete idiot" and the degree to which she is still sad and anxious about it. Noting significant change, the therapist asks Ms. A to summarize her new conclusion and her homework—to talk to the instructor.

After Ms. A had begun functioning better and had learned the tools to respond to her distorted thinking, her therapist started to focus on her belief about inadequacy. To counter this belief, her therapist had Ms. A keep logs of experiences in which she functioned adequately or better. She also learned to see improvements in her mood and functioning as the result of her own efforts. Early on, Ms. A had shown a tendency to rely on her therapist, saying, "If I had had you there, I know you could have helped me feel better." The therapist pointed out that there was nothing special about the questions and techniques used by the therapist and that she was, in fact, learning to use the techniques on herself. Ms. A surprised herself by doing several behavioral experiments that turned out well, counter to her predictions: being assertive with her boss, getting her taxes finished on time, and suggesting social activities to friends.

Toward the end of therapy, Ms. A and her therapist concentrated on relapse prevention. Ms. A collected her therapy notes, noted the tools that had helped her the most, and devised a system for reviewing what she had learned. She and her therapist discussed her early warning signs of depression, and she wrote down a plan of action should they recur. They discussed potential problems that could arise in the next year and engaged in advanced problem solving. Ms. A's therapist also elicited her automatic thoughts about ending therapy, and Ms. A was able to use the skills she had learned to respond to them and decrease her anxiety.

Ms. A was seen for a total of 13 sessions, with the final 4 sessions spaced at 2-week, and then 4-week, intervals. At the end of that time, her depression was in full remission.

Conclusion

Cognitive therapy has been shown to be an efficacious and efficient form of treatment for a wide range of psychiatric disorders. Developed as a treatment for unipolar depression in adults, it has now been extended to and tested for a range of psychiatric disorders, including (as an adjunct to medication) bipolar disorder and schizophrenia, and for many medical problems as well. The therapy is based on a largely empirically supported theory. Treatment proceeds from a cognitive formulation of the disorder and a cognitive conceptualization of the individual patient and emphasizes the modification of distorted and dysfunctional cognitions to bring about enduring cognitive, emotional, and behavioral change.

References

Antony MM, Swinson RP: Phobic Disorders and Panic in Adults: A Guide to Assessment and Treatment. Washington, DC, American Psychological Association, 2000

Baucom D, Sayers S, Sher T: Supplementary behavioral marital therapy with cognitive restructuring and emotional expressiveness training: an outcome investigation. J Consult Clin Psychol 58:636–645, 1990

Beck AT: Thinking and depression: idiosyncratic content and cognitive distortions. Arch Gen Psychiatry 9:324–333, 1963

Beck AT: Thinking and depression: theory and therapy. Arch Gen Psychiatry 10:561–571, 1964

Beck AT: Depression: Clinical, Experimental, and Theoretical Aspects. New York, Harper & Row, 1967

Beck AT: Beyond belief: a theory of modes, personality, and psychopathology, in Frontiers of Cognitive Therapy. Edited by Salkovskis P. New York, Guilford, 1996, pp 1–25

Beck AT, Emery G: Anxiety Disorders and Phobias: A Cognitive Perspective. New York, Basic Books, 1985

Beck AT, Rector NA: Cognitive therapy of schizophrenia: a new therapy for the new millennium. Am J Psychother 54:291–300, 2000

Beck AT, Steer RA: Manual for the Beck Hopelessness Scale. San Antonio, TX, Psychological Corporation, 1989

Beck AT, Steer RA: Beck Anxiety Inventory Manual. San Antonio, TX, Psychological Corporation, 1990

Beck AT, Weishaar ME: Cognitive therapy, in Current Psychotherapies, 6th Edition. Edited by Corsini RJ, Wedding D. Itasca, IL, Peacock, 2000, pp 241–272

Beck AT, Rush AJ, Shaw BF, et al: Cognitive Therapy of Depression. New York, Guilford, 1979

Beck AT, Freeman A, and Associates: Cognitive Therapy of Personality Disorders. New York, Guilford, 1990

Beck AT, Steer RA, Brown GK: Beck Depression Inventory—Second Edition Manual. San Antonio, TX, Psychological Corporation, 1996

Beck JS: Cognitive Therapy: Basics and Beyond. New York, Guilford, 1995

Beck JS: Cognitive approaches to personality disorders, in American Psychiatric Press Review of Psychiatry, Vol 16. Edited by Dickstein L, Riba MB, Oldham JM. Washington, DC, American Psychiatric Press, 1997, pp I-73–I-106

Beck JS: Complex cognitive therapy treatment for personality disorder patients. Bull Menninger Clin 62:170-194, 1998

Beck JS, Beck AT: Beck Youth Inventories Manual. San Antonio, TX, Psychological Corporation, 2001

Butler AC, Beck JS: Cognitive therapy outcomes: a review of meta-analyses. Tidsskrift for Norsk Psykologforening [Journal of the Norwegian Psychological Association] 37:1–9, 2000

Clark DA, Beck AT, Alford B: Scientific Foundations of Cognitive Theory and Therapy of Depression. New York, Wiley, 1999

Craske MG, Mohlman J, Yi J, et al: Treatment of claustrophobias and snake/spider phobias: fear of arousal and fear of context. Behav Res Ther 33:197–203, 1995

DeRubeis RJ, Crits-Christoph P: Empirically supported individual and group psychological treatments for adult mental disorders. J Consult Clin Psychol 66:37–52, 1998

DeRubeis RJ, Gelfand LA, Tang TZ, et al: Medications versus cognitive behavior therapy for severely depressed outpatients: mega-analysis of four randomized comparisons. Am J Psychiatry 156:1007–1013, 1999

Emmelkamp PMG, Visser S, Hoekstra RJ: Cognitive therapy vs exposure in vivo in the treatment of obsessive-compulsives. Cognitive Therapy and Research 12:103–114, 1988

Fairburn CC, Jones R, Peveler RC, et al: Three psychological treatments for bulimia nervosa: a comparative trial. Arch Gen Psychiatry 48:463–469, 1991

Strunk DR, DeRubeis RJ: Cognitive therapy for depression: a review of its efficacy. Journal of Cognitive Psychotherapy: An International Quarterly 15:289–297, 2001

Tarrier N, Pilgrim H, Sommerfield C, et al: A randomized trial of cognitive therapy and imaginal exposure in the treatment of chronic posttraumatic stress disorder. J Consult Clin Psychol 67:13–18, 1999

Taylor S: Meta-analysis of cognitive behavioral treatment for social phobia. J Behav Ther Exp Psychiatry 27:1–9, 1996

White JR, Freeman AS (eds): Cognitive-Behavioral Group Therapy for Specific Problems and Populations. Washington, DC, American Psychological Association, 2000

Woody GE, Luborsky L, McLellan AT, et al: Psychotherapy for opiate addicts. Does it help? Arch Gen Psychiatry 40:639–645, 1983

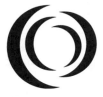

Brief Behavior Therapy

Elizabeth A. Hembree, Ph.D.
Deborah Roth, Ph.D.
Donald A. Bux Jr., Ph.D.
Edna B. Foa, Ph.D.

In this chapter, we describe an approach to psychotherapy that has produced a vast body of literature in recent years. In particular, numerous treatment outcome studies have generated considerable knowledge about the efficacy of behavioral interventions. Although a review of the treatment efficacy literature is beyond the scope of this chapter, the behavioral treatments described in this chapter are among those that have amassed strong empirical support.

We begin with a general description of the behavioral approach to psychotherapy. Next, because thorough assessment is a crucial first step in behavioral interventions, we briefly review some of the evaluation techniques commonly used by behavior therapists. We describe two types of behavior therapy that have received much empirical support, particularly for their efficacy in the treatment of pathological anxiety: a commonly used form of anxiety management training called *stress inoculation train-*

ing (SIT) and *exposure therapy*. After introducing these techniques, we present detailed descriptions of two exposure-based treatment programs that have been developed and extensively studied at the Center for the Treatment and Study of Anxiety (CTSA) at the University of Pennsylvania in Philadelphia. These are the Exposure and Ritual Prevention (EX/RP) program for the treatment of obsessive-compulsive disorder (OCD) and the Prolonged Exposure (PE) Therapy program for the treatment of chronic posttraumatic stress disorder (PTSD). Each type of treatment is illustrated by a detailed case example. In addition, the chapter contains many other clinical examples of the interventions we describe.

As is suggested by the preceding overview, our presentation of the application of behavior therapy to psychological problems focuses primarily on the treatment of anxiety disorders. Although behavior therapy is commonly used for a wide variety of other disorders and problems in individuals of all ages (e.g., mood disorders, marital and family problems, child behavior disorders, impulse-control disorders, personality disorders), we restrict our focus to adult anxiety disorders for two reasons. The first is that our expertise and our clinical experience lie primarily in the study and treatment of disorders in this diagnostic category. The second reason is that the large body of literature in the anxiety disorders domain supported our aim of presenting theoretically and empirically grounded brief therapeutic interventions.

General Description of Behavior Therapy

Behavior therapy is notable for its empirical approach to developing intervention techniques and evaluating their efficacy in the treatment of a range of psychological problems. This spirit of empiricism has a strong influence on the tone that is set in behavior therapy. *Psychoeducation* is a major component of behavior therapy treatment programs. Patients are educated about the behavioral approach to understanding and treating their particular problems. Therapeutic techniques are directly related to the way in which disorder etiology and maintenance are conceptualized.

The goal of psychoeducation is twofold. First, patients will be more likely to comply with therapy if they understand why they are being asked to do particular exercises. Second, our aim as therapists is for patients to become experts in their own treatment. In doing so, they will be able to continue applying what they have learned long after treatment has ended. This likely plays a role in the good long-term efficacy of behavior therapy across a range of disorders (see Mavissakalian and Prien 1996).

The duration of behavioral treatment often differs from that of more traditional forms of psychotherapy. Traditional psychodynamic therapy is typically long term, with no set end point. At the initiation of behavior therapy for a specific problem, clinicians usually have a good estimate of how many sessions will be required. Some specific phobias can be treated effectively in a matter of hours; even severe cases of other anxiety disorders can be treated in fewer than 20 sessions.

Significant gains are often made quite quickly in behavior therapy because it is *problem focused* and *present focused*. Focus is usually placed on one problem, and a great majority of the treatment time involves dealing with that problem. Clinicians initiate a course of behavior therapy knowing not only how the treatment as a whole will progress but also what each treatment session should entail. As is outlined later in this chapter, the treatment program for OCD used at the CTSA consists of 17 sessions. It begins with 2 sessions of psychoeducation and information gathering and progresses to 15 sessions of EX/RP. Each EX/RP session begins with a review of homework, is followed by in vivo and/or imaginal exposures, and is closed with assignment of homework.

Another unique aspect of behavior therapy is that little attention is dedicated to figuring out the origins of the patient's problem. Some time is spent during psychoeducation speaking very generally of why people might develop a particular disorder, but this conversation is general to the disorder more than it is specific to the patient. Behavior therapy patients often find the present-centered or here-and-now focus of attention to be quite refreshing. Many of our patients with anxiety disorders know that insight is often helpful, but figuring out *why* they have a particular problem does not necessarily change their current situation. For this reason, behavior therapy focuses on making changes in current behavior and on how to maintain these changes in the future.

With this focus on making changes in current behavior, behavior therapy is a very active treatment. Once assessment, treatment planning, and psychoeducation have been accomplished, most sessions of behavior therapy involve participation in active behavioral techniques, including exposure, relaxation, problem solving, and role-playing. There is very little unfocused talking and a lot more active doing. This active approach carries over to the time between sessions; an integral component of behavior therapy is *homework*. Practicing skills between sessions increases patients' proficiency with them and also promotes a sense of mastery and confidence. For the exposure-based treatments (described later in this chapter), homework practice increases the likelihood that patients will habituate to or experience a decrease in the anxiety that arises in feared but "safe" situations. It also provides patients with more opportunities to have corrective learning experiences within their feared situations (e.g., "I rode the subway every day this week, and although I felt the symptoms of panic, I managed just fine"). Homework also provides important opportunities for patients to learn that they can use their newly acquired skills to manage alone (i.e., without the therapist) and in real-life settings outside the therapist's office. Doing homework also gives them an opportunity to "be their own therapist," a role in which we would like patients to feel comfortable at the end of treatment. Given these positive aspects of homework, it comes as no surprise that homework compliance is a good predictor of treatment outcome (e.g., De Araujo et al. 1996; Leung and Heimberg 1996).

The relationship between behavior therapist and patient is highly collaborative. The therapist has expertise and experience that may help the patient with his or her problems, but the therapist seeks the patient's full and knowledgeable participation in treatment planning and decision making. As in most forms of psychotherapy, a strong therapeutic alliance is critical. The therapist begins to establish this alliance at the very first meeting by acknowledging the patient's courage in entering treatment and supporting his or her desire to learn new ways to cope with problems. When the therapist provides education in the early sessions of therapy about the patient's disorder and recommendations for treating it, the therapist communicates his or her understanding of the patient's unique situation by including specific examples from his or her particular experience and symptoms. As treatment progresses, decision making about the frequency of sessions, target problems, and homework assignments is collaborative, with the therapist making recommendations but taking into consideration the patient's preferences and judgment.

Another critically important component of behavior therapy is the presentation of a *clear and credible treatment rationale.* The patient must "be on board" or accept the rationale in order to follow the therapy plan both in and out of session. To accomplish this, the therapist usually describes the conceptual model underlying the treatment as clearly as possible, with the goal of helping the patient see that it makes sense and "fits" with the patient's experience. The reasons that the therapist thinks particular skills or specific therapy procedures will help the patient's problems are made clear.

The use of metaphors or analogies can be helpful in presenting a convincing rationale by illustrating the treatment model and giving the patient and the therapist something to refer to as therapy progresses. For example, in PE therapy for treatment of PTSD, we sometimes liken the process of confronting and describing painful trauma memories to the cleaning of a wound that has scabbed over but is not healed and remains sensitive to touch. PE is the process of opening up and cleaning that wound and healing it thoroughly, and even though it still may leave a scar, it will not hurt when something touches it.

In summary, behavior therapy is empirically based, time-limited, problem-focused, present-centered, active, collaborative, rationale-supported, and often very effective.

Behavioral Assessment

Conducting a thorough assessment and establishing an accurate diagnosis is a critical first step in treatment planning. Jumping into treatment without first having a very clear sense of the patient's problems can be frustrating (and even detrimental) for both patient and therapist. The process of assessment and diagnosis is best accomplished with a clinical interview. Although some clinicians prefer to use an unstructured interview format, structured clinical interviews (e.g., Structured Clinical Interview for DSM-IV [First et al. 1997], Anxiety Disorders Interview Schedule for DSM-IV [Brown et al. 1994]) are useful tools. Structured interviews that are disorder specific, including the Yale-Brown Obsessive Compulsive Scale (Goodman et al. 1989) and the PTSD Symptom Scale (Foa et al. 1993), are commonly used. These focused interviews are very helpful for treatment planning and for tracking changes in disorder-specific symptoms over the course of treatment.

Self-report measures (e.g., quality of life, difficulties with anger), which can provide useful information in addition to the clinical interview, serve as another way to track progress over time. Antony et al. (2001) recently edited an excellent volume aimed at helping clinicians to select empirically based assessment measures for anxiety disorders.

Regardless of the specific tools used, the goal is the same: to identify the primary problem that should be the focus of treatment and also assess other factors that might be relevant to the clinical picture. A diagnosis rarely can be made solely on the basis of the patient's simple description of a presenting problem. For example, consider a patient who presents to the clinic with a fear of flying. Knowing only this information does not establish a diagnosis or a treatment plan. The patient might fear being in an airplane crash, suggesting the presence of a specific phobia of flying. The patient might have actually been on an airplane that made an emergency landing because of engine failure and might have since been experiencing nightmares and flashbacks. This history would be more suggestive of a diagnosis of PTSD. Or the patient might fear having a panic attack while on an airplane and be uncomfortable with the idea of not being able to leave the situation if this were to occur. This patient would most likely have panic disorder. These distinctions are important because although behavior therapy for the various anxiety disorders certainly shares common features, the treatment approach for each of these causes of fear of flying would be quite different.

It is also important to obtain a full or complete description of the characteristics of feared situations. Typically, subtle variables influence the clinical picture of each patient. For example, a patient with panic disorder who (among other situations) fears flying might be fine on a 1-hour airplane ride. Longer flights, however, might be a problem. Similarly, this patient might feel confident flying with a companion but might be very frightened of flying alone. Getting a sense of the overt avoidance practiced by the patient (e.g., not taking long flights and not flying alone) and more subtle avoidance (e.g., having a few drinks before getting on the airplane) is very important for the process of treatment planning. Patients are often amazed when clinicians ask questions about these subtle nuances. This type of questioning conveys the therapist's understanding of the patient's disorder and his or her particular symptoms. This makes the patient feel understood and enhances the establishment of a strong therapeutic alliance.

In the process of assessment, patients are also asked about other problems or difficulties that they might be experiencing. Comorbidity is common with many disorders, and although treatment should focus on one disorder at a time, clinicians should be aware of the bigger picture. Additional diagnoses may play a role in the maintenance of a primary disorder (e.g., a person with social anxiety who drinks alcohol as a means of alleviating anxiety in social situations) and also can influence the targets and progress of therapy (e.g., a person with PTSD and very severe depression accompanied by suicidal ideation may benefit from treatment aimed at amelioration of depression before focusing on the PTSD).

Behavior therapists also assess the patient's general functioning and how it has been affected by the presenting problem. Important areas to assess include occupational or educational and social functioning. This serves as a useful metric for the severity of the disorder and helps in the process of establishing rapport by looking at the whole person rather than focusing on only symptoms. Furthermore, knowing what the patient hopes to gain from a decrease in symptoms can be helpful later in treatment when he or she is faced with challenging tasks in therapy. For example, when giving up rituals is extremely difficult for patients with OCD, being reminded of how their lives will improve with less OCD interference (e.g., returning to work, having more time to spend with the family) can be very motivating.

Although behavioral tests are not essential, they can be used in the assessment process. During clinical interviews and when completing self-report measures, many patients have difficulty reporting on the thoughts, behaviors, and feelings that they experience when they are faced with their feared object or situation. Other patients avoid their feared object or situation to such an extent that they may not have a clear recollection of how they reacted in the past when confronted with these feared stimuli. In these instances, having patients undergo a behavioral test in the presence of the assessing clinician can provide valuable information for diagnosis and treatment planning.

Behavioral tests often involve having patients engage in a feared behavior, such as asking a patient with a fear of public speaking to give a speech in front of several strangers. Role-playing a social interaction with a patient can give the assessor a good sense of the patient's strengths and weaknesses in social skills or assertive behavior. Behavioral tests also can involve assessing how far a patient can progress through a series of actions leading up to a feared behavior. For instance, a person with agoraphobia who can no longer go to work may be asked to progress as far along his or her route to work as possible (e.g., leaving the house, getting in the car, driving through traffic, arriving at the office). The major variable of interest in this type of behavioral test is how far along the fear hierarchy the patient can progress; this also can be used as a good measure of treatment outcome.

Being observant of subtleties in behavior can help formulate a clearer clinical picture. Patients with OCD may arrive at sessions very late because they were held up at home with their rituals, or compulsions may be evident right in the session. For example, a patient whose primary ritual was making things "come out even" was quite distressed in her first exposure session to have only one exposure planned by the therapist for that session. Her compulsion compelled her to insist on doing two of the exposures on her hierarchy. Another patient automatically straightened sheets of paper on the therapist's desk that were off center; another was reluctant to use the therapist's pen to fill in self-report measures, because of contamination fears.

Interventions

In this section, we describe two types of treatment that are frequently used interventions of the behavior therapist: anxiety management training and exposure therapy.

Anxiety Management Training (Stress Inoculation Training)

The conceptual model underlying anxiety management training stems largely from theories of stress and coping. One of the most commonly used forms of anxiety management training—SIT (Meichenbaum 1984)—is firmly rooted in this framework. In Meichenbaum's description of the conceptual underpinnings of SIT, stress is viewed not just as an environmental event or as the individual's emotional and behavioral response to the event but rather as an interaction between the person and the environment. Stress is experienced when the person views the environment as straining his or her coping resources and thus threatening his or her safety or well-being. In this model, stress is a dynamic, inevitable aspect of life and cannot be eliminated. Anxiety is a normal response to stress. The goal of the stress inoculation treatment is to teach patients to understand the dynamics of stress and to develop or enhance their intrapersonal and interpersonal skills for managing stress.

SIT has been used in numerous settings and with various populations, including female rape victims with PTSD, medical patients undergoing painful procedures, workers in high-stress job settings (e.g., police officers and firefighters), and athletes enduring the stress of intense competition. Meichenbaum's well-studied SIT program begins with an *initial conceptualization phase* in which the patient's presenting problems are analyzed from the transactional perspective, the patient is enlisted as a collaborator, and the rationale or conceptual groundwork for the skills training is laid down. The next phase includes *training and practice of coping skills*. These typically include breathing and relaxation training to aid in the reduction of physiological arousal and tension, structured problem solving, cognitive restructuring, guided self-dialogue, assertiveness training, behavioral rehearsal or covert modeling, and role-playing. Some of these skills are described in the following subsections:

Breathing Training

The therapist explains that the goal of the breathing retraining is to slow respiration rate and reduce oxygen intake. The therapist gives specific instructions for how to slow down breathing and pair it with a cue for calming and relaxing the mind (e.g., silently and slowly drawing out the word *calm* while exhaling very slowing—"caaaaaaaaaaaaallllllllllllmmm"). The therapist models this slow breathing pattern and then observes as the patient tries and provides appropriate feedback. Finally, for use at home, an audiotape is made of the therapist guiding the patient through 10–15 such respiratory cycles. The patient is encouraged to practice the skill several times daily in order to develop its use for managing anxiety.

Relaxation Training

A very commonly used method of relaxation training is the progressive muscle relaxation exercise. During progressive muscle relaxation training, the patient is taught to systematically tense and then relax specific muscle groups throughout the body, while focusing his or her attention on the tension–relaxation contrast. The goal of this training is to learn to identify what muscles feel like when they are tense and tight and thus be able to eliminate excessive muscle tension when it is detected. The therapist teaches the relaxation exercises in session, and an audiotape is usually made of the instructions for the patient to practice with every day at home. Once proficient at identifying and eliminating excess muscle tension, the patient is often taught abbreviated or shortened forms of relaxation. For example, therapists often teach patients in this stage to relax by "focusing in" on each muscle group and "letting go" of tension, preceded and followed by slow, calm breathing.

Structured Problem Solving

The patient learns to define and solve problems by following a series of steps. Most problem-solving strategies require the patient to systematically 1) define the problem in concrete terms; 2) set a realistic goal and steps to the goal; 3) generate a list of possible solutions or alternative courses of action; 4) evaluate the pros and cons of each possible solution; 5) choose a solution and determine the steps necessary to implement it, which may include behavioral or imaginal practice of the steps with the therapist; 6) implement the plan; and 7) evaluate the outcome, including reinforcing himself or herself for attempting to solve the problem.

Guided Self-Dialogue

In guided self-dialogue, the patient learns to focus on his or her internal dialogue or on what he or she "is saying to himself or herself." The overall aim is to replace irrational, unhelpful, or negative self-dialogue with rational, facilitative, and task-enhancing dialogue. The patient is taught to prepare for stressful situations by asking and answering a series of questions. In a version of Meichenbaum's SIT program adapted by Veronen and Kilpatrick (1983) for rape survivors, coping with stressors consists of four stages: 1) preparation, 2) confrontation and management, 3) coping with feelings of being overwhelmed, and 4) reinforcement. For each stage, the patient and therapist generate a series of questions and statements that encourage the patient to 1) assess the actual probability of a negative event happening, 2) manage avoidance behavior, 3) control self-criticism and self-devaluation, 4) engage in the desired behavior, and 5) reinforce himself or herself for attempting the behavior and for following the plan.

Behavioral Rehearsal

Two common methods of rehearsing new and developing behaviors are covert modeling and role-playing. *Covert modeling* is imaginal practice of a desired behavior and is essentially role-playing in the imagination (i.e., covert). Typically, the therapist first describes a scene involving a difficult situation for the patient in which he or she confronts and successfully works through the situation (i.e., modeling). Next, the patient visualizes himself or herself coping successfully with the situation. Scenes used for covert modeling are sometimes those later used for role-play practice with the therapist.

Role-playing is the rehearsing of speech and actions while pretending to be in a particular situation or in a set of circumstances. During the role-play training, the patient and therapist actually act out scenes in which the patient confronts a difficult or stressful situation. Role-playing is a means of learning new behaviors and words and provides a chance to practice the new behaviors before the real-life event occurs. Like a dress rehearsal, the repetition of a behavior reduces anxiety and makes it more likely that a new behavior will be used when it is called for.

During role-play, it is common for the therapist to first play the patient's role and model appropriate social skills. Then, roles are reversed so that the patient plays himself or herself. The patient and therapist discuss the experience after each role-play. The patient is encouraged to point out positive aspects of his or her performance as well as areas that could be improved, and the therapist also gives feedback. Role-plays are repeated, with the goal of shaping desired behavior and developing better skills through practice.

As noted in our introduction to behavior therapy, homework and repeated practice of newly acquired skills are integral to this approach. The more that a patient practices the new tools outside of sessions, the more proficient he or she becomes and the more data he or she has to bring into sessions for continued fine-tuning of the skills. At the same time, increased proficiency in successful management of stress promotes increased confidence and self-efficacy in the patient. The anxiety and other negative emotions (e.g., anger, sadness) that are associated with high levels of stress typically diminish as the patient's skills for managing stress improve. Another very effective means of decreasing anxiety is learned in the process of exposure therapy.

Exposure Therapy

Excessive and persistent fear is a core feature of anxiety disorders. Yet fear is certainly a normal and appropriate response to dangerous or threatening situations. What distinguishes normal or appropriate fear from pathological fear? How can we conceptualize clinically significant fear, and how can it be modified? According to Foa and Kozak (1986), pathological fear is distinguished from normal fear by its disruptive intensity; by the presence of inaccurate associations among stimuli, response, and meaning elements; and by its resistance to modification.

Consider the example of a man who is bitten by a stray dog one day and subsequently develops a fear of all dogs. The sight of a dog walking down the street reminds him of the dog that bit him (stimulus–stimulus association), and he immediately associates this unfamiliar dog with danger (inaccurate association of stimulus with meaning of danger). This association triggers extreme fear (disruptive intensity) in the man. His heart rate and respiration accelerate rapidly, his muscles tense and his body trembles, and he breaks out in a sweat. He immediately runs to the nearest building (association between harmless stimuli and avoidance responses), not leaving until he is sure that the dog will be gone. He has a hard time believing that this particular dog is friendly and safe and has never bitten anyone, despite repeated reassurance (resistance to modification). This scenario is repeated every time the man encounters a dog, even at a distance. His fear, continually reinforced by this persistent and pervasive avoidance of dogs and any place a dog might be encountered, makes him begin to just stay at home. The avoidance ultimately causes so much interference in the man's life that he finally seeks treatment for his phobia. How can the clinician help this patient to decrease this pathological fear?

Foa and Kozak (1986), building on the work of Rachman (1980), proposed that in order for treatment to successfully modify a pathological fear structure, intervention must 1) activate the fear structure and 2) provide new information that is incompatible with the existing pathological elements so that they can be corrected. Exposure therapy has proven to be a very effective means of accomplishing both of these objectives. Exposure procedures activate the fear structure through direct or imaginal confrontation with the feared situation or object. This confrontation provides an opportunity for corrective information (i.e., new learning) to be integrated into the person's representation or memory of this situation, thus lessening the fear associated with it. For example, if the man with the dog phobia repeatedly approaches and pets dogs that wag their tails and do not bite him, then he will learn that some dogs are safe.

In exposure treatments, patients are encouraged to confront the feared and avoided situations or objects in two main ways: 1) imaginal exposure, which requires the patient to vividly imagine the feared situation and its consequences and to not avoid or escape the resulting anxiety; and 2) in vivo exposure, which entails systematic and gradual confrontation with objects, situations, places, or activities that will trigger fear and urges to avoid.

Imaginal Exposure

In imaginal exposure, the patient vividly imagines himself or herself coming into contact with the feared situation or stimulus. The imaginal scene typically includes a detailed description of events as well as the thoughts, feelings, and physical sensations the person imagines would result from that contact. Imaginal exposure is most commonly used in the treatment of PTSD and OCD.

Imaginal exposure for treatment of PTSD. In PTSD treatment, imaginal exposure or reliving is used to help the patient to emotionally process and organize his or her traumatic memory. Before initiation of imaginal exposure, the therapist provides a thorough rationale for its use in ameliorating PTSD symptoms. The therapist explains to the patient that imaginal exposure to the trauma memory promotes emotional processing of the traumatic experience. This results in increased coherence and organization of the memory, habituation of distress when thinking about the trauma, realization that the memory itself is not dangerous and that anxiety does not last forever, and increased confidence in one's competence and ability to cope.

In imaginal exposure, the patient is instructed to close his or her eyes and describe aloud what happened during the trauma, while visualizing it as vividly as possible. The patient uses the present tense to describe the thoughts, emotions, and sensory experiences that occurred during the traumatic event. Imaginal exposure is continued for a prolonged period (usually 30–45 minutes) and includes multiple repetitions of the memory if necessary. The goal is to help the patient access and emotionally engage in the trauma memory. Immediately following the imaginal exposure, the patient and therapist discuss the experience. Once begun, the imaginal exposure is conducted in multiple treatment sessions, until the anxiety and distress associated with the memory have subsided. For homework, the patient is asked to listen to audiotapes of the imaginal ex-

posure on a daily basis, which continues the work of emotionally processing of the trauma.

Imaginal exposure for treatment of OCD. In OCD treatment, imaginal exposure is used primarily as a means of exposure to the feared consequences of obsessions or of not performing compulsive behavior. Before beginning the imaginal exposure, the therapist and patient together develop
the details of the imaginal scenario, which is written in the present tense
and includes a great deal of elaborate sensory and affective detail to enhance
the vividness of the story. Next, the patient engages in the imaginal exposure by vividly imagining this event and its consequences while describing
aloud the scene he or she is visualizing. The session is tape-recorded, and
the patient is instructed to listen to the scenario over and over and to imagine the events described as though they were happening "right now." Imaginal exposure is conducted over a prolonged interval and over several suc-
cessive days to achieve habituation and extinction of the fear.

The following is an example of an imaginal exposure script for Mr. B,
an OCD patient with harming obsessions. Note that the imaginal narrative clearly aims to promote engagement with the OCD patient's feared
consequences (killing innocent children through his careless handling of
chemicals and going to jail for life for this). Imaginal exposure is often an
effective means of confronting feared situations and their unrealistic or
excessive consequences.

> I fill up the sprayer with pesticides and go out into the garden to spray the
> yard. I decide to give everything an extra-heavy coating because it's been
> so long since I did it last. I notice the fluid collecting on the leaves of the
> shrubs and on the grass, coating every surface until it drips onto the
> ground. The sight of the poison dripping from the leaves triggers a mo-
> ment of fear as I think about how it could be dangerous or deadly to
> someone and that maybe I should put up signs to warn people. Instead, I
> decide it's not worth the trouble and do not bother.
>
> As I'm finishing and putting the equipment away, I hear the sound of
> children from behind me, and I turn to see two kids running through the
> yard where I just finished spraying. They are playing a game and are dart-
> ing in and out through the bushes. I feel a twinge of anxiety as I think
> about the pesticides and worry again that it could be dangerous to the
> kids. I consider telling the kids to stay away, but I don't have the energy
> to yell that loudly, so again I shrug it off and turn to go into the house.
>
> Later that night, I hear a loud disturbance and see flashing lights out-
> side. When I go out to investigate, I see police cars and ambulances on the
> street in front of the neighbors' house, the same house where the children
> live. Once again, I think of the pesticides the kids had been running
> through, and it occurs to me with a sudden rush of dread that if they have
> been poisoned, the emergency team will need to know this. I find the
> children's parents and feel a knot of fear growing in my stomach as they

tell me that the children have fallen mysteriously ill with severe rashes and stomach pain and that they may die. I am now certain that the kids are poisoned from the pesticides, and I am very worried, but I don't say anything, thinking that I don't want to be held responsible and hoping that the doctors will know what to do.

The next morning, I am awakened by a loud banging on the door, and when I open it, I see the children's parents with tearstained faces, flanked by several stern-looking police officers, who promptly place handcuffs on me and inform me that the children died during the night and that I'm under arrest for manslaughter because of my reckless behavior. I feel completely helpless and terrified as I am led away, and I turn to see my wife looking at me in shock, saying, "Is it true? Did you really kill those poor children? How could you?"

My case quickly comes to trial, and in front of the entire courtroom, witness after witness testifies to how I recklessly sprayed a deadly pesticide all over my yard and knowingly allowed children to play in it. I look around from where I am seated and see the angry, disgusted expressions on the faces of the jury, the audience, and even my own family. I realize that I am completely alone in that courtroom, that not one person is on my side. I am quickly found guilty and sentenced to life in prison. As I am led away, I see my family looking at me with disgust, and I know that I will never see them again. I think of what my future holds: living in a dark, damp, smelly cell, filthy with urine and waste, among hardened criminals and being forced to endure a lifetime of violence and brutality. This is how I will spend my last years.

In Vivo Exposure

In vivo exposure refers to real-life confrontation with feared stimuli as opposed to confrontation in imagination. The first step in implementing in vivo exposure is to create an exposure hierarchy: the patient and the therapist work together to generate a list of situations or activities that the patient either endures with great discomfort or avoids completely. Once the list is generated, patients are asked to assign a subjective units of distress rating (ranging from 0 to 100) to each item as a means of arranging the items in a hierarchical order. A well-constructed hierarchy includes a range of items spanning from those that generate moderate anxiety to those that generate the most anxiety a patient can imagine (see Table 3–1). In general, it is best to confront the items in a systematic way, beginning with items that have been assigned moderate subjective units of distress ratings and working up through the list to more feared items. This approach allows patients to gain confidence and self-efficacy through early success experiences and is also more palatable than starting exposure exercises with the most anxiety-provoking items on the hierarchy.

The first exposure typically takes place during a treatment session so that the therapist can demonstrate the process of exposure and lend sup-

Table 3–1. Sample hierarchy for specific phobia of dogs

Item	Subjective units of distress rating
Look at *Dogs Illustrated* magazine	30
Watch movie about wild dogs	35
Go to mall and look at dogs through front plate-glass window of pet store	50
Sit in therapist's office with small dog (on leash)	55
Pet small dog with therapist holding on to leash	60
Sit on floor of office with dog walking freely around office	65
Refrain from crossing to other side of street when people walk by with dogs on leashes	65
Go to pet store where people walk around with their pets on leashes	75
Go to pet store and ask to pet and hold specific dogs	80
Visit friend who has large, rambunctious dog who likes to jump on people	85
Go to dog park in city where dogs have to be on leashes	90
Go to dog park in city where dogs can run freely	100

port and encouragement for this challenging task. In-session exposures are not limited to the clinician's office but rather take place where the anxiety "lives." If a patient fears riding elevators in skyscrapers, a good early exposure would certainly be to ride the elevator in the therapist's office building. Yet treatment will be most effective if a later session is held in a skyscraper to directly confront the patient's specific fear. It is also essential that patients begin to do exposures on their own in between sessions as soon as the first in-session exposure is completed. Some patients discount success experiences that occur during in-session exposures. In the case of social phobia, patients may credit success experiences to the benevolence of the therapist or others involved in the exposure. In the other anxiety disorders (e.g., OCD, panic disorder), clinicians are seen as "safe" people, and it is important for patients to see that they can confront their feared situations on their own and effectively manage their anxiety.

Duration of exposure to feared situations is an important factor. Exposure should last long enough for anxiety to habituate. As such, treatment sessions should rarely be less than an hour and might even need to last for several hours. If an exposure is by nature very short in duration (e.g., asking a stranger a question), the exposure should be repeated numerous times. For example, if a patient with social phobia fears saying hello to people (a behavior that takes just a few seconds), he or she could go to the mall and say hello to the clerk in every store. For additional guidelines on how to conduct effective exposures, readers are referred to Antony and Swinson (2000, see p. 199).

In vivo exposure for treatment of phobias.   In vivo exposure is preferable to imaginal exposure in the treatment of phobias. However, if patients are extremely fearful at the beginning of the exposure phase of treatment, it might be appropriate to spend one session (or part of a session) doing imaginal exposure. For example, our patient who is very afraid of dogs can be asked first to imagine petting a dog before moving on to actually doing it in vivo. Imaginal exposure also can be used for phobic stimuli that occur infrequently (e.g., thunderstorms) or that are logistically difficult to implement on a regular basis (e.g., flying).

Even in these situations, however, in vivo exposure must be a part of treatment. If a patient who lives in the North presents for treatment of a phobia of thunderstorms during the winter, it would be best to advise him or her to come back for treatment during the spring or summer. Similarly, patients who are being treated for a fear of flying must be committed to taking at least one flight at some point in treatment. In the case of social phobia, in vivo exposure is always preferred to imaginal exposure, particularly because the feared situations of people with social phobia are amply available.

Flexibility and creativity on the part of the clinician are necessary when setting up exposures for the treatment of phobias. A patient who has a fear of public speaking can practice an impromptu speech in front of the therapist and office staff. Role-plays can be set up in which patients practice asking people out on dates, having casual conversations, or going for a job interview. Therapists also can accompany patients with social phobia as they return an item of clothing to a store or attend a public event, such as a book reading, where they can ask questions in front of strangers.

In vivo exposure for treatment of panic disorder.   As in the case of social phobia, imaginal exposure is rarely used in the treatment of panic disorder. Situations feared by patients with panic disorder are typically readily available. People with panic disorder frequently fear enclosed places, so even sitting in the clinician's small office with the door closed can be a useful exposure. Other common exposures include riding the elevator, standing in lines, riding the subway, driving during rush hour, and going to crowded supermarkets.

Some patients with panic disorder have difficulty transitioning from in-session exposures in the presence of the "safe" therapist to doing homework unaccompanied. In such cases, it can be helpful to add intermediate steps to the hierarchy. For example, the therapist and patient can ride in separate cars of the same subway train and arrange to get off at a particular station. This exercise might make it easier for the patient to then ride the subway alone. Similarly, patients sometimes do exposure homework accompanied by a friend or family member. This is helpful early in treatment, but such safety nets are gradually phased out as treatment continues.

In vivo exposure for treatment of OCD.   In vivo exposure is an essential component of treatment for most patients with OCD. Specific to OCD is the use of exposure combined with prevention of rituals or compulsions (EX/RP). The goal of EX/RP is for patients to expose themselves to feared situations and to learn that anxiety will habituate without the use of compulsive behavior. It is particularly important in OCD treatment to be aware of subtle rituals that patients might use to alleviate anxiety. For patients who use mental rituals or whose behavioral rituals are very subtle, therapists should remind them of the importance of complete ritual prevention before the exposure begins as well as during the exposure itself.

Exposures for patients with OCD vary greatly given the heterogeneity of symptoms seen in the disorder. For a patient who fears getting ill from germs, an exposure might involve touching doorknobs and other objects around the office and then refraining from washing before eating food. For a patient who fears making others ill by spreading contamination, a better exercise is to touch the doorknobs and light switches and then shake hands with office staff or offer them a snack that the patient must handle.

Home visits are often an important component of treatment of OCD. If patients have difficulty leaving the house because they worry about forgetting to lock the door, the therapist goes to the patient's home for a session and helps him or her to leave the house without checking the locks. For patients with contamination fears whose homes are considered "safe" places, it is beneficial to have a session at home that is focused on contaminating objects there.

In vivo exposure for treatment of PTSD.   Trauma survivors often avoid places, people, and objects that remind them of the trauma. Certainly, exposure to feared stimuli that are realistically dangerous or high risk is not appropriate or beneficial. There is no need for victims to confront the perpetrator of a crime or to go to the place where the trauma occurred if that place is objectively considered unsafe (e.g., going to an empty parking garage alone late at night). With this caveat in mind, other in vivo exposures are very beneficial in the treatment of trauma. For example, a patient who survived a car crash may avoid driving his or her car whenever possible. A reasonable goal of treatment is to get the patient back behind the wheel. If a patient was assaulted in a hotel and now avoids being in any hotel, it is reasonable to incorporate that into treatment. Certain objects also might come to be associated with fear. During a kidnapping, one of our patients tried unsuccessfully to use a telephone to call for help, and the assailant tried to strangle her with the telephone cord. Following the trauma, she would only use cordless telephones. Her in vivo exposure exercises included making calls from telephones with cords, which are, of course, not dangerous.

Interoceptive Exposure

Interoceptive exposure is a technique most often used in the treatment of panic disorder. In this form of exposure, patients do things that will deliberately induce feared physical sensations (e.g., running in place, breathing through a straw, hyperventilating). The goal of interoceptive exposure is to help patients learn that although some physical sensations might be uncomfortable, they need not be feared or viewed as a sign of imminent catastrophe. Given that panic has been conceptualized as a fear of bodily sensations (Clark 1988), it is quite reasonable to help patients learn to be less afraid of these sensations.

Symptom induction exercises should be used that tap into the patient's specific concerns. Roth, Antony, and Swinson (see Antony and Swinson 2000, p. 212) identified which physical symptoms are most strongly experienced during particular symptom induction exercises. Patients who are fearful of the sensation of dizziness or light-headedness, for example, could be asked to spin around in a swivel chair, shake their head from side to side, or hyperventilate.

Common Concerns and Caveats in Conducting Exposure Therapy

The conducting of exposure therapy often provokes anxiety in novice therapists, particularly because it requires the therapist and the patient to confront a degree of risk with which neither may be entirely comfortable. However, the therapist must convey confidence in and comfort with the exposure model and with exposure exercises, lest his or her own hesitation instill doubt in the patient and undermine treatment. In the following subsections, we discuss common sources of such discomfort and our suggestions for dealing with them; as a general rule, we strongly suggest that exposure therapy be conducted under close supervision with an experienced exposure therapist.

Risk to the patient. In vivo exposure for simple phobia (e.g., dogs), OCD (e.g., contamination), PTSD (e.g., parking lots or other public places), and panic disorder (e.g., driving) may entail some degree of risk to the patient (i.e., being bitten, becoming ill, being assaulted, or having an accident). Therapist and patient alike must contend with the reality that very few activities in life are completely free of risk. For most of us, living requires making informed decisions about everyday risks and learning to accept small risks, rather than attempting the impossible task of completely eliminating danger. The general rule of thumb we use in deciding what constitutes appropriate exercises is to consider whether the proposed activity is something most people would do or consider reasonable. For instance, walking on a crowded, busy street in the daytime might be considered a reasonable in vivo exercise, whereas walking on a dark, deserted street in a dangerous neighborhood would likely be considered unacceptably risky. In vivo exposure for patients with PTSD often involves helping to return to former levels of behavior or activity. In the case of designing exposure exercises for OCD, however, we have found that exposure often needs to go beyond what "most people" typically do, and thus we usually apply a different standard for ascertaining "acceptable" risk; that is, would a reasonable person do the exercise if circumstances necessitated it? For example, although most people might not routinely put their hands into a toilet in the normal course of events, if one were to drop something important into the toilet, most people would do so. Because these judgments are often difficult to make without the benefit of experience in conducting this form of therapy, the beginning behavior therapist is strongly encouraged to use supervision for help in making such judgments.

Risk to the therapist. Sometimes therapists express hesitation to assign certain in vivo exposure exercises because they fear risk to themselves or because they would not themselves be willing to complete the assignment. Therapists may, for example, hesitate to accompany someone who has a driving phobia on an in vivo exposure exercise for fear of an accident or may be reluctant to conduct certain harm- or contamination-related in vivo exposures for OCD because they fear being harmed or made ill themselves. The best remedy for these doubts is experience; after training and practice with such techniques, the therapist becomes much more comfortable with them. In some cases, therapists might even want to do an exposure on their own a few times before doing the exposure with the patient. For example, if a therapist is not particularly fond of spiders and is getting ready to treat a person with a specific phobia of spiders, he or she might want to spend some time getting used to spiders (e.g., touching them, letting them crawl on his or her hand) so that confidence rather than discomfort or fear is modeled for the patient. At our clinic, therapists often notice that their own anxiety about certain activities habituates after guiding patients through them several times.

Risk to others.   Certain forms of OCD often raise particular concerns among professionals—namely, those involving harming obsessions or obsessions of a sexual nature. When assessing OCD patients with harming obsessions (e.g., the fear that one may suddenly and impulsively harm another person, perhaps by grabbing a knife and stabbing him or her) or sexual obsessions (particularly pedophilic obsessions), many professionals may reasonably worry whether these patients pose a risk to others. This dilemma is basically one of differential diagnosis (i.e., OCD vs. homicidal ideation or pedophilia).

Several features distinguish harming obsessions from homicidal ideation. Harming obsessions are experienced as involuntary intrusions that are inconsistent with the patient's self-image (i.e., are ego-dystonic), whereas homicidal ideation tends to be volitional and goal directed. In OCD, the principal affective response to harming intrusions is fear or distress, whereas true homicidal ideation is more often accompanied by anger, rage, or satisfaction. Although homicidal ideation may be accompanied by fear, this is more likely when the fear is the product of some real or imagined threat from another person, and the homicidal thoughts are driven by a desire for self-protection. Moreover, some behavioral or mental ritual intended to neutralize the impulse usually accompanies harming obsessions. Finally, OCD patients with harming obsessions very seldom have any history of violence or of having taken steps toward implementing their intrusive impulses. If anything, they make great efforts to avoid cues that might increase the likelihood of acting on these unwanted and feared impulses (e.g., removing all knives from the house).

When distinguishing between OCD with pedophilic content and true pedophilia, an important distinction is whether the pedophilic intrusions are accompanied by sexual arousal and a desire to act on them. If sexual arousal is part of the clinical picture, true pedophilia is more likely (although not necessarily certain), and exposure should be terminated if the exercises consistently provoke sexual arousal. Certainly, a careful assessment, including a thorough history, is always indicated in advance of treatment planning, and close supervision is critical for less experienced therapists.

Another source of concern involves the use of confederates in exposure treatment, especially when intended to provoke harming obsessions. For example, when a patient in our clinic, accompanied by the therapist, offers one some kind of unwrapped food to eat, it is likely that this patient is offering food that he or she fears is contaminated. Being helpful colleagues, we eat a bit of the food regardless of whether we are hungry.

Confederates who are unfamiliar with the patient's particular fears (and thus in the patient's eyes more likely to be caught unawares by the patient's "harmful" behavior) are very useful in treating harming obsessions. When enlisting a particular person as a confederate, however, the therapist should ensure that the person understands the rationale for EX/RP. The involvement of loved ones in exposure therapy for harming obsessions may be essential when the patient's core fear is of harming those closest to him or her. The loved one needs to be fully informed as to the nature and intention of the exercise and given the opportunity to decline any part with which he or she is not comfortable. For example, an exposure exercise, such as the patient holding a sharp knife while sitting next to a loved one, would be conducted only if the family member understood the point of and agreed to participate in the exercise.

Two Exposure-Based Behavioral Treatment Programs

In this section, we present two of the exposure-based treatment programs developed and extensively studied at the CTSA: EX/RP for treatment of OCD and PE for treatment of PTSD.

Exposure and Ritual Prevention Treatment Program for Obsessive-Compulsive Disorder

EX/RP is the psychotherapy treatment of choice for OCD. As described earlier in this chapter, EX/RP involves systematic, voluntary exposure to stimuli that provoke anxiety (e.g., handling garbage to confront fears of contamination by germs). Ritual prevention, the other key component, is the voluntary suppression of the usual ritualistic response or compulsion (e.g., washing hands, using disinfectant, wearing gloves, checking something repeatedly).

Research has shown that combining exposure and ritual prevention produces more overall improvement than either component individually. Although less research has addressed the question of the optimal level of ritual abstinence needed for successful outcomes, it is generally accepted that total abstinence from rituals is optimal and that patients who retain much of their ritualistic behavior during and after treatment are at greater risk for relapse (Kozak and Foa 1997; Riggs and Foa 1993), as was the case with Mr. C.

> Mr. C, a 26-year-old man, presented with severe OCD, primarily involving fears of contamination, especially with the AIDS virus or carcinogens.

He had relatively poor insight, meaning that he remained unconvinced throughout treatment that his fears were unrealistic. Throughout his intensive (daily therapy) treatment course, he completed exposure exercises diligently, often going beyond what the therapist expected he would have been capable of (e.g., sharing a drink with a male confederate Mr. C believed to be homosexual; touching objects and surfaces in an adult peep show). However, on most of these occasions, Mr. C was observed to engage in covert or near-covert rituals, such as repeating the phrase "minimal risk" under his breath to reassure himself that the exercise would not result in harm. At the end of treatment, Mr. C's distress resulting from obsessions was improved, but approximately 2 months after completing treatment, he had relapsed to his pretreatment level of severity.

Although it is most common for patients undergoing EX/RP to be instructed to abstain from rituals completely from the beginning of treatment, this "cold turkey" approach is sometimes unrealistic for patients with severe OCD. In such cases, rituals may be eliminated on a graded schedule, as illustrated in the case of Mr. D.

Mr. D was a 50-year-old man with severe contamination-related OCD; his avoidance and rituals (including washing, showering, and using disinfectants) were so pervasive and extreme that he was neither able nor willing to comply with complete abstinence from rituals. Therefore, Mr. D and his therapist instead incorporated gradual ritual prevention in specific situations into his exposure hierarchy. Thus, for example, one week he refrained from washing his hands after urinating, substituting instead a simple rinse of the hands. After successful implementation of this change, Mr. D then refrained from rinsing his hands after urinating. Similarly, Mr. D experienced such intense anxiety after defecating that he was unable to refrain from showering; eventually, however, he was persuaded to give up this particular ritual as one of his weekly exposure exercises.

An interesting question concerning implementation of EX/RP is whether treatment must include actual physical contact with feared stimuli (in vivo exposure) or whether imaginal exposure is sufficient to achieve symptom reduction. Research generally suggests that exposure in vivo is more effective in reducing OCD symptoms, although initial imaginal exposure appears to improve the effectiveness of subsequent in vivo exposure. On a related issue, the addition of imaginal exposure to the feared consequences of subsequent in vivo exposure appears to produce better long-term outcomes. The case of Mr. B, introduced earlier, illustrates this point.

Mr. B, a 67-year-old man, presented with harming obsessions that involved causing illness or death to others by inadvertently poisoning them with household or industrial chemicals. In vivo exposures included activities such as handling household chemicals in proximity to food or using pesticides in his yard. These exercises were greatly enhanced by the addition of imaginal exposure. For example, a script was developed in which children in his neighborhood became ill and died as a result of his having sprayed pesticides in his garden (see the earlier subsection "Imaginal Exposure for Treatment of OCD" for an example of an imaginal exposure script). As a result of listening to this scenario numerous times, Mr. B's distress when actually using pesticides was significantly diminished.

Certainly in some cases, in vivo exposure is impractical or unethical (e.g., exposure to naked children for a patient with obsessive fears of being a pedophile); in such cases, imaginal exposure may be sufficient to activate the patient's fear network and accomplish habituation.

Stan was a 15-year-old boy with OCD whose symptoms included intrusive sexual images and thoughts that he was homosexual. In vivo exposures were conducted in situations that Stan avoided because of these fears (e.g., speaking face-to-face with a male peer, looking at magazines that contained attractive male models, or watching television shows with attractive male actors); however, because of the ethical and legal problems inherent in conducting in vivo exposure to sexual stimuli, many of Stan's exposure exercises were conducted in imagination. For example, Stan was encouraged to purposely expose himself in imagination to the sexual images he reported experiencing spontaneously, often in combination with the in vivo exercises he was engaged in.

Taken together, treatment outcome studies suggest that the optimal behavior therapy for OCD involves both exposure and ritual prevention components, with therapist-supervised exposure sessions including both imaginal and in vivo elements, using exposures of long duration over consecutive days, and instructing the patient to completely resist rituals. In keeping with these findings, the OCD behavior therapy program typically conducted at our center, consisting of 17 sessions in total, has the following structure: The first 2 sessions are devoted to detailed information gathering and treatment planning. These assessment and planning sessions are followed by fifteen 2-hour, therapist-supervised exposure sessions that are conducted either in the office or in whatever setting (e.g., home, driving in cars, public bathrooms) might be necessary to maximize the effectiveness of the exposure exercises. The sessions begin with homework review, are typically followed by 45 minutes of imaginal exposure and then 45 minutes of in vivo exposure, and end with homework assignment. At the end of this treatment phase, if home visits have not already been conducted during the course of therapy, a 1- or 2-day home visit is sometimes scheduled to ensure generalization of treatment gains to the home environment.

The intensive treatment program offered at our center involves 3 consecutive weeks of daily, 2-hour sessions. Although intensive treatment is powerful in that patients see change in their behavior very rapidly, it can be logistically difficult. It is most commonly provided to individuals with very severe and sometimes crippling OCD who are unable to work or attend school because of the interference of the symptoms or to those who come from out of town just for treatment. For those patients whose symptom severity does not warrant daily treatment or who are unable to devote such a concentrated amount of time, OCD treatment at the center is conducted in less intensive formats. A commonly used format consists of two 2-hour sessions per week. To illustrate the EX/RP program, we present the following detailed case description of an OCD patient treated with the twice-weekly session format.

Case Example: Ms. E

Ms. E, age 53, presented for treatment with symptoms consisting principally of harming obsessions. She feared that she would impulsively and purposefully injure or kill another person. The means by which she feared doing so varied considerably but included stabbing, poisoning, arson, and pushing someone in front of a train. She also feared impulsively poisoning her pets and breaking valuables. At the time she entered treatment, she reported that she had discarded all knives from her home, was avoiding travel by train and subway, was avoiding ordering steak or other foods that might require use of sharp utensils in restaurants, and was avoiding contact with household chemicals. She also avoided close contact with loved ones for fear of harming them, which had led to a significant estrangement from her son, parents, and sisters, with whom she had previously been very close. Despite these and other attempts to minimize contact with stimuli that might trigger her obsessions, Ms. E had frequent, intrusive images and impulses involving harm to other people and experienced distress to the point of tearfulness on a daily basis in response to her fears.

Ms. E's compulsions were primarily mental, involving the use of ritualistic imagery that would temporarily neutralize her fears (e.g., imagining herself standing in a purifying white light). She also reported frequently checking various areas for safety (e.g., stoves, locks), seeking reassurance from others that she had not actually caused harm, and frequently expressing her love for others to reassure herself that she would not actually harm them.

After living with OCD in various forms for many years, Ms. E had experienced an acute exacerbation of her symptoms approximately 1 year previously, which ultimately led her to admit herself to a hospital on the advice of a psychologist who was concerned that she might pose a threat to others. She presented for behavior therapy in our treatment center several months after her discharge. Her intake evaluation indicated a moderately severe level of OCD.

As described earlier in the chapter, treatment of OCD begins with a careful and detailed assessment of the patient's symptoms, including a detailed examination of all people, places, objects, and situations that trigger obsessional fears, particularly those stimuli that are actively avoided. This information is then used to construct a hierarchy for exposure that forms the basis for the treatment. Ms. E's exposure hierarchy is presented in Table 3–2.

Table 3–2. Partial exposure hierarchy for Ms. E, a patient with obsessive-compulsive disorder

Situation	Subjective units of distress rating
Standing behind someone on subway platform	55
Buying a knife	65
Handling knife in office in front of therapist	90
Carrying knife in purse; keeping knife at home	90
Handling household chemicals	80–90
Lighting matches and candles	99
Handling knives; riding subway with son	99
Choosing the "dark side"	100

Because the ultimate goal of EX/RP treatment is to assist the patient in confronting and successfully habituating to his or her greatest fear, it is essential to identify the patient's feared consequence of exposing himself or herself to this situation. This is because often in OCD treatment, many in vivo situations represent proxies for still greater underlying fears. For example, Ms. E's fear that handling knives in the presence of her son might cause her to murder her son led to a whole chain of feared consequences: she would then be arrested, shunned by her loved ones, and left to rot in prison for the rest of her life. Many of the in vivo exercises were therefore preceded by exposure to various imagined scenarios in which she actually carried out her intrusive impulses. For feared consequences that were not associated with any particular environmental trigger, imaginal exposure was conducted in isolation. This was the case for the top item on Ms. E's hierarchy: the idea that she might "turn over to the dark side" and embrace evil forever.

In addition to construction of the in vivo hierarchy, Ms. E was instructed to monitor carefully all compulsions on a daily basis to heighten awareness of them, to identify environmental triggers that might have been overlooked in the initial assessment, and to begin the process of ritual abstinence. The monitoring of rituals is highly detailed and requires that the patient note not only the specific ritual engaged in (e.g., washing, checking, asking for reassurance from others) but also the amount of time spent, the stimulus that triggered the ritual, and the peak level of distress experienced before engaging in the ritual. Because Ms. E's rituals were primarily covert (mental) rather than overt (behavioral), they were initially difficult for her to monitor and control. Monitoring of and then abstinence from mental rituals require a degree of self-awareness that patients achieve with varying degrees of success; in Ms. E's case, self-monitoring was relatively easily accomplished.

The planning stage of Ms. E's treatment was completed by the end of session 2, and exposure exercises were initiated in session 3. As determined by her exposure hierarchy, Ms. E's first in vivo exercise involved standing on the subway platform to confront her obsessive fear that she might push someone into the path of an oncoming train. The therapist therefore accompanied Ms. E to a subway station, and they stood at the edge of the platform, with the patient standing behind the therapist. Initially, Ms. E's distress was extremely high, and she was reluctant to stand close to the therapist, but after several minutes, she was able to stand directly behind the therapist as he stood at the edge of the platform. She and the therapist continued in this fashion for approximately 35 minutes, after which she had experienced only minimal reductions in distress. In the next session, this exercise was therefore repeated during the evening rush hour (with trains appearing about once every 90 seconds), for a total of about 60 minutes. During this session, Ms. E's distress peaked at approximately 90 subjective units of distress and declined to approximately 40 by the end of the session. As a follow-up to this exercise, Ms. E was instructed to ride the subway daily and to stand near other passengers on the platform while waiting for the train, as a covert means of provoking her obsessional fears. By the next session, she reported substantially reduced anxiety on the subway and was ready to proceed to the next item on her hierarchy.

Session 5 involved the therapist and patient visiting a kitchen supply store to shop for knives (as mentioned earlier, Ms. E had no knives in her house). Because of the public nature of this exercise, it was important for Ms. E to covertly augment the exercise with imaginal exposure, so she was instructed before entering the store to imagine her worst fear throughout the visit: losing control and impulsively stabbing the therapist or shopkeeper. She was encouraged to select and handle several large and dangerous-looking knives and to test the blade and tip for sharpness to enhance the vividness of the exercise. The exercise terminated with Ms. E purchasing one large and one small knife; however, because it appeared that having the knives in her home would be too difficult for her to accomplish at this stage, it was agreed that she would leave the knives with the therapist until the next session.

In the next session, imaginal exposure was again paired with in vivo

exposure; this time Ms. E was encouraged to handle a knife in close proximity to the therapist, including pointing the knife at the therapist,
touching the point to his chest, and making stabbing motions in the air
behind his back. Ms. E mentioned that she derived some comfort from
the knowledge that the therapist was aware of her obsessions and thus
might be prepared to defend himself should she "snap" and actually attack. Therefore, she repeated this last exercise with a confederate of the
therapist who was not informed as to the nature of her obsessions and
whose back remained to her throughout the exercise. These exercises resulted in a reduction in distress from a peak of 98 to a low of 49 at the
end of the session. At this point, Ms. E felt "ready" to take the knives
home, and she was instructed to use them regularly and to store them in
the open in her kitchen so that they would always be in sight, thereby ensuring constant exposure and habituation to having knives in the house
again.

Several subsequent sessions focused on this same theme of harming,
in which various other people and stimuli of gradually increasing threat
were used, including Ms. E's close friend, sister, and college-age son, and
various household chemicals were used around food, followed by handling food directly. As described earlier, Ms. E first approached these exercises through the use of imaginal exposure and then eventually followed up with in vivo exposure with each of the scenarios involved. In
later sessions, she was encouraged to do in vivo exercises, such as 1) inviting separately a friend and then her son to her home and using her new
knives in their presence and 2) inviting her sister to sleep overnight and
then lighting candles after her sister went to sleep, to trigger her obsession
about causing a fire. As treatment approached the top of Ms. E's hierarchy, she was instructed to ask her son to accompany her to two sessions
so that he might act as a confederate in several exercises. In these sessions,
Ms. E and the therapist first provided her son with a careful explanation
of OCD and of the treatment rationale, so that he could provide informed consent to his involvement in the procedures. The exercises conducted in these sessions closely resembled those conducted with the therapist, including standing on the subway platform and handling knives in
her son's presence.

The final sessions of treatment consisted of Ms. E's constructing and
then implementing a script for imaginal exposure to her most feared consequence—that she would "turn over to the dark side" and become evil.
This exercise required that Ms. E elaborate extensively on her notions of
what it would mean to be evil and what the consequences would be for
herself and her relationships if this occurred. Because Ms. E had experience with several scripts prepared by the therapist, she was encouraged
to develop her own script in this case, in preparation for her taking over
responsibility for maintenance of her treatment gains after completion of
therapy.

By the end of treatment, Ms. E's OCD symptom severity was greatly
reduced and fell within the normal range for nonclinical samples. She reported having completely given up her rituals, including the highly automatic mental rituals she had engaged in with such frequency. Although

Ms. E continued to experience occasional intrusive impulses and images that caused some distress, she responded to these by either ignoring them or, if this proved unsuccessful, contriving some kind of imaginal or in vivo exposure exercise to combat them. She reported that this strategy was highly successful, and she enthusiastically reported a high degree of confidence that she would continue to be able to manage her OCD effectively.

Prolonged Exposure Treatment Program for Posttraumatic Stress Disorder

Our current PE therapy program for treatment of chronic PTSD consists of 10 individual 90-minute sessions. The goal of the treatment program is to help the patient acquire and master specific skills that are used to ameliorate PTSD symptoms. The core components of PE are education about PTSD symptoms and common reactions to trauma, breathing retraining, in vivo exposure, and imaginal exposure. As always in behavioral programs, homework practice of these skills is an essential part of the treatment.

Treatment begins in session 1 with a discussion of the effect of traumatic experiences and the development of PTSD, and the therapist explains the rationale underlying exposure therapy. It is stressed that posttrauma difficulties are primarily maintained by two factors:

1. Avoidance of thinking about the trauma and avoidance of trauma reminders, although effective in the short term at reducing or blocking anxiety, have prevented the event from being emotionally processed and integrated.
2. The presence of unhelpful and often erroneous beliefs and thoughts is brought about by the trauma (e.g., especially prominent are the beliefs that the world is extremely dangerous and that the trauma victim himself or herself is extremely incompetent).

A clinical interview is also conducted in session 1 to acquire extensive information about trauma history and how the patient views his or her PTSD symptoms.

The slow-breathing skill is taught at the end of the first treatment session and is thereafter assigned each week for homework. Daily practice is strongly encouraged. Session 2 begins with an in-depth discussion of common reactions to trauma, followed by the introduction of in vivo exposure and the construction of an in vivo hierarchy. Items on the hierarchy are ranked on the basis of the patient's expectation of the amount of distress he or she would experience if confronting the situations. Once in vivo exposure is introduced, the patient chooses in vivo assignments for homework between sessions each week. The patient is instructed to remain in each situation for 45–60 minutes or until his or her anxiety decreases considerably (by at least 50%). Imaginal exposure is the last procedure to be introduced. It begins in session 3 and is conducted in each treatment session thereafter. Imaginal homework consisting of daily listening to audiotapes of the imaginal exposure continues the work of emotionally processing the traumatic experience.

Sessions 4–10 follow a standard agenda. Each session begins with a detailed review of the preceding week's in vivo and imaginal homework. Patterns of habituation are discussed, and decisions are made about where to focus exposures next. Imaginal exposure is then conducted for about 30–45 minutes, followed by a period of postexposure "processing," during which the therapist and patient discuss the patient's reaction to the reliving and any insights or feelings that have emerged from it. The next week's homework is assigned. In the tenth and final treatment session, the therapist and patient review progress and what the patient has learned from using the therapy. In most successful outcomes, the patient has adopted a whole new orientation in managing his or her PTSD symptoms: avoidance maintains fear, whereas confrontation with trauma memories and reminders promotes recovery and mastery.

The following is a detailed case example of a woman treated with PE for rape-related chronic PTSD.

Case Example: Ms. F

Ms. F, a 35-year-old white woman, was referred to our PTSD program by a marriage counselor. Ms. F had married for the second time about 3 years prior to this and had one child, a 6-month-old daughter. She had an associate's degree and had left her job as a paralegal to stay home with her infant.

Ms. F's trauma history consisted of multiple sexual assaults. At around age 8 years, she was fondled by a much older male cousin, and she was fondled again by an adult male stranger at age 13 years. At age 16 years, she experienced what was in her view the worst and what remained the most upsetting sexual assault. While visiting a 16-year-old male acquaintance in his house, Ms. F was sexually assaulted by this boy and two others ranging up to age 20. During the assault, Ms. F was threatened, struck in the face, smothered by hands over her mouth, and vaginally raped by two of the assailants. She disclosed this assault to no one until her early 20s and received no help or treatment at the time. Three years after the rape, at age 19 years, Ms. F was raped again and did not disclose the assault or seek help.

The initial evaluation found that Ms. F had moderately severe PTSD. Her history included one episode of major depression, beginning after the gang rape at age 16 and lasting at least 1 year. In addition, Ms. F had struggled for many years with bulimia nervosa, which also developed shortly after the rape at age 16. No other diagnoses were given.

Ms. F sought treatment for the first time at age 26, when she entered couple therapy. She described receiving "a good deal of therapy"—both individual and group—off and on for years. Much of her therapy was focused on the effect of the sexual assaults and her struggles with poor self-esteem and binge eating. Treatment history also included an inpatient stay in a 28-day eating disorders program in her early 30s. Her bulimia had been under control for about 18 months prior to our treatment. She did not use alcohol or drugs and had no history of alcohol or substance abuse or dependence.

Ms. F said that her assault-related problems had waxed and waned over the 20 years since her first rape but had never been resolved. The catalyst for seeking treatment in our program was the birth of her daughter 6 months earlier. Ms. F reported that a lot of feelings and memories of her past assaults had been stirred up by the birth. She was experiencing frequent intrusive thoughts and images of the first rape, intense emotional distress when reminded of it, avoidance of thoughts and situations that triggered assault memories, nightly sleep disturbance, and chronic irritability. In addition, she was experiencing fear and worry about her daughter's safety and future. She wanted to resolve these problems and fears "before it affects my daughter, too."

It was apparent early in treatment that Ms. F was feeling extreme shame and guilt about her assault history. She had long-standing and deeply held beliefs about being abnormal, damaged, and "bad." She commented several times: "It's one thing to be raped once, but something is wrong with someone who gets raped more than once." Ms. F also had strong guilt and shame related to the belief that she had not done enough to fight off her assailants at ages 16 and 19; she reported: "I did absolutely nothing. My body just shut down, and I let them do whatever they wanted." These feelings and thoughts were prominent in her imaginal exposure from the beginning.

Imaginal exposure initially focused on the gang rape at age 16 because this was the most distressing and most frequently reexperienced trauma. After five sessions, Ms. F began processing the second rape at age 19, also using imaginal exposure. Her in vivo exposure hierarchy included items such as going to the area where she had met the boy the day she was raped (an objectively safe place), interacting with men of the same race as her assailants, interacting with unfamiliar men in church or in other settings (e.g., asking men for directions or for assistance in a store), going out after dark, and sleeping in her bed with the curtains open when her husband was away. Ms. F was highly motivated, worked hard in her therapy, and was faithful in following through with homework assignments and practicing the skills between sessions.

Ms. F showed effective emotional engagement with the traumatic memories during her imaginal exposures. She reported initially high distress (subjective units of distress) levels and then showed progressive habituation of anxiety within and between subsequent sessions. Her affect during exposure was congruent with her self-reported distress level. Successful emotional processing of the traumatic experiences was seen in several other ways as well. Immediately after her third imaginal exposure, she spontaneously said: "I've been listening to myself say over and over, 'I'm doing nothing to stop them,' and it's beginning to hit me.... What did I think I could do? I was scared to death." She reported in the next session that for the first time, she felt "at peace" with herself about her behavior during the rape.

This acceptance was enhanced by her recall of a few parts of the assault that she had not really thought much about before. For example, her distress about "not doing anything" to resist her assailants also was diminished when she recalled that early in the assault, one of them had put his fist to her face, threatening to "let her have it" and terrifying her into submission. After the imaginal exposure in the following session, she spontaneously said: "You know, I'm beginning to realize that all these years I've blamed myself for the rape, but it's really not about me, it's about them. They raped me." This was quite a significant shift in her view of the assault and her culpability for it.

The treatment produced a significant reduction in Ms. F's PTSD symptoms and in her depression and anxiety. Assessments were conducted before, immediately after, and up to a year following therapy. Ms. F's PTSD severity decreased by 70% from pre- to posttreatment, and 12 months after treatment ended, the severity had declined by 90% from the pretreatment level. Comparable decreases in depression and anxiety were observed.

Ms. F continued to maintain her treatment gains. She spontaneously called her therapist 2½ years after treatment ended to report that she had recently run into one of the men who had raped her so many years ago. He engaged her in a conversation, which she allowed, and in the course of it, he acknowledged that he had "treated her very badly" when they were younger. Ms. F agreed that he had and calmly accepted his apology. As she related this story to the therapist, she said that what pleased her the most about this conversation was that "it just didn't matter to me...I don't care that he apologized, I didn't need it, and it doesn't change how I feel OK today about the past." She felt that this was final proof of how thoroughly the therapy had helped her to resolve the traumatic experiences of her past.

Summary

Behavior therapy is an extensively validated and effective treatment for a variety of disorders, including anxiety, posttraumatic stress, depressive, impulse-control, and personality disorders, as well as for marital and family problems. It pays little attention to gaining insight into the origins of the problems, because insight does not necessarily lead to change. It seeks instead to make changes in current behavior and to maintain these in the future. Therapy is time limited, collaborative, and focused on the present. A thorough initial assessment, which is critical, leads to a treatment plan and psychoeducation regarding the problem and the rationale for behavior therapy. Therapy then becomes very active—active behavioral techniques such as relaxation, exposure, problem solving, and role-playing are used in sessions and practiced after sessions as regularly prescribed homework. The approaches presented here—SIT and two specific forms of exposure therapy, EX/RP for OCD and PE therapy for PTSD—are best learned under supervision and should allow therapists to successfully treat many of the patients seen in a brief therapy practice.

References

Antony MM, Swinson RP: Phobic Disorders and Panic in Adults: A Guide to Assessment and Treatment. Washington, DC, American Psychological Association, 2000

Antony MM, Orsillo SM, Roemer L (eds): Practitioner's Guide to Empirically Based Measures of Anxiety. New York, Kluwer Academic/Plenum, 2001

Brown TA, DiNardo PA, Barlow DH: Anxiety Disorders Interview Schedule for DSM-IV, Lifetime Version. San Antonio, TX, Psychological Corporation, 1994

Clark DM: A cognitive model of panic attacks, in Panic: Psychological Perspectives. Edited by Rachman S, Maser JD. Hillsdale, NJ, Lawrence Erlbaum, 1988, pp 71–89

De Araujo LA, Ito LM, Marks IM: Early compliance and other factors predicting outcome of exposure for obsessive-compulsive disorder. Br J Psychiatry 169:747–752, 1996

First MB, Spitzer RL, Gibbon M, et al: Structured Clinical Interview for DSM-IV Axis I Disorders, Clinician Version (SCID-CV). Washington, DC, American Psychiatric Association, 1997

Foa EB, Kozak MJ: Emotional processing of fear: exposure to corrective information. Psychol Bull 99:20–35, 1986

Foa EB, Riggs DS, Dancu CV, et al: Reliability and validity of a brief instrument for assessing post-traumatic stress disorder. J Trauma Stress 6:459–473, 1993

Goodman WK, Price LH, Rasmussen SA, et al: The Yale-Brown Obsessive Compulsive Scale (Y-BOCS): past development, use, and reliability. Arch Gen Psychiatry 46:1006–1016, 1989

Kozak MJ, Foa EB: Mastery of Obsessive-Compulsive Disorder: A Cognitive-Behavioral Approach. San Antonio, TX, Psychological Corporation, 1997

Leung AW, Heimberg RG: Homework compliance, perceptions of control, and outcome of cognitive-behavioral treatment of social phobia. Behav Res Ther 34:423–432, 1996

Mavissakalian MR, Prien RF (eds): Long-Term Treatments of Anxiety Disorders. Washington, DC, American Psychiatric Press, 1996

Meichenbaum D: Stress Inoculation Training. New York, Pergamon, 1984

Rachman S: Emotional processing. Behav Res Ther 18:51–60, 1980

Riggs DS, Foa EB: Obsessive-compulsive disorder, in Clinical Handbook of Psychological Disorders: A Step-by-Step Treatment Manual, 2nd Edition. Edited by Barlow DH. New York, Guilford, 1993, pp 189–239

Veronen LJ, Kilpatrick DG: Stress management for rape victims, in Stress Reduction and Prevention. Edited by Meichenbaum D, Jaremko ME. New York, Plenum, 1983, pp 341–374

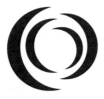

Solution-Focused Brief Therapy

Doing What Works

Brett N. Steenbarger, Ph.D.

Have you ever noticed how authors of journal articles and book chapters rarely introduce themselves at the start of their writing? In a social context, of course, this would constitute unspeakable rudeness. Scholars, however, hardly dare write from the first-person perspective. To do so would be like pulling the curtain from the Wizard, piercing the veil of objectivity.

With this introduction, I have already spoiled any possibility of your ignoring the man behind the curtain, so I might as well allow yellow brick readers a full view. My students refer to me simply as Brett; I teach in an academic health center, where I supervise psychology interns, graduate students in counseling, and psychiatry residents. I also direct a program of counseling for medical, nursing, graduate, and health professional students. If there is a singular passion in my professional life, it is the issue of change: understanding how people change and how we can become ever more effective and efficient as change agents.

Now, I assume that you have acquired this book in order to assist yourself in developing your skills as a brief therapist. Perhaps you are a graduate student or resident learning short-term approaches to therapy for the first time. Alternatively, you might be an experienced counselor or therapist looking to hone your talents and add to your repertoire. In any event, you probably come to this text with several assumptions. You assume that I, as a chapter author, have certain experience and expertise in the field of solution-focused brief therapy. You also assume that I will attempt to share this background with you in the chapter and that you will be able to absorb some of these ideas and apply them to your practice. This, of course, entails yet another assumption: that you have certain holes in your training and experience that need to be filled.

Notice how these very natural and basic assumptions structure our relationship. You, the reader, are the vessel waiting to be filled by me, the expert. I am in the active role of delivering ideas and skills; you are in the role of absorbing these. That does not sound like a very promising start to our fledgling relationship, does it? So, while we are getting acquainted, let us turn these assumptions on their head and see what happens.

Please recall a recent occasion in which you helped a person make a change in his or her life. It does not have to be an earth-shattering change, and it does not even have to be a therapeutic change. It could be as simple as assisting a friend through a loss or helping your child with a conflict at school. I want you to vividly replay that helping episode in your mind, focusing on what you did and said to help the other person make the change. Imagine the nonverbal elements—your look, your tone of voice, the way you sat or stood beside the person—as well as your specific messages. Try to put yourself in the other person's shoes and form an image of what he or she would have experienced in his or her interaction with you.

Although the details of your scenario will be unique, I strongly suspect that there will be some universal elements. The odds are good that you began your helping by attentively listening to the other person, expressing concern and interest. Quite likely, in tone or words, you expressed a degree of encouragement, making it clear that all was not hopeless. Perhaps most important of all, you probably helped shift that person's perspective, providing him or her with a novel way of viewing the situation and perhaps some new ways of responding to the challenge. If your friend came to you with a loss, you might have helped him or her see that all was not lost; if your child was experiencing conflict, you may have modeled a strategy for resolution. Regardless of the details, however, you are likely to have accomplished three things in your helping: 1) the establishment of a trusting bond, 2) the introduction of hope and optimism, and 3) the creation of a novel perspective, experience, and/or skill.⌐

If you were able to achieve these ends with another person in the course of a single helping interaction, then you already know quite a bit about how to do brief therapy. Because that is what brief work is all about, whether it is behavioral, cognitive, psychodynamic, solution-focused, strategic, or interpersonal. Moreover, if you can catalog enough examples of your successful helping in personal and professional settings, you probably will find that you know more about short-term work than you think because you will have a template for the kinds of brief helping that *you* do best.

My goal in this chapter is not to enable you to conduct brief therapy in the manner of recognized practitioners. I also do not intend to encourage you to do therapy my way. Instead, I wish you to *consider becoming more of the effective helper that you already are when you are at your best.* Identify what you are already doing when you are an efficient, effective facilitator of change, and then do those things more consistently and intentionally.

Essence of Solution-Focused Brief Therapy

By now, you have probably figured out my game. The introductory paragraphs were my solution-focused brief therapy (SFBT) with you. As a reader, you, like most clients, might come to this text focused on your problems and deficits. You acquired this book to fill the holes in your training, and so your perspective is hole centered. I can imagine that a mouse that saw only holes would never find Swiss cheese. Similarly, clients who are locked into their problems frequently are starved for solutions. SFBT, like the earlier paragraphs, stands the usual assumptions of therapy on their head. Instead of focusing on what people lack, it looks for occasions in which they are able to think, feel, and act in ways that move them toward their goals. Analyzing the past and developing insight into conflicts are thus not a part of SFBT, nor are behavioral analyses or the keeping of problem-based journals. Instead, SFBT emphasizes goals and ways in which clients are already (if inconsistently and incompletely) achieving these.

Interestingly, it was my parenting experiences that first interested me in SFBT. As the father of two adopted children, I quickly learned that they came into this world with temperaments and behavior patterns far different from my own. Any Pygmalion-inspired hope I may have harbored about creating them in my image was dashed at the outset. I realized that if I were going to be at all successful as a father, I would have to learn who these little people were and then help them become the best individuals they could be, given their personalities, skills, and interests. When I first encountered SFBT, I recognized this same attitude. If I can be a model for my clients, that is wonderful, but my role is not to mold others to my preconceived image. Each individual comes to therapy with his or her own tools, problems, and exceptions to these problems. My job is to learn as much as I can about my clients and find out how they are already doing some of the things that they want to be doing in their lives. Then I have an opportunity to help them become more of who they already are.

Assumptions of Solution-Focused Brief Therapy

The underpinnings of SFBT can be traced to the pioneering work of the Bateson research group on schizophrenia in the 1950s, which examined the role of communication processes in emotional disorders. Many of the group members—most notably, Jay Haley—were familiar with the innovative brief therapy practice of Milton H. Erickson, who used hypnosis, metaphoric communication, and directed tasks to alter problem patterns. Haley's efforts to understand Erickson's work, followed by the efforts of Richard Bandler and John Grinder and of Steven Lankton, inspired strategic and single-session therapies. These approaches, which emphasize the self-reinforcing nature of problems and attempted solutions, seek minimal interventions to break these vicious cycles. Clients with insomnia, for instance, become increasingly concerned with their problem, trying everything possible to fall asleep. These efforts, however, only heighten the sleeplessness because the process of trying to fall asleep interferes with the necessary relaxed state of mind.

Strategic therapists emphasized that people are suffering not so much from their problems as from the ways in which their attempted solutions maintain these problems. Instead of analyzing and working through these problems, change simply requires an interruption and shift of these attempts at solution. A SFBT practitioner, for example, might have clients with insomnia explore what is happening at those times when they *are* able to feel a little bit drowsy, such as when they are engaging in routine, boring tasks. Instead of trying to fall asleep, the client is encouraged to forget about sleeping and perform some of the routine tasks that have been associated with drowsiness in the past. In this way, sleepiness can emerge naturally, without the interference of effort and frustration.

The strategic focus led de Shazer and colleagues at the Brief Family Therapy Center in Milwaukee, Wisconsin, to develop an approach to therapy that was explicitly solution focused. In a series of efforts to map the structure of therapy, de Shazer (1985, 1988) identified exceptions to presenting problems as fundamental to this solution-focused approach. Instead of exploring the initial complaints of clients and maintaining a problem focus, de Shazer instituted a variety of strategies for inquiring about and reinforcing examples of solution: those instances in which clients behaved in ways consistent with their desired ends. By circumventing traditional procedures of evaluating and exploring past problems, and by targeting specific, desired patterns as objectives, solution-focused therapy was able to address the concerns of clients in a brief fashion, generally in fewer than 10 sessions. Subsequent writings by O'Hanlon and Weiner-Davis (1989) and Walter and Peller (1992) have elaborated on the SFBT model, making it one of the most popular brief approaches to therapy.

From a theoretical vantage point, SFBT draws heavily on constructivism: the notion that the problems experienced by clients are not intrinsic to them but the result of the ways in which they construe themselves and their world. Constructivism is a philosophical tradition that emphasizes perception as the result of active, interpretive processes mediated by people's experience, values, and beliefs. A problem, such as the insomnia mentioned earlier, only becomes a problem when it is so construed by an individual. Once people construct the notion that they have insomnia, they engage in various behaviors to address this problem, often reinforcing the very concern that they are trying to address. The real problem, according to the SFBT practitioner, is not so much the pattern of behavior that brings the client to therapy but the construal that reifies this pattern as a problem. Maintaining a problem focus in therapy by exploring and targeting unwanted patterns only reinforces the mode of construal that troubles the client in the first place. Accordingly, SFBT seeks to construct alternatives to problem-based construals. These can be identified from implicit goals brought to therapy by clients and from exceptions to problem patterns that are similarly implicit. Such solutions, once identified, can anchor new adaptive efforts, as clients are encouraged to do more of what might work for them.

The crucial assumption made by SFBT is that therapy is more of an epistemological activity than a medical or therapeutic one. "We live in a world of meaning and language that is creational, social, and active," Walter and Peller (1996, p. 11) stressed. Common complaints such as depression, anxiety, anger, diminished self-esteem, and interpersonal conflicts are seen as things that people *do*, not as things that they *have*. Once the person diagnoses himself or herself as someone "with" depression, anxiety, or interpersonal problems, this identification cements the status of the problem. The SFBT practitioner is thus more concerned with the factors that maintain problems than with initial causes. Indeed, a problem such as insomnia may be initiated by any of a variety of factors, from situational stress to a severe cold. It is the person's identification with the problem, however, that is necessary for its maintenance. de Shazer (1988, p. 8) observed that "problems are problems because they are maintained. Problems are held together simply by their being described as 'problems.'" Once this identification is broken, the individual gains the ability to do something different and discover new, constructive patterns that become solutions.

Simon (1996) and O'Hanlon and Weiner-Davis (1989) made the important point that, despite its name, SFBT is less about solutions than about goals and possibilities. The client enters therapy with problems in the foreground of perception. SFBT attempts to shift this focus to the life that clients want to be living, and it places this in the foreground. Walter and Peller (1996) used the term *goaling* to describe the ways in which individuals continually develop life possibilities. The objective of therapy, from this perspective, is less of an end point than a process of evolving meaning, jointly guided by the participants. Much of the "stuckness" that we observe in therapy—and in our own personal lives—can be seen as the result of "probleming" overtaking "goaling." The emphasis on problems blocks the creative search for alternatives, stifling healthy development.

An appealing aspect of SFBT is its emphasis on client strengths and assets. Gingerich and Eisengart (2000), in their review, noted that "solution-focused therapists assume clients want to change, have the capacity to envision change, and are doing their best to make change happen. Further, solution-focused therapists assume that the solution, or at least part of it, is probably already happening" (p. 478). This latter point is especially important. Solutions are not therapist-driven framings of problem patterns. Rather, they are grounded in the adaptive efforts of clients already under way. Even when distinct exceptions to problem patterns cannot be identified, it is usually possible to encourage people to imagine what such an alternative might look like. A couple may be so mired in arguing that they cannot think of a single recent time in which they have interacted positively. Still, they might be able to identify elements of such positive interaction from their days of dating, their professional interactions, or their communications with members of their extended families. The operative assumption is that somewhere there is a context in which clients do not enact their problems. Once this can be identified, it is a candidate for a constructed solution.

Case Example: Mr. and Mrs. G

A good example of the ways in which SFBT intervenes in the meaning-making of clients can be found in my counseling with Mr. and Mrs. G, a couple who sought counseling for marital problems.

> Mr. and Mrs. G, both medical students, found that their studies caused them to spend decreasing time with each other, leading them to feel more like roommates than romantic partners. They reported being too tired at night to talk, go out, or make love. Their days, when not filled with classes and study, were taken up with the routine tasks of maintaining a home, such as paying bills and doing grocery shopping. Matters came to a head when Mrs. G began spending more time with Mr. H, a study partner from her class. Mrs. G began feeling an attraction to Mr. H, and during one late-night study session, she kissed him. She guiltily confessed her transgression to Mr. G, who became both angry and concerned for the marriage. Both agreed to seek marital counseling that week.

The preceding information came from the first interview, in which both members of the couple participated actively. Both affirmed that they wished the marriage to continue and expressed a desire to avoid divorce at all costs. Mr. G acknowledged his anger over Mrs. G's relationship with Mr. H but also indicated that he appreciated her honesty after the fact. Mrs. G expressed more resignation than Mr. G, lamenting how they had "grown apart" during their rigorous years of school. Although she did not want to leave the marriage, she could not see how it would be possible to make things right, given the demands of their education. Mrs. G voiced her greatest concern that the two of them would wind up like her parents: a couple who lived together but showed little mutual affection.

Rather than explore the relationships of Mr. and Mrs. G's parents or the detailed history of their own relationship, I attempted to use Mr. and Mrs. G's motivation as a lever in the search for solutions. "I'm not sure I can help you," I explained to them, "although I would like to. Counseling can certainly help a couple work out difficulties between them, but it can't replace love that isn't there. I'm just not hearing much about the *love* in your marriage."

At this, Mr. and Mrs. G emphatically stated that they did love each other and spontaneously produced several examples of their dedication to each other. One such example centered on an episode in which Mrs. G became ill and Mr. G made a heroic effort to nurse her to health, while helping her keep up with her course work. Although she had been quite ill, Mrs. G said that she had enjoyed this time in medical school most of all because of their feeling of being "a team." Another instance of love surfaced when Mr. G described the ways in which they would study together before examinations. When one of them became fatigued or discouraged, the other usually was very willing to put down his or her work and offer a hug, a kiss, and some encouragement. Each of them was willing to accept a lower grade for himself or herself to help the other one pass.

I then introduced a modified version of the scaling question and asked Mr. and Mrs. G to give themselves a report card grade on their marriage, ranging from A to F. When they both rated their marriage as a "D" and asserted that they would never settle for such a grade in school, I suggested to them that they make their couples counseling a medical school elective, complete with expectations of attendance, homework, and a grade at the end. Both members of the couple warmed to this idea and indicated that they wanted an "honors" grade for "our" course. I asked what would have to happen between the two of them for a grade of "honors" to be earned, and they provided many ideas, mostly building on the idea of teamwork and togetherness. Most concretely, they committed to spending one night together per week and 1 hour together per day in a mode that was free of schoolwork and home tasks. Both could agree that they were willing to accept possible lower scores on their medical school tests to help each other pass the elective course we had established.

We held a total of four sessions, scheduled intermittently. These focused on their efforts at teamwork and togetherness and grading each other's work. A particular breakthrough occurred when both of them raised their scores on examinations, even after spending considerable time together in a nonwork mode. This convinced them that the best way to be at their peak for their studies was to be happy with their marital life. It also spawned a variety of creative strategies for enjoying their time together, including taking day trips to area parks, staying overnight at a bed-and-breakfast inn, and signing up for a several-session weekend adult education course on techniques of massage. Mr. and Mrs. G reported greater emotional and physical intimacy as a result of their time together, lessening any lingering concerns Mr. G had about Mr. H. Mrs. G discontinued her studying with Mr. H and instead joined Mr. G for study sessions at a local college library, where they took study breaks together. By the end of the fourth session, both were able to give each other an "honors" mark for their progress.

The example of Mr. and Mrs. G is as notable for what was not undertaken as for its affirmative strategies. We did not explore family histories of dysfunction or their own personal relationship histories. Nor did we dwell on the events that drove the couple apart or that led to the attraction to Mr. H. We spoke of Mr. G's reaction of jealousy and concerns regarding trust, but not as central themes in the sessions. Rather, from the outset, the focus was on the love between them and how this was manifested. The assumption was that the couple, while feeling estranged, were still in love and doing loving things while not even noticing it. It took a subtle threat—the statement of "I don't know if I can help you"—to galvanize the couple into an acknowledgment of the assets they already possessed. There was essentially no teaching of skills in the sessions. Rather, our focus was on helping them do more of what they already had been doing to sustain the marriage.

Compressed Duration of Solution-Focused Brief Therapy

Let us step back a moment and examine the characteristics of SFBT that qualify it as a brief therapy. The major brief therapies share several elements (Steenbarger 1992), including

- Maintenance of a tightly circumscribed focus
- Efforts to establish an early, positive therapeutic alliance
- Efforts to facilitate change in a time-effective manner
- Therapist activity
- Efforts to involve clients in change efforts through within-session experiences and between-session homework
- Relative de-emphasis on the past and emphasis on generating novel experiences, understandings, and skills

The various approaches to brief therapy embody these elements differently and thus differ in their use of time (see Steenbarger et al., Chapter 1, in this volume). SFBT falls on the briefest end of this continuum. Reviews of SFBT generally have found an average number of sessions ranging between three and five (McKeel 1996). Such brevity is attributable to several factors:

- SFBT establishes its solution focus early, eliminating much of the time associated with problem talk and diagnosis. A tight focus for intervention is generally established in the first session, based on the individual's stated goals.
- SFBT views its objective as initiating change rather than seeing clients through an entire change process. People are seen as continually changing and capable of change. Once they have established a useful direction and an appreciation for what they are already doing that is

bringing them closer to their goals, they can sustain change efforts independently.

- SFBT stresses client definitions of goals and, hence, places little time and emphasis on resistances and work to overcome these.
- The SFBT therapist is active from the outset, helping to structure the solution talk. SFBT also emphasizes client activity between sessions, with direct suggestions of "doing something different" if current strategies are not working and doing more of what works.

Elsewhere (Steenbarger 1994), I have proposed that brief therapy achieves much of its brevity by generating novel experiences under conditions of heightened emotional experiencing. Through the use of active interpretations, in-session exercises, and homework tasks, the techniques of brief therapy bring individuals closer to the anxieties, resentments, and losses that trouble them. Then, in the context of this enhanced experiencing, brief therapists introduce new ways of viewing problems, new skills for coping, and/or new experiences of oneself. Just as experiences during periods of trauma tend to imprint themselves on the psyche, the novel experiences of brief therapy tend to "stick" in emotionally charged circumstances.

SFBT achieves this novelty through its redefinition of presenting complaints. Clients come into therapy seeking help for their problems and leave with a focus on their assets and solutions. The real change occurs, however, when clients actually begin doing more of what works and see that it really does work. This is a direct, immediate confirmation of their adaptive capacities. With support and encouragement—a bit of cheerleading—from the therapist, the client begins to internalize a new sense of self: one that emphasizes competence and the capacity for control.

The brevity of SFBT raises concerns that perhaps the work is too brief. Some may view SFBT as "solution-forced" counseling, concerned that clients' normal need to talk about their concerns could be truncated by therapists hell-bent on brevity and solution-talk. These are real pitfalls, to be sure. Research conducted to date and outlined later in this chapter suggests that SFBT is effective, but relatively little work has been done with long-term follow-up to determine rates of relapse. Highly abbreviated therapies may have a better track record initiating change than sustaining it (Steenbarger 1994), raising questions about the appropriateness of three- to five-session therapy for clients with chronic problems such as major depressive disorder. Also, many clients enter therapy not only for reasons of self-change but also for ongoing social support. These individuals are apt to be dissatisfied with any brief modality, SFBT or otherwise.

Effectiveness of Solution-Focused Brief Therapy

A small but growing literature documents SFBT as an effective therapy. Outcome studies generally presume that clients come to therapy with real problems, which then can be followed up over time to assess objective improvement. If the improvement shown by therapy clients significantly exceeds that of persons receiving a placebo intervention, an alternative therapy, or no help whatsoever, the therapy can be said to have been effective.

Many practitioners of SFBT rebel against such outcome assessment because of its grounding in epistemological realism. The constructivist bent of SFBT questions the notion that people enter therapy with objective, diagnosable problems and illnesses. Change, they insist, comes from recognizing that there was no real problem, that clients were already doing what they needed to be doing to become unstuck from their patterns.

Is it necessary to abandon the DSM framework and outcome assessment in order to practice SFBT? As Held (1996) argued, clients do make real changes in their lives as a result of SFBT. Attempts to objectively assess and measure such changes need not collide with a therapist's commitment to explore and expand existing adaptive efforts. As a result, we are now seeing studies not only of SFBT outcomes but also of the component processes that may be contributing to success in SFBT.

Gingerich and Eisengart (2000) offered a particularly useful review of the SFBT outcome research, dividing studies into three categories: well controlled, moderately controlled, and poorly controlled. Through 1999, the authors located 15 controlled outcome studies of SFBT, 5 of which met the criteria for well-controlled research. These 5 studies supported the efficacy of SFBT for problems such as moderate depression, parenting skills, rehabilitation of orthopedic patients, recidivism of prisoners, and antisocial adolescent behavior. Only 1 of the 5 directly compared SFBT with another therapeutic approach, and this found no significant difference between the two. Thus, although "these five studies provide initial support for the efficacy of SFBT" (Gingerich and Eisengart 2000, p. 493), they do not establish that SFBT is uniquely effective relative to other brief forms of therapy.

In his review, McKeel (1996) noted that some of these outcome studies did compare the effects of SFBT with those of existing services within school and prison settings, establishing the effectiveness of SFBT above and beyond the existing services. McKeel (1996) also summarized process-oriented studies of SFBT, examining the effectiveness of typical

SFBT interventions such as the formula first session task. The formula first session task, which encourages clients to focus between sessions on what is happening in their lives that they would like to continue, was found to enhance client cooperation. Clients completing the formula first session task also were significantly more likely to report improvement and optimism than were those not performing the task. McKeel (1996) also cited evidence that most clients do report pretreatment changes— improvements that have occurred between the time of calling for an appointment and attending that appointment. These changes are significantly more likely to emerge in therapy if targeted by the therapist in the first session. This suggests that a focus on positive change can be viable for most clients, if therapists think to ask the questions.

DeJong and Hopwood (1996) summarized outcome research at the Brief Therapy Family Center in Milwaukee, Wisconsin, and found that approximately 80% of the clients reported satisfaction with their therapy 7–9 months after their counseling. Moreover, at this follow-up period, 49% of the clients reported that their therapy goals were fully met, and another 37% indicated that they had made "some progress." These outcomes did not appear to vary as a function of client race or the gender mix of the therapeutic dyads. Interestingly, the clients received an average of only three sessions of therapy, suggesting that a high level of satisfaction with services—and significant perceived success—can be achieved and sustained in a time-effective manner.

A series of studies reported by Beyebach and colleagues (1996) examined the processes contributing to success in SFBT. Their investigations highlighted the role of communications between therapists and clients as an ingredient of success. Dyads that showed a competitive battle for control of session topics obtained less favorable outcomes than did those without such control struggles. Interestingly, in the successful cases, therapists tended to be more directive, providing instructions, whereas an excessive amount of agreement between therapists and clients led to increased relapse. Sequential analyses found that controlling "one-up" and "one-down" communications in therapy tended to elicit subsequent controlling communications from the other party. "One-across," noncontrolling communications, conversely, yielded further noncontrol.

Beyebach et al. (1996) examined SFBT outcomes and found that the sole significant predictor of success was client internal locus of control, which reflects the degree to which individuals perceive that they are in control of their lives. The internal locus was positively correlated with favorable pretreatment reports of change and subsequent goal formation in counseling. "These results show that locus of control is variable and becomes more internal over the course of successful therapy," the authors noted. "This lends support to the notion that the task of solution-focused therapists is to foster situations in which clients experience a better sense of control over their own lives" (Beyebach et al. 1996, p. 325).

Such an analysis suggests that SFBT may work for reasons other than those postulated in the theory. Specifically, the nature of client–counselor communications and the ability to support and extend reports of pre-therapeutic change may be every bit as important as the specific tasks initiated by therapists. This conclusion finds support in the qualitative research reported by Metcalf et al. (1996), who found that clients and therapists in SFBT view the events of therapy quite differently. In general, therapists tended to see themselves as relatively nondirective, whereas clients pointed to direction as a central helping element. Therapists also were likely to attribute success to goal-oriented interventions in therapy, whereas clients emphasized the role of the helping relationship. Given that nonspecific factors tend to be of importance across psychotherapies (see Greenberg, Chapter 8, in this volume), such findings are not surprising.

Practice of Solution-Focused Brief Therapy

By now, you have some idea of what SFBT is, how it fits into the larger scheme of brief therapy, and where it stands relative to issues of brevity and efficacy. The manner in which I presented the studies undoubtedly made my own biases known, which are that SFBT is an effective and innovative therapy that probably works for reasons other than those typically postulated. In particular, I find the notion that solution-focused therapists are nondirective to be well wide of the mark. Practitioners may be confusing the process of guiding therapy (which therapists direct toward solutions from the outset) with the content of counseling goals (which rightly come from the client). Strategic therapists, more directly connected to the work of Erickson, are generally appreciative of the role of persuasion and interpersonal influence in change processes. O'Hanlon, on reviewing transcripts of his SFBT sessions with clients, was said to have been surprised by the degree to which he spoke for clients (McKeel 1996). In the terms of Beyebach et al. (1996), SFBT may be more successful when it involves complementary control than when it involves noncontrol. When clients have control over goal specifics and counselors exercise control over the process of focusing on and attaining goals, both parties can feel appreciated and in the driver's seat.

As a rule, directive therapies, such as systematic desensitization, are easier to manualize than are more exploratory therapies. The directive interventions are largely technique driven and often depend on using the techniques in a particular sequence. Exploratory therapies, by their very nature, can go in any of a number of directions, given the concerns of the client at the time. It is much easier to describe how to do relaxation training than how to turn a countertransference reaction—a therapist's reaction to a client—into an effective intervention.

The practice of SFBT, thanks to the interests of its founder, Steve de Shazer, can be described relatively straightforwardly and even mapped out (de Shazer 1988; Walter and Peller 1992). de Shazer was interested in capturing the process by which people change in therapy and distilling this process to its essence. He found that problems and their discussion were not essential to change. What was essential was a goal and an idea of how to achieve that goal. As a result, de Shazer's maps describe procedures for eliciting goals and either existing or hypothetical ways by which clients can pursue these.

Certain specific techniques distinguish SFBT as a modality. In their review, Gingerich and Eisengart (2000) described seven distinctive criteria for SFBT:

1. A search for presession change
2. Goal setting
3. Use of the miracle question
4. Use of scaling questions
5. A search for exceptions
6. A consulting break
7. A message including compliments and a task

These seven criteria constitute the SFBT road map of change. Let us examine each in turn and then explore the map as a whole.

Search for Presession Change

We are accustomed to beginning therapy with the first session, once the client has entered the office. The solution-focused therapist, however, may view the initial call for an appointment as the actual start of SFBT. During that call, the therapist might encourage the client to be on the lookout for changes that occur during the time between the telephone call and the first meeting. This subtly makes use of regression to the mean as a therapeutic tool. Most clients call for their initial session when they are at their point of maximum discouragement, having failed in their prior attempts to solve their problems. The natural ebb and flow of problems suggests that these might abate to some degree after the initial call, if only as a return to a normal baseline. Such variation becomes an opportunity for inquiring about what the client is doing differently when the problems abate, aiding the construction of potential solutions.

Questions about presession change establish the solution focus very early in therapy and quickly engage the client in the active process of thinking about solutions between sessions. The language in which the discussion of presession change proceeds is important: it frames such change as something the client is doing rather than as something happening to the client. What is being constructed, as a result, is not only solution talk but also a greater sense of internal locus of control. Clients often feel out of control with respect to their problems; this is why they seek help from a professional. By pointing to those occasions when the individual is doing something that produces desired change, the therapist highlights the control that clients may have but may not recognize.

Goal Setting

Walter and Peller (1992) indicated that goal setting occurs very early in SFBT and is distinguished by several characteristics:

- *Goals come from the client*—Goals are stated in the language of the client and reflect the desired ends of the clients. Goals do not emerge from analyses by the therapist, which are then interpreted to clients or otherwise recommended to them via a treatment plan. Anchoring therapy in client goals minimizes the likelihood of resistance by ensuring that the participants in counseling are working toward common ends.
- *Goals are stated in positive form*—Many times clients describe their goals in negative terms, such as "I would like to feel less depressed." Such statements, although a start in establishing a direction for therapy, say little about what clients affirmatively want for themselves. As a result, therapists might follow up with questions such as "What do you see yourself doing when you're not depressed?" or "What will be different in your life if you're not depressed?" A positively stated goal might then emerge, such as "I will reach out to others when I feel depressed."
- *Goals are stated in active form*—The goals of therapy should be stated in the active terms of what the client would like to be doing rather than as some future end state. If the client says, "I would like to do well in my classes," then the therapist might reply by asking, "What do you see yourself doing differently when you are doing better in your classes?" The active framing of goals helps to translate them into con-

crete tasks for therapy. A goal stated in active form could then be "I will break my work into manageable chunks before I study."

- *Goals are stated in here-and-now terms*—Many times a client goal might be stated as a future state of affairs, such as "I would like to be in a successful relationship." This leaves the client stymied, for there is no obvious bridge between his or her current state of affairs and his or her stated ideal. When this occurs, the therapist is apt to solicit a reframing of the goal statement by asking, "What might you be doing right now if you were on track toward developing a successful relationship?" The idea of being "on track," described by Walter and Peller (1992), emphasizes the process of change, creating a present-day bridge between real and ideal. Such a goal might be framed as "I will put myself into two situations this week in which I have to introduce myself socially."

- *Goals are stated in specific, attainable terms*—It is not unusual for clients to state that they would like greater self-esteem or to feel better about themselves. This, Walter and Peller (1992) noted, leaves them in little control of goal attainment because they cannot change their feelings about themselves through a mere act of will. By asking a question such as "What, specifically, would you be doing right now if you were developing better feelings about yourself?" the therapist facilitates a crucial translation to goals that empower the client and foster the sense of internal control. Such a self-esteem goal, stated specifically, might be "I will take care of myself by exercising each day."

More than 15 years of having supervised psychology interns and psychiatry residents in brief therapy has convinced me that such work generally runs aground when goals are insufficiently salient to clients and therapists. A useful exercise in therapy is simply to ask the client to restate the goals of the therapy. Many times, a vague and even confused response is elicited—and many times a different response from the therapist! Perhaps only behavior therapy rivals SFBT in the degree to which the goals of therapy are defined in highly explicit terms and then pursued in a systematic manner. Accordingly, clients in a high state of readiness for change (Prochaska and DiClemente 1986) may find the active goal orientation of SFBT more helpful than those who are in early phases, only just beginning to contemplate the commitment to change.

Use of the Miracle Question

One of the most common ways of eliciting goals in SFBT is through the miracle question. This was described by de Shazer (1988, p. 5) as follows: "Suppose that one night, while you were asleep, there was a miracle and this problem was solved. How would you know? What would be different? How would your husband know without your saying a word to him about it?"

The miracle question, de Shazer (1988) noted, is actually a series of questions designed to elicit descriptions of specific behaviors that can serve as useful goals for therapy. "Through the use of the miracle question," de Shazer noted, "the therapist and client are able to have as clear a picture as possible of what a solution will look like even when the problem is vague, confused, or otherwise poorly described" (p. 6).

The framing of the question as a "miracle" allows the client to step outside current constraints that might be inhibiting the search for solutions. For example, a client might indicate a desire to begin dating but complain that this is impossible, given his or her current lack of funds. The miracle question allows the client to look beyond the lack of funds and define what would be happening if he or she were on track to developing dating relationships. This could easily lead to solutions that allow for meeting people in ways that do not involve the spending of money, such as through religious groups or community organizations.

The question "How would your best friends (e.g., family, spouse) know that you had solved this problem?" also is helpful in encouraging clients to frame goals in observable, concrete terms. This is particularly useful in couples counseling, where such a question frequently elicits specific, interpersonal behaviors that can become initial goals for therapy.

Use of Scaling Questions

A scaling question in SFBT, as in behavioral work, is a request for client self-report. It also can be an effective tool in eliciting client goals. Such a question might be "On a scale from 1 to 10, where 1 is "constantly arguing" and 10 is "getting along perfectly," on average, how would you rate your relationship over the past month?" If the clients give the marriage an average rating of 5, follow-up questions might be "So, with an average of 5, does that mean sometimes you are really arguing badly and other times not so much? What is happening differently at the times when you're arguing less than a 5?" Another approach would be to ask, "A 5 rating? That is better than many couples starting counseling. What are you currently doing that keeps you from being a 1 or a 2?"

Note that the scaling question can be asked to introduce the notion of variability into the definition of problems and solutions. By asking about the "average" rating, the therapist can then naturally inquire about those occasions that are above average and what makes these different. Such scaling may be conducted throughout therapy, both as a way of tracking progress and as a way of focusing on the specific actions that can account for improvements over time. The latter forms the basis for between-session tasks in counseling.

Search for Exceptions

The search for exceptions is the intervention perhaps most commonly associated with SFBT. Clients come to therapy focused on their problems and often frame their presentations in ways that suggest that they have identified with these problems. For example, clients will say that they "always" argue or that they are "always" feeling depressed. Such presentations are then reinforced if therapists adopt a subsequent problem focus.

The search for exceptions emphasizes client strengths by soliciting those instances when clients have *not* been enacting their problem patterns. A therapist might say, for example, "None of us is perfectly consistent, and I can't believe you have a perfect record of arguing every hour of the day. Tell me what you are doing differently on those occasions when you are not arguing." Alternatively, a client may spontaneously mention a sphere of life in which the problem pattern does not occur, as in "I don't know why I feel anxious during examinations. When I am with my friends or out on a date, I never feel nervous." The therapist can then respond with the inquiry "So, tell me what you are doing differently with your friends that you are not doing in the examination situation."

I have found it helpful, at certain times, to elicit exceptions from clients by initially agreeing with their extreme self-presentation. For instance, when Mr. and Mrs. G entered therapy and indicated that they were growing too far apart, I replied that perhaps they could not benefit from counseling if their relationship were so devoid of love. Both members of the couple became agitated at this remark because they did not wish to divorce and immediately gave examples of occasions when they manifested love and closeness. Such exceptions can then be used to identify what each party was doing differently in the "close times," so that each could do more of it between sessions and observe the results.

A Consulting Break

At the Brief Therapy Family Center in Milwaukee, Wisconsin, therapist teams conduct collegial consultations during sessions to evaluate what has occurred and construct promising interventions. Not all therapists work in training settings, of course, and thus not all can make use of such consultation. Nonetheless, the notion of a consulting break still has value in SFBT if the therapist thinks of the client as a collaborator. The consultation, conducted toward the end of the session, wraps up what has been discussed so far and tries to establish consensus between therapist and client.

Such a consulting break might take the following form: "Okay, let's summarize what's been going on. Both of you came in feeling frustrated with the marriage and feeling like you might be headed toward divorce. When I asked about love in the marriage, however, you both told me that there were times—even now with the distance—when you do some loving and close things together. You told me that those have been some of the best times in your marriage. For you, Mrs. G, it sounds as though the close times occur when you and Mr. G are alone and have time to talk together and share what you're doing at school. Mr. G, for you, the close times seemed to happen when you took time off from studies and took vacations together. Does that sound right to you?"

Clients may then add to the therapist's observations, agree with them, or otherwise reformulate them. For example, "Well, we also have felt closer when we've done projects together. Remember when we remodeled the basement together? That was a headache, but we had a good time doing it together."

Such a consultation crystallizes solution behaviors and provides a natural bridge to between-session tasks during which clients can try more of what has worked for them. The consultation also ensures that the solution focus pursued by the counselor is indeed one that is user-friendly for clients.

A Message Including Compliments and a Task

Very often the solution-focused therapist will conclude the session with compliments, affirming the strengths of the client. For instance, "I am impressed by the degree to which both of you have held on to your love for each other despite the stress you've been under. You obviously want your marriage to work out, and I applaud you for that." Not infrequently, I will also add a message of hope: "If we can learn from what you're doing right in the marriage, I think we might be able to make some real strides toward your goal of rebuilding the loving times." The compliment is designed to convey several messages: 1) You have real strengths. 2) These strengths are manifested even now, when things seem to be at their worst. 3) We can build on these strengths to achieve your goals. No small amount of initial client improvement in mood can be attributed to the internalization of such messages.

In keeping with the goal focus of SFBT, the compliment is followed by a concrete task to be attempted between sessions. This task must be doable and must draw on the exceptions and solutions noted during the meeting. Very often the task will be to note what happens when the client tries to do more of what has worked for him or her recently or to do something new that he or she imagines might work. Following the first meeting, the client is often assigned the formula first session task, which de Shazer (1985) described as follows: "Between now and the next time we meet, we would like you to observe, so that you can describe to us next time, what happens in your family that you want to continue to have happen" (p. 137).

This task extends the search for solutions and encourages clients to observe solutions that may not have been discussed during the prior meeting. Most important, it maintains the solution focus between sessions, reinforcing a new way of thinking about oneself.

Mapping the Practice of Solution-Focused Brief Therapy

Both de Shazer (1988) and Walter and Peller (1992) offered useful flowcharts that map the practice of SFBT, helping therapists facilitate the construction of solutions. The following discussion will draw on these maps to describe SFBT as a series of steps and options.

Step One: Search for a Difference

Option one: explore for presession change. As a rule, favorable change that is already occurring and that is already within the client's awareness represents a promising first focus for SFBT. Research suggests that such change is most likely to be reported if requested by the therapist; clients will not necessarily report improvements in their state before entering counseling, even when these have occurred.

It is ideal if the task of noticing presession change can be given at the time the appointment is first made. This is difficult to achieve in larger clinics where appointments are made by a secretary and easier in settings where therapists set their own appointments. In my student counseling practice, where I see an average of 20–25 students a week, I always set my own appointments. Hearing the initial presentation helps me determine whether the need for meeting is routine, urgent, or emergent and allows me to structure an initial task if this seems appropriate. (In an urgent or emergent situation, when the client has significant presenting distress, I am unlikely to suggest such a task, preferring instead to offer reassurance and a quick appointment.)

Many times, however, the busy schedules of clients and therapists do not permit detailed contact prior to the first meeting. The search still can be conducted in the first session, however, simply by asking clients to identify positive changes that have occurred since the initial telephone call. It is helpful to make this a presuppositional question, such as "Many people notice that they feel a little better by the time of their first meeting. Have you noticed any positive changes since setting up our appointment?" One, of course, should always exercise discretion in making such an inquiry. If, for instance, the client is very tearful at the start of a first session, a query about presession improvement could seem insensitive and hinder the development of rapport.

A different way to assess presession change is to request that clients complete a sine-wave chart. The peaks of the chart represent occasions when they have been closest to their goals during the past 2 weeks, and the valleys represent the occasions when they have been most distant from their goals. The chart generally takes little time to complete and is useful in establishing the notion of goals and the idea of variability in behaviors and outcomes.

A review of the peaks of the chart generally shows presession changes that can anchor solution talk in the session. This is particularly the case when two or more peaks describe similar changes. Often, however, the peaks will describe internal states that need to be investigated more concretely. For instance, a student with test anxiety may describe peaks in which "I got some work done without procrastinating" and "I felt confident about my work." Follow-up questions would focus on "What, specifically, were you doing to get your work done without procrastinating?" and "What, specifically, were you doing when you were feeling confident about your work?" Multiple follow-up questions may be needed to frame the changes in action-oriented terms. In such situations, a single solution pattern often underlies the multiple peaks, as in "I tackled a doable amount of work, instead of the entire assignment." This presession change may then form the basis for a "do more of what is working" task between the first and second meetings.

It is not unusual for clients to experience difficulty with the sine-wave chart and other inquiries about presession change. In SFBT, this is not viewed as resistance and should never be a source of frustration for the therapist. Remember, the client has been absorbed by his or her problem and, by definition, has been locked into a problem-based mind-set. It may take considerable encouragement, modeling, and coaching to turn this mind-set around.

Option two: identify exceptions to the problem. If the client cannot identify presession changes, or if these cannot readily anchor solutions at the present time, the therapist changes "frames" (de Shazer 1988; Walter and Peller 1992) and begins the search for exceptions to presenting problems. This exercise is especially helpful in situations in which clients are mired in problem talk and cannot identify goals or presession changes.

A presession change is a self-report of a positive behavior that is consonant with client goals. When clients describe presession changes, they are engaged in solution talk. Exceptions to problems, on the other hand, are a step behind this from a solution-focused perspective. When the therapist asks about exceptions to problem patterns, the talk at that point is still problem focused. The inquiry into exceptions, indeed, is a strategy for shifting problem talk into solution talk.

A client, for instance, may report no presession change, indicating, "I'm feeling worse than ever." Once again, this is taken as a genuine expression of the individual's experience, not as a manifestation of a desire to avoid change. In such circumstances, the search for exceptions may focus on instances when things were better "even a little bit" (Walter and Peller 1992). A couple, for example, may state that they have not been able to get along for the past several months and have made no recent changes in a positive direction. When they report no good days as well, a scaling question might be used to capture their average degree of fighting. If the couple reports fighting of 8 on a 10-point scale, exceptions could be solicited as "What, specifically, are you doing on those occasions when your fighting is less than an 8?" I have found it helpful to ask clients to give a separate scaling rating for their best days and worst days, acknowledging that there may not yet be any truly "good" days. This then leads naturally to exception questions of "What are you doing differently when your fighting is a 5 rather than an 8?"

The search for exceptions can be especially helpful in couple therapy and in therapy for children brought by their parents. Very often, an adversarial situation has developed between members of a couple or between parents and children. Each party has been focused on the shortcomings of the other, with considerable emphasis on blaming and defending. When the therapist asks for exceptions, each participant in therapy may be able to identify solution behaviors used by the others, building a sense of appreciation and cooperation. For example, in a recent session, the husband indicated that he felt closest to his wife when she did not nag him about getting chores done around the home and instead just wrote the items down on a refrigerator to-do list. The wife, in response, exclaimed that she no longer felt the need to nag because he was now spending enough time at home to read the refrigerator list! This led us to construct an initial task in which each party agreed to do more of what worked for the other. The shift toward solution talk helped to defuse the resentments that had accumulated and start a rebuilding of trust between the parties.

de Shazer (1988) made the distinction between deliberate and spontaneous exceptions. When, in the course of therapy, clients try to do something different and thereby bring themselves closer to their goals, the therapist enters a "cheerleading" mode and encourages further enactment of the solution. On other occasions, a client may spontaneously stumble on an exception. This then becomes an opportunity to explore what, specifically, the client was doing on the exceptional occasion so that it can be constructed as a potential solution. Indeed, even random efforts at "doing something different" are apt to produce spontaneous exceptions that can then become deliberate, underscoring the importance of tasks that encourage novelty on the part of the client.

As mentioned earlier, the language used to frame exceptions is crucial in using these in therapy. Many times, the client may describe the exception as something that "just happened" or that occurred as the result of someone else's actions. Questions that reframe the exception in active terms can elicit useful information that assists with the construction of solutions. For example, the client might report that he or she felt less depressed on a particular day because of a nice thing that someone said to him or her. A follow-up question might be "Do you always feel better when someone says something nice to you? What might you have been doing to be more open to positive remarks on this occasion?" The key is to help clients see that exceptions may not be random events but could, indeed, be the result of actions that are reproducible.

Option three: generate hypothetical solutions. On occasion, clients cannot identify presession change and are unable to identify exceptions to problem patterns. These are most likely to be situations in which the individual is very much stuck in a problem focus. In such situations, the search for hypothetical solutions can generate ideas that form the basis for between-session solution-based tasks.

Let us say that our couple cannot think of any exceptions to their pattern of fighting or that the exceptions they generate are equally problematic ("We didn't argue because we were ignoring each other"). In the hypothetical frame (Walter and Peller 1992), the therapist might ask, "Imagine that the problems between the two of you have been solved. What will each of you be doing differently?" or "If, by a miracle, your problem were solved, what would you be doing differently?" When a client's imagination has been lacking, I sometimes have had success asking for the name of a person he or she admires greatly. I then inquire what

that admired person might be doing or saying in the problematic situation. Using an admired person to generate hypothetical solutions has the
disadvantage of not rooting the initial search in the client's direct experience but does very much stay within the values and priorities of the client. This can be especially helpful in multicultural counseling with
international clients and clients from racial, religious, or ethnic groups
different from the therapist's. The focus on an admired person often generates culture-specific solutions that are uniquely valid for the client (see
Echemendía and Núñez, Chapter 9, in this volume). In one memorable
counseling session several years ago, the client reported that her grandmother was a revered figure because of her wisdom and strength of character. Solution-focused responses to incidents of campus racism consisted
of role-playing the hypothetical responses of the grandmother, invoking
her spirit and enacting her virtues.

As Walter and Peller (1992) noted, inquiring about hypothetical solutions in counseling creates a bridge from imagined responses to concrete,
here-and-now tasks that can be enacted between sessions. Toward that
end, such inquiries encourage clients to identify occasions when the hypothesized solution has been happening just a little bit. This notion of "a
little bit" frees the client to focus on pieces of solutions that can become
a basis for initial counseling tasks. The therapist is most likely to elicit
such examples when questions have a presuppositional quality. Instead of
asking, "Have you done anything like this recently?" the counselor might
instruct, "Tell me of a time when you have done a little of this recently."
The presupposition is that a little piece of the hypothetical solution has
been occurring already, cueing the client to scan for such occasions.

Step Two: Assign Tasks

The preceding three options—identifying presession changes, exceptions, and hypothetical solutions—are ways of shifting problem talk to
solution talk in counseling and defining practical, here-and-now goals.
Much of the actual work of SFBT, however, occurs between sessions,
when the client attempts to make use of the solutions constructed in
therapy.

Bridging the exploration of solutions in session and their enactment
between sessions is the assignment of tasks. Walter and Peller (1992) described three kinds of therapeutic tasks arising from a solution focus.
When exceptions are identified that are deliberate, the homework task
typically takes the form of "do more of it" (p. 64). When the exceptions
are spontaneous, the initial task may be to have the client figure out how
the exception occurred, by watching for it in the future. Once this infor-

mation is obtained, the spontaneous exception can become deliberate. If the client develops a hypothetical solution, then the assigned task calls for the client to enact a small piece of this solution. In each case, the client is asked to make use of the solution talk within sessions during the time between sessions. The performance of these tasks then typically becomes the initial topic for the next session.

Option one: do more of it.　　The most clear-cut tasks to assign as homework emerge when clients are already aware of steps they are taking to bring them closer to their goals. This can occur as the result of either noticing a presession change or identifying an exception to problem patterns. When these steps have been the result of deliberate efforts to break old patterns, the therapist has some reassurance that the solution pattern is within the conscious control of the client and therefore is doable as a task. Many times, the specific task will take the form of extending actions that already have been taken: "I notice that standing up for yourself worked very well in your work setting. You let your supervisor know exactly what you were thinking and feeling in a cooperative, constructive way. Perhaps that is something we could try with your co-workers as well and see what happens."

Crucial to such "do more of it" task assignment is that clients recognize their solution patterns, and recognize that those patterns had favorable outcomes and that the patterns are within their control. Clients often feel that they have no control over their emotional responses and thus feel helpless. By highlighting that they do have control over actions that generate new feeling states, therapists help to instill a greater sense of internal control, which is then reinforced by the between-session tasks.

Option two: figure out how to do it.　　When an exception is spontaneous, clients may be puzzled as to how they were able to avoid their usual problem patterns. A couple might notice that they felt close on a particular evening but could be unable to verbalize what each person was doing differently on this occasion. The initial task, then, would be to have the couple be on the lookout for future close occasions and note carefully the preceding actions and interactions.

I have found journal writing or the use of the sine-wave chart to be a helpful tool for tasks involving the exploration of solution patterns. Clients are asked to "take your emotional temperature" several times during the day and notice those occasions when they are feeling especially good. Journal entries then include the actions and thoughts accompanying these good-feeling times, helping clients identify what they are doing constructively. Once the positive action patterns can be singled out, they can form the basis for a subsequent "do more of it" task.

Option three: try a small piece of the solution. When the client has identified a hypothetical solution, there may be considerable doubt about its value. There also may be doubt as to whether it can be enacted on demand. To allay these concerns, the therapist may simply ask the client to enact a small part of the solution pattern and observe the results. Generally, this small part will be a solution element well within the client's control. In a recent session, a student imagined that she would not have an anxiety attack if she were with her friends and family members. She lamented that all of these people lived far away and could not be with her. We constructed a task in which she could touch base with them through an online instant messenger service and by telephone and achieve a little of the sense of interpersonal connection. This helped her feel that she could be with supportive others at any time of the day or week, contributing to a greater sense of security.

It is important that such tasks be defined as clearly and specifically as possible, making use of the client's language and drawing on the client's experience. For instance, if the client hypothesizes a solution in which he or she might overcome anxiety by moderating his or her work expectations, the assigned task could be to identify an upcoming assignment and create reasonable expectations for working on this. Particular care should be taken to make the task doable; the therapist should not require the client to create reasonable expectations for *all* upcoming work. Many times, I make the task "something I would like you to try during the week." In the following session, it might then be possible to contrast those occasions when the client attempted the solution with those when he or she did not, to determine whether this is indeed something worthy of further enactment.

If, in the next session, clients indicate that they were not successful in implementing any of these tasks, a scaling question is often quite useful. Many times, clients will expect perfection at the outset and report failure when, in fact, they have successfully performed much of the defined task. The scaling question might then be "On a scale of 1 to 10, where 1 is "totally unreasonable expectations" and 10 is "totally reasonable ones," how would you rate those times when you tried to do something different? How would you rate those times when you continued to do things the old way?" If a scaling difference is reported, the subsequent conversation can explore what, specifically, occurred that made the little bit of difference and how this might be extended.

However, if clients report that they implemented the task as discussed in the prior session but found no results, then it is generally useful to reassure them that change does not typically happen all at once or right away. As Walter and Peller (1992) noted, however, sometimes a change may have occurred without the client's recognition. For instance, the client might indicate that his or her anxiety was still very high immediately before taking the test but, with the use of the scaling question, that there were periods during the studying when anxiety was markedly reduced. The follow-up inquiry can then focus on "What might you be doing during your studying that we can bring into the examination room?" One client in this very situation sheepishly admitted to me that he studied at home with his Bible open because it gave him inspiration and strength. He knew that I did not share his religion and was concerned that I might look down on this use of his faith.

Interestingly, I noticed that as he was talking to me about the use of his Bible, he actually seemed to become more relaxed in our interaction. Once it was clear that I did not challenge his faith, he opened up considerably about his beliefs and the ways in which these reassured him. I then asked him to rate his comfort level in the session with me, and, indeed, he acknowledged feeling much less anxiety than at the start of our session. This, then, became the basis for our solution task, as he decided to see if bringing his Bible to class and risking the reactions of classmates could yield similar relief. To his surprise, two classmates actually sought him out when they noticed his Bible, and together they formed an extra-curricular group on campus. Armed with his faith during examinations, he found that his anxiety declined noticeably.

This student's therapy illustrates how solutions can be constructed from a variety of sources, including positive interactions with the therapist. Although SFBT does not typically feature an examination of interactions between clients and therapists in the manner of short-term psychodynamic work, occasions when the client attempts to do something different in the helping relationship can form the basis for helpful solutions. Indeed, it is possible to reframe much of such psychodynamic work in solution-focused terms, as clients break their problem patterns by enacting adaptive solutions in the helping relationship and then generalizing these to other interpersonal contexts.

Step Three: Provide Feedback

Walter and Peller (1992) used the term *cheerleading* to capture the positive support and encouragement provided by therapists when clients move closer to their goals by enacting solutions. Such feedback might be offered early in a session, as in "You're looking and sounding much more lively than last week; what were you doing this past week that was different from before?" or feedback could occur in response to a client's reported progress. Feedback of this kind often acknowledges that a client has not completely attained his or her goal—for example, "You've made an excellent start"—thereby building momentum for attempting further progress.

Some of the feedback is more of the reassuring variety, especially when client progress has been modest. Finding small steps of progress, even amid general discouragement, can anchor efforts to extend these modest steps into larger strides. When clients come to a session with renewed problem talk, perhaps out of discouragement over a setback, the feedback is both reassuring and sympathetic. Walter and Peller (1992) emphasized the importance of normalizing setbacks, letting clients know that success is not a simple, linear path. The focus on solutions should in no way interfere with basic empathy for the discouragements that clients may experience. Even when problems are overwhelming, it is generally possible to ask clients what they are doing to stay sane in the situation and to elicit positive coping efforts. The tenacity with which the therapist remains grounded in assets and strengths often becomes contagious, allowing clients to define solutions even in the most trying circumstances.

With this feedback, clients can often enact solutions on their own, reducing the need for weekly sessions. I rarely, if ever, talk in terms of "termination," preferring instead to transition meetings to an "as needed" basis. It is not unusual for individuals to make steady progress, only later to face a situation that elicits the old problem-based modes. Single "booster" sessions are often helpful in such circumstances. Such intermittent intervention allows therapy to be an ongoing developmental resource for clients rather than a one-time treatment.

Summary Case Illustration: Ms. I

Ms. I, a medical student, came to our first session complaining of an "out of control" problem with her eating. Ms. I was in the third year of her medical curriculum and had just begun her clinical work. By all accounts, she was a motivated, talented student who interacted well with patients and whose fund of knowledge exceeded expectations. Ms. I was also attractive and personable and had many friends on campus. To an outside observer, Ms. I led a charmed life.

This, however, was not Ms. I's experience of herself. She reported occasional bulimic episodes since her early years in college. During these periods, she criticized herself unmercifully, generally focusing on her body and her weight. She spent many hours in front of a mirror in this self-critical mode, scanning her body for imperfections and convincing herself that she was ugly and grotesque. Her greatest fear was that she would never be able to maintain a romantic relationship with a man.

In a desperate attempt to control her weight and improve her body image, Ms. I would withhold food from herself for an extended time, eating only enough to avoid passing out. As her self-criticism and depressed mood deepened, however, she found herself voraciously turning to food for relief and gratification. These bingeing episodes left her feeling profoundly guilty, triggering further self-criticism.

In the days prior to contacting me, Ms. I had spent an unusually large amount of time in front of the mirror. Her binge eating had returned, disrupting her efforts at studying. She presented herself as a woman out of control, completely disgusted with herself. She did acknowledge, however, that she was able to refrain from purging the food, because she found that repulsive.

Information that I gathered in the initial session suggested that Ms. I did not meet formal diagnostic criteria for an eating disorder and was not experiencing a diagnosable mood disorder. This raised my confidence that BSFT might be appropriate. I searched for presession change during our first meeting by asking Ms. I to identify any occasions since setting up the appointment with me in which she felt more "in control." Ms. I readily responded that she felt good about herself when she was working with patients. She knew that she was effective with other people, and she had already developed confidence in understanding her patients' medical conditions. As Ms. I spoke of her clinical experiences, her mood brightened noticeably, and she became more animated in her speech.

"Suppose I were a fly on the wall of your apartment," I suggested to Ms. I. "What would I observe if you were on your way toward feeling in control, the way you do in medicine?"

"I guess I would like myself better," she responded hesitantly.

I needed her to be more specific. "And how would I know that you were feeling better about yourself? What would I be seeing if I were that fly on the wall?"

"I wouldn't be so hard on myself," Ms. I offered.

"And instead of being hard on yourself, you would be doing what? What would I observe?"

"I would just be eating normally," Ms. I said with feeling. "I would just eat when I was hungry, without giving myself a big guilt trip about it."

"OK," I followed. "Looking over the last few weeks, how would you rate your eating? If you imagine a 10-point scale, where 1 represents being completely in control of your eating and 10 means having no control whatever, where would you stand?"

"Maybe an 8," Ms. I answered. "It's been really bad lately. The only okay times were after I had a great day on the floors."

This struck my interest. "And what happened on those great days in the hospital that made the eating better than usual?"

"I don't know," Ms. I responded. "The time I'm thinking about, the patient called for me before being discharged and told me how much I had helped her and what a great doctor I'll become. I felt great. Afterward, I went home and ate some leftover food and then realized that I hadn't even made a big deal about the eating. I didn't even think about it."

"So when you felt like Dr. I," I offered, "you didn't beat up on yourself. You could value yourself for who you are, what you do, and what you know. When you come home and you're just plain Ms. I, it's a lot harder to hold on to those good feelings."

Ms. I agreed. "After a big test, I never have any problem eating. Usually I feel good about being done with the test, and I'm just happy to go out with friends and enjoy myself."

"These are your medical school friends?" I inquired. Ms. I nodded. "And you eat well when you go out with them?"

Ms. I laughed. "Too well! The last clerkship was really hard, and we went out for pizza afterward. It was disgusting."

"But you didn't feel guilty?" I asked.

"A little bit the next day, maybe," she responded. "But we had fun after the test."

"Hmmm…it sounds as though Dr. I knows how to eat pretty well!"

Ms. I laughed again. "That's funny. We had a couple of lunches sponsored by the drug representatives, and I ate plenty." By this time, her tone was quite lively and animated, much as I assumed it was during her working day.

"What specialty are you thinking of entering?" I suddenly asked.

Ms. I's response was swift. "Pediatrics. I love working with kids. It's what I've always wanted to do."

"I have a feeling you'd be good with kids," I offered. "They respond so well to nurturing, someone who cares about them. It's very scary for children in a doctor's office and especially in the hospital, all those strange people, not knowing what's wrong with them, or if it will ever get better. They feel so helpless; they don't have control over anything happening to them. A good doctor who can be reassuring and fun and caring can make all the difference in the world."

Ms. I seemed attentive.

"Do you think you'd be open to trying a little experiment with me?" I asked.

"Sure," Ms. I replied. She seemed much calmer than at the outset of our meeting.

I asked Ms. I to close her eyes and focus her thoughts on her deep and slow breathing. I suggested that she imagine that she had a little girl assigned to her as a patient. The little girl's name was Marie [Ms. I's first name]. She was very scared and nervous and didn't want to eat anything. But she needed to eat to stay healthy. "Can you see little Marie in your mind's eye?" I asked. "Can you imagine yourself helping her, reaching out to her?"

Ms. I seemed deep in reverie. "What are you imagining?" I asked.

"She's in bed and almost all the way under the covers," Ms. I replied. "She seems so small."

"And what are you doing with little Marie?" I asked.

"I'm sitting at the side of her bed looking down at her. I want to help her. I'm holding her hand with one hand and giving her a little food with the other."

"And what are you saying to little Marie?"

Ms. I's voice cracked. "It's OK, it's OK," she whispered. "I love you. It'll be OK."

For a few moments, Ms. I was silent, a few tears welling in her eyes. When she looked at me directly, I complimented her sensitivity. "It sounds as though you'll be very good to your patients. You really make them feel secure." Ms. I agreed. "Do you think you can be your own patient now? Do you think you could take care of yourself the way you imagined taking care of the little child?"

"How do you mean?" Ms. I asked quizzically.

"When you come home at the end of each day, I want you to keep your white coat on. Make sure you have your stethoscope with you and all your pens and books. I want you to stay as Dr. I when you get home, because you have a patient to take care of at your house. Her name is Ms. I, and she's been having a hard time feeling good about herself. She takes it out on her body, and she takes it out on her eating. Your job, first thing in the morning when you put on your white coat, and when you get home from your clinical rotation, is to feed Ms. I and take care of her. I don't want you to think about eating. I want you to think about taking care of your patient Ms. I and offering her some food and support."

The idea intrigued Ms. I, and she agreed to give it a try. The following week, she reported no episodes of binge eating. The exercise came to her with some difficulty at first but became easier when she imagined herself as a little child before sitting down for a meal. Interestingly, based on one of her imagery sessions, she was able to recall a lullaby her mother had sung to her when she was young. Playing that lullaby in her head, she found, was helpful in her assigned task of taking care of "patient Ms. I." She found that being in the role of a nurturing physician caring for a child in pain was easier for her than taking care of an adult. Thinking of herself as a vulnerable child enabled her to mobilize her physician-self and the caring responses associated with that role.

In subsequent weeks, Ms. I reported that eating in a healthy way still required some forethought but that it was coming more naturally. A major step of progress came when she was criticized during a clinical rotation and returned home feeling miserable. She caught herself starting to examine herself in the mirror but instead kept her white coat on and decided to take care of her patient Ms. I by offering a small snack. Afterward, she felt no lingering guilt, reinforcing a new sense of control.

Shortly after this episode, Ms. I began a dating relationship—the first in more than a year—and reported feeling much better about herself. I emphasized to Ms. I that I had not taught her to do anything new. She had always been a good, caring person; a capable physician; and someone who had been well nurtured as a child. I simply helped her apply those talents and experiences to herself.

Conclusion

Readers will recognize many elements of SFBT in the case example of Ms. I, including the search for presession change, the use of the miracle and scaling questions, and the emphasis on exceptions to the problem pattern. From the outset, the goal of the therapy was not to explore the historical and contemporary roots of her eating complaints. We did not refer to an "eating disorder" or "eating problems" at all. Rather, I borrowed her phrase of being "in control" as an anchor for her positive goals. We did not explore her negative feelings about herself, in their personal or sociological contexts. Rather, we structured the conversation in a way that identified and reinforced her strengths as a physician-to-be.

A key nonverbal element in Ms. I's therapy was the shift in her tone of voice from the very start of our session—when she was problem-focused—to the portion of the session when she described her work as a medical student and her love of pediatrics. My working hypothesis was that this brightened tone reflected a greater sense of perceived control and an enhanced experience of self. The key, then, was to mobilize this "doctor-self" in the context of eating. If food could be viewed as a medication—something to be administered by a caring physician—eating would now fit into her strengths. Reframing eating as a clinical activity allowed her to take a solution from her training and "do more of it" in her personal life. Ultimately, it was her solid sense of herself as a student-physician and her willingness to enact the solution on a daily basis that allowed for the relatively rapid change.

Readers will recognize elements from other approaches to therapy in the example as well. My work owes more than a little inspiration to the strategic therapists, who emphasize minimal interventions to interrupt problem patterns, and to practitioners such as Erickson and Lankton, who used imagery and shifts in client experiencing to anchor new behavior patterns. Such elements may strike the reader as lying outside the purview of SFBT proper, but I think not. In an insightful observation, de Shazer (1988) noted that many of his solution-focused interventions with clients were paced in an Ericksonian manner and even elicited trancelike responses (p. 139). Such shifts of state appear to be powerful tools in helping clients shift from problem to solution talk.

In conclusion, I would like to congratulate you, the reader, on your desire to move toward your goals as a brief therapist. You have taken an excellent step by exposing yourself to a variety of short-term approaches. Between now and when we should run into each other again, I would like to suggest a task. Rather than view SFBT as a completely separate and unique therapy, examine all therapies and identify the ways in which they introduce and reinforce solutions: departures from old, problem patterns. Determine how you are solution focused in your best moments as a therapist, in your own unique way. Once you discover how you are best at cultivating change, try doing more of that in your upcoming sessions. Perhaps your clients will be more likely to find their solutions once you have targeted your own.

References

Beyebach M, Morejon AR, Palenzuela DL, et al: Research on the process of solution-focused therapy, in Handbook of Solution-Focused Brief Therapy. Edited by Miller SD, Hubble MA, Duncan BL. San Francisco, CA, Jossey-Bass, 1996, pp 299–334

DeJong P, Hopwood LE: Outcome research on treatment conducted at the Brief Family Therapy Center, in Handbook of Solution-Focused Brief Therapy. Edited by Miller SD, Hubble MA, Duncan BL. San Francisco, CA, Jossey-Bass, 1996, pp 272–298

de Shazer S: Keys to Solution in Brief Therapy. New York, WW Norton, 1985

de Shazer S: Clues: Investigating Solutions in Brief Therapy. New York, WW Norton, 1988

Gingerich WJ, Eisengart S: Solution-focused brief therapy: a review of the outcome research. Fam Process 39:477–498, 2000

Held BS: Solution-focused therapy and the postmodern: a critical analysis, in Handbook of Solution-Focused Brief Therapy. Edited by Miller SD, Hubble MA, Duncan BL. San Francisco, CA, Jossey-Bass, 1996, pp 27–43

McKeel AJ: A clinician's guide to research on solution-focused brief therapy, in Handbook of Solution-Focused Brief Therapy. Edited by Miller SD, Hubble MA, Duncan BL. San Francisco, CA, Jossey-Bass, 1996, pp 251–271

Metcalf L, Thomas FN, Duncan BL, et al: What works in solution-focused brief therapy: a qualitative analysis of client and therapist perceptions, in Handbook of Solution-Focused Brief Therapy. Edited by Miller SD, Hubble MA, Duncan BL. San Francisco, CA, Jossey-Bass, 1996, pp 335–350

O'Hanlon W, Weiner-Davis M: In Search of Solutions: A New Direction in Psychotherapy. New York, WW Norton, 1989

Prochaska JO, DiClemente CC: The transtheoretical approach, in Handbook of Eclectic Psychotherapy. Edited by Norcross JC. New York, Brunner/Mazel, 1986, pp 163–200

Simon D: Crafting consciousness through form: solution-focused therapy as a spiritual path, in Handbook of Solution-Focused Brief Therapy. Edited by Miller SD, Hubble MA, Duncan BL. San Francisco, CA, Jossey-Bass, 1996, pp 44–64

Steenbarger BN: Toward science-practice integration in brief counseling and therapy. Couns Psychol 20:403–450, 1992

Steenbarger BN: Duration and outcome in psychotherapy: an integrative review. Prof Psychol Res Pr 25:111–119, 1994

Walter JL, Peller JE: Becoming Solution-Focused in Brief Therapy. New York, Brunner/Mazel, 1992

Walter JL, Peller JE: Rethinking our assumptions: assuming anew in a postmodern world, in Handbook of Solution-Focused Brief Therapy. Edited by Miller SD, Hubble MA, Duncan BL. San Francisco, CA, Jossey-Bass, 1996, pp 9–26

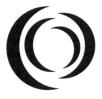

Brief Interpersonal Psychotherapy

Scott Stuart, M.D.

Interpersonal psychotherapy (IPT) is a time limited, dynamically informed psychotherapy that aims to alleviate patients' suffering and improve their interpersonal functioning. IPT focuses specifically on interpersonal relationships to bring about change, by helping patients to either modify their interpersonal relationships or change their expectations about them. IPT also assists patients in improving their social support network so that they can better manage their current interpersonal distress.

Empirical Support for Efficacy

Originally developed as a research treatment for major depression, IPT was codified in a manual in 1984 (Klerman et al. 1984). Since then, IPT has been shown to be superior to placebo and as effective as the antidepressant imipramine and cognitive-behavioral therapy for mild to moderate depression over a 16-week course (Elkin et al. 1989). Neither therapy was as effective as imipramine for severe depression. In a 3-year follow-up study of patients with recurrent depression (E. Frank et al. 1990), patients remained depression free for 120–130 weeks with imipramine and for 75–80 weeks with IPT, as compared with about 40 weeks with placebo. A current opinion is that recurrent depression should be treated with maintenance antidepressant medication (E. Frank and Spanier 1995; Kupfer et al. 1992), with IPT as a viable alternative for patients who do not want or who cannot tolerate medication.

IPT has been shown to be efficacious in several psychiatric disorders, including geriatric depression, adolescent depression, depression in HIV-positive patients, dysthymic disorder, the depressed phase of bipolar disorder, and eating disorders. IPT is also effective for perinatal depression, including postpartum (O'Hara et al. 2000) and antenatal depression. Current research is examining the effectiveness of IPT in depression associated with cardiac disease, social phobia, and somatization disorder. Finally, the use of IPT has been described with groups, with couples, and in a family practice setting. Excellent reviews of this research have been conducted by Weissman and colleagues (2000) and Stuart and Robertson (2003).

In addition, as clinical experience with IPT has increased, its use has broadened to include not only a variety of well-specified DSM-IV-TR (American Psychiatric Association 2000) diagnoses but also a variety of interpersonal problems (Stuart and Robertson 2003). IPT reflects the best of both empirical research and clinical experience and continues to incorporate changes that improve the treatment. Rather than being designed to be applied in a strict manualized form in which the clinician is required to precisely follow a specified treatment protocol, IPT encourages clinicians to use their clinical judgment to modify treatment in order to maximally benefit patients. Thus, the practice of IPT should be based on equal measures of empirical research and experience-based clinical judgment.

Essential Characteristics

IPT is characterized by three primary elements: 1) IPT focuses specifically on *interpersonal relationships* as a point of intervention; 2) IPT is *time limited* when used as an acute treatment; and 3) the *interventions used in IPT do not directly address the transference relationship* as it develops in therapy (Stuart and Robertson 2003).

Interpersonal Relationships

IPT is based on the premise that interpersonal distress is intimately connected with psychological symptoms. Thus, the foci of treatment are twofold. One focus is the difficulties and changes in relationships that patients are experiencing, with the aim of helping patients either to improve communication within those relationships or to change their expectations about those relationships. The second focus is helping patients to build or better use their extended social support networks so that they are better able to muster the interpersonal support needed to help them deal with the crises that precipitated their distress.

For example, this approach is extremely well suited for the treatment of women who may be experiencing an episode of postpartum depression (O'Hara et al. 2000). Many perinatal women state that their distress is linked to difficulties in their relationships with their partners or in making the transition from working woman to mother. A therapist using IPT would help the patient to resolve conflicts with her partner over issues such as division of child-care labor and also would assist the woman to garner more support from her social network (e.g., connecting with and asking for support from other friends who have had children, from extended-family members, or from colleagues at work). Resolution of the particular interpersonal conflicts, along with improved interpersonal support while the role transition is being negotiated, would then lead to symptomatic improvement.

IPT therefore stands in contrast to treatments such as cognitive therapy (Beck et al. 1979) and psychoanalytically oriented psychotherapy. In contrast to cognitive therapy, in which the focus of treatment is the patient's internally based cognitions, IPT focuses on the patient's interpersonal communications with others in his or her social sphere. In contrast to analytically oriented treatments, in which the focus of treatment is on understanding the contribution of early life experiences to psychological functioning, IPT focuses on helping patients improve their communication and social support in the present. Past experiences, although clearly influencing current functioning, are not a major focus of intervention.

This latter point leads to a corollary of the IPT approach: by virtue of its time limit and its focus on here-and-now interpersonal functioning, IPT seeks to resolve psychiatric symptoms rather than to change underlying dynamic structures. Although ego strength, defense mechanisms, and personality characteristics are all important in assessing suitability for treatment, change in these constructs is not presumed to occur in IPT. Rather, they are taken as a given for a particular patient, and the question that drives the therapist's interventions is "Given this particular patient's personality style, ego strength, defense mechanisms, and early life experiences, how can he or she be helped to improve here-and-now interpersonal relationships and build a more effective social support network?"

Case Example: Mrs. J

Mrs. J, a 27-year-old woman, presented with symptoms of depression at 9 weeks' postpartum. She described feelings of worthlessness, guilt, low energy, crying spells, anhedonia, and low mood. The child was her first, and her pregnancy and delivery were unremarkable. She reported no history of psychiatric illness.

Mrs. J spontaneously identified that her distress was related to two issues. First, she had an escalating conflict with her husband: prior to the arrival of their child, he had agreed to assist with child care, but he had actually been working longer hours since the birth and had left Mrs. J with nearly all of this work. Second, she identified that she was having a great deal of conflict about returning to work; her maternity leave was ending in 3 weeks, and although she did want to return to work eventually, she did not feel prepared to do so quite so soon.

A contract to meet for 12 sessions of IPT was established, during which these two issues would be addressed. Mrs. J's expectations regarding her husband were explored, as well as her attempts to enlist him in child-care activities. Although her expectations about what he could and should contribute appeared to be realistic, it became apparent that rather than directly asking her husband for help, Mrs. J was expecting him to "know" what help she wanted without her having to ask. She would typically withdraw in silence when he failed to anticipate her needs.

Work on communicating more effectively with her husband was a major part of the treatment, which included a great deal of communication analysis and role-playing. Mr. J also participated in several sessions, during which both Mr. and Mrs. J were able to give each other more direct feedback about their expectations. As Mrs. J's communication improved, Mr. J was able to respond and meet her needs more effectively.

Her work situation was addressed in three ways. First, her ambivalence about returning to work was framed as a normal experience encountered by many new mothers. Initially concerned about losing her social contacts at work if she were to take more time for maternity leave, she began contacting her friends from work and found that they were quite willing to maintain contact with her outside of work. Several of her colleagues who had children shared their similar experiences of ambivalence about returning to work, which she found very supportive. Second, she began developing new social supports in a "new mothers" group, which included some women who had chosen to stay at home with their children rather than return to work. Third, after consulting with her husband about the financial consequences of the decision, she elected to take an additional 6 months of maternity leave without pay.

As Mrs. J's communication with her husband improved, and as she began to resolve her conflict about returning to work, her symptoms improved quite rapidly. She also identified that maintaining her social support from colleagues at work along with the new support she had developed with the new mothers group was extremely helpful.

Time Limit

The second characteristic of IPT is that it is time limited in the acute phase of treatment. In general, for the acute treatment of depression and other major psychiatric illnesses, a course of 12–20 sessions tapered over time is effective (Stuart and Robertson 2003), such that weekly sessions may be used for 6–10 weeks, followed by a gradual increase in the time between sessions as the patient improves.

A contract should be established with the patient to end acute treatment after a specified number of sessions. Having a definitive end point often pushes patients to make changes in their relationships more quickly (Klerman et al. 1984; Stuart and Robertson 2003) and also influences both patient and therapist to maintain their focus primarily on here-and-now interpersonal problems rather than working on issues from the patient's past. Finally, the time frame is helpful in preventing the therapy from moving from a symptom-focused treatment to one that is based on the development of the transference relationship.

Case Example: Mr. K

Mr. K, a 37-year-old computer programmer, came for help after having been laid off from his job. His depressive symptoms had gradually increased as he realized that he was going to have to seek new employment. He reported a lifelong pattern of social avoidance and was fearfully anticipating the interviewing process for a new job. He had not been able to even put together a resumé prior to entering therapy.

Mr. K reported that his two brothers and parents all lived some distance away. He had occasional telephone contact but saw them only during holidays. When employed, he had little contact with colleagues at work and very little social support in other settings. He reported dating rarely, and he was not in a romantic relationship. He was clear, however, that he had enjoyed his job, particularly because it was intellectually challenging with little need for personal contact, and felt quite happy with his life before his layoff.

The therapist took particular care to be empathic and to ensure that a good therapeutic alliance was established given Mr. K's avoidant style. Detailed descriptions of Mr. K's work interactions were examined for communication patterns, with the therapist strongly reinforcing Mr. K's examples of good communication. Later in the therapy, role-playing, particularly of potential job interviews, was used, with the therapist giving direct constructive feedback to Mr. K about his interpersonal communication.

Although Mr. K reported reduced anxiety, he continued to be very reluctant to apply for jobs and go through the interview process. Despite conversations in therapy about the need to do this, he had not, by session 5, applied for any jobs. The therapist, empathic to Mr. K's difficulties, nonetheless emphasized that he and Mr. K had agreed that the therapy would last 12 weeks. Given that time frame, the therapist thought that Mr. K would benefit most from the treatment if he had completed several interviews by the time IPT ended: role-playing was helpful, but there was no substitute for the real thing. Both agreed on a deadline of getting job applications out within the next week.

Despite his anxiety, Mr. K did send applications out to several computer firms. He was well qualified and received several interview offers. By session 8, however, he still had not scheduled any interviews. The therapist once again noted that although Mr. K was improving, he would not obtain maximum benefit from treatment without having completed several interviews. With only four sessions left, it was imperative that Mr. K begin the interview process.

By session 10, Mr. K had completed one interview and had scheduled two additional interviews. The therapist used the opportunity to examine in great detail Mr. K's communication and the management of his anxiety during the completed interview. The therapist gave Mr. K positive feedback for the productive ways in which he communicated, and they used more role-playing to examine different approaches that he might have used. Although Mr. K had not yet been offered a job at the conclusion of treatment, he reported a great deal of symptom relief and increased confidence about being interviewed. He also acknowledged that he would likely not have applied for jobs and gone through the interviews without the therapist's "gentle" push.

The Transference Relationship

The third characteristic of IPT is the absence of interventions that address the transference aspects of the therapeutic relationship. This trait is shared with cognitive-behavioral therapy and solution-focused therapies, but it clearly distinguishes IPT from most dynamically oriented therapies.

An explanation of the use of transference in IPT is necessary to fully appreciate the nature of the treatment. It is acknowledged that transference is a universal phenomenon in all psychotherapy. In IPT, the therapist's experience of transference is crucial in understanding the patient's interpersonal world and attachment style and in formulating questions about the patient's relationships outside of therapy. However, the transference relationship is not addressed directly by the therapist. The transference experience also should inform the therapist about potential problems in therapy and help predict the likely outcome of treatment.

As an illustration, consider a patient who forms a dependent relationship with the therapist, manifested as difficulty in ending sessions, calls to the therapist between sessions, or use of more subtle pleas to the therapist for help or reassurance. This transference relationship should inform the therapist that the patient is likely to 1) relate to others in a similar dependent fashion, 2) have difficulty in ending relationships with others, and 3) have exhausted others with persistent calls for help. The continual reassurance-seeking of a hypochondriacal patient would be an excellent example of this kind of behavior.

This information is then used by the therapist to formulate hypotheses about the patient's difficulties with others and should lead the therapist to ask questions about how the patient asks others for help, ends relationships, and reacts when others are not responsive to his or her needs. Furthermore, the therapist might hypothesize that the patient's dependency is likely to cause a problem when concluding treatment, and the therapist may begin discussing the ending of therapy much sooner than with less dependent patients. The therapist also should emphasize to a dependent patient the need to build a more effective social support network, so that the patient's needs are more fully met outside of therapy rather than within a dependent or regressive therapeutic relationship. Appropriate modifications also would be made with patients who are avoidant or who manifest other personality characteristics.

In summary, transference is an extremely important part of IPT but is not addressed directly in therapy. To do so detracts from the focus on symptom reduction and rapid improvement in interpersonal functioning, the basis of IPT, and typically lengthens the course of treatment. The goal in IPT is literally to work with the patient quickly to solve his or her interpersonal problems before problematic transference develops and becomes an additional focus of treatment.

Case Example: Mr. L

Mr. L, a 54-year-old man, presented with marital problems that had been increasing over the last year. At that time, he had been given a diagnosis of type 1 diabetes mellitus following numerous consultations for chronic fatigue. He described being very frustrated with his physicians and their lack of attentiveness to his distress. He was also angry with his wife of 30 years because she had begun refusing to help him administer his insulin shots and had told him to "stop being a baby." Mr. L felt that she did not understand how much he was suffering and was refusing to be supportive. Although he did not endorse any psychiatric symptoms, he reported numerous physical problems, such as headaches, limb pain, and fatigue.

Mr. L had no psychiatric history, but his medical history indicated frequent visits to physicians for various physical complaints. He often thought that something was physically wrong and recognized that he needed a great deal of reassurance at times, both from physicians and from his wife. The diagnosis of diabetes had exacerbated his fears about other physical problems. Despite reassurance from his physicians that he had not developed any complications, he had returned repeatedly to his family doctor with concerns about his vision, limb pain, and fatigue. He had been encouraged by his family doctor to seek counseling. Mr. L was insightful enough to realize that he was "wearing out his welcome" with his doctor and that his wife was getting annoyed with him as well.

Following an assessment, a contract was established for 12 sessions of acute treatment with IPT. The therapist recognized that Mr. L was likely to develop a dependent therapeutic relationship, particularly if treatment was continued for more than several months. Although examining this dependency in longer-term therapy was one option for treatment, dealing with Mr. L's acute distress and helping him to manage his diabetes more effectively seemed to be goals more in line with what Mr. L wanted and would tolerate.

Mr. L's communication with Mrs. L was examined in detail. His typical method of engaging her was to complain of a physical problem and to complain that she did not understand how much pain and suffering he was experiencing. For a time after the diabetes diagnosis, she had responded to this by literally caring for him, giving him his shots and monitoring his diet; more recently, she would either ignore his requests or angrily tell him that he needed to "deal with it yourself." Mrs. L, invited to session 3, confirmed this pattern, adding that Mr. L had always been somewhat dependent but that the diabetes had increased this trait beyond her tolerance.

In subsequent sessions, the therapist explored what Mr. L intended to communicate to his wife and what he really wanted from her. When queried in detail, he was able to articulate that he really wanted reassurance from both his wife and his doctors. This reassurance from his wife was best delivered as emotional support. Mr. L was able to recognize that his current communication was alienating his wife and that he needed to ask her more directly for the specific kind of support he wanted. By session 6, he had made several attempts at more direct communication, to which his wife had responded well.

Anticipating that concluding therapy might be difficult given Mr. L's dependent traits, the therapist brought up the topic during session 7. Mr. L quickly responded that the therapy had been very helpful but he was concerned about having to finish because he felt that the therapist was "the only person who really understood my suffering." Rather than addressing the looming dependency in the context of the therapeutic relationship or addressing the transference implications of this comment, the therapist asked Mr. L if others in his social network could provide similar support. Mr. L's immediate response was that he could think of no one. The therapist then suggested that Mr. L attend a program for patients with chronic illnesses at the local hospital, both as a means of extending his social support in general and as a means of identifying others who might understand his experience.

At the next session, Mr. L reported that his initial reaction to the therapist's suggestion was to feel angry and rejected, "as if the therapist were sending me out so that he didn't have to take care of me." He had reluctantly attended the group but found to his surprise that many of the people he had met had experiences similar to his own, and he found it quite useful. The therapist used this as an example of Mr. L's typical pattern of response to well-intended offers of help and quickly moved to a discussion of how this pattern played out with his wife. Mr. L gradually recognized that his wife was attempting to help him by encouraging his independence, although it had seemed as if she were rejecting him, too. The therapist chose this intervention using transference to inform the questions about likely problems in relationships outside of therapy, but the relationship between the therapist and patient was not directly addressed.

Mrs. L attended several of the later sessions, and both Mr. and Mrs. L reported that their relationship was greatly improved. Furthermore, Mr. L continued to attend the support group, which he found quite helpful and supportive. When discussing the conclusion of therapy, the therapist continued to emphasize that Mr. L would benefit greatly from continuing his involvement in the group as a means of obtaining social support to deal with his illness.

Theoretical Framework

IPT is grounded in both attachment theory and interpersonal communication theory.

Attachment Theory

Attachment theory, as described by Bowlby (1988) among others, rests on the premise that people have an instinctual drive to attach to one another (i.e., to form and maintain meaningful relationships in which they receive and provide care). When crises occur, individuals seek care from those important to them; they seek emotional proximity. Interpersonal communication is intrinsic to this process, and individuals who cannot effectively ask for care, and consequently cannot obtain the physical and psychological care they need, will suffer as a result. When interpersonal support is insufficient or lacking during times of stress, individuals are less able to deal with crises and are more prone to develop symptoms (Bowlby 1988; Stuart and Robertson 2003).

The hallmark of good mental health is the capacity to form flexible attachments, which allow people both to ask for care and to provide care when appropriate. Mental health is compromised when people have a fixed attachment style in which they are persistently seeking care but are unable to provide it to others or in which they persistently provide care but are unable to ask for help.

Bowlby (1988) described three attachment styles that drive interpersonal behavior. People with *secure attachment* are able to both give and receive care and are relatively secure that care will be provided when it is needed. Because securely attached individuals are able to communicate their needs effectively and provide care for others as well, they typically have good social support networks that are responsive to their needs. Thus, they are relatively protected from developing problems when faced with stressors.

People with *anxious ambivalent attachment*, in contrast, behave as if they are never quite sure that their attachment needs will be met. Consequently, such individuals seek care constantly. When their demands for care are not met, the urgency of the demands is increased in order to ensure that care is provided. Anxious ambivalent individuals usually form insecure relationships, with typical dependent behavior (Stuart and Noyes 1999). They often lack the capacity to care for others because getting their own attachment needs met outweighs all other concerns. Consequently, they have a poor social support network, which in combination with their difficulties in enlisting help leaves them quite vulnerable to interpersonal stressors.

People with *anxious avoidant attachment* typically believe that others will not provide care in any circumstances. As a result, they avoid becoming close to others. Avoidant, schizoid, and antisocial interpersonal behaviors are common. Poor social connections, along with avoidance of asking for help during crises, leave these individuals quite prone to difficulties.

In essence, attachment theory states that people with less secure attachments are more prone to psychiatric symptoms and interpersonal problems during times of stress. A persistent belief that care must be constantly demanded from others, or that care will not be provided by others under any circumstances, typically leads insecurely attached individuals to have more difficulty generating social support during times of crisis, leading to an increased vulnerability to illness. In addition, severe disruptions of important attachment relationships, such as the death of a significant other, will lead to an increased vulnerability to psychiatric symptoms. If the stressor is great enough, even individuals with secure attachments may have difficulties.

Interpersonal Communication Theory

IPT is also based on communication theory, as described by Kiesler and Watkins (1989) and others, because attachment needs are communicated (well or poorly) within relationships. Many securely attached individuals are able to communicate their needs effectively, whereas those more insecurely attached individuals communicate in ways that are indirect or even counterproductive. Rather than eliciting a caregiving response, their unclear or ambivalent requests for help may instead elicit a neutral response or even hostility. The persistent care-seeking behavior and maladaptive communication of an anxiously attached or hypochondriacal individual, for instance, although initially drawing a caregiving response from others, will, over time, tend to exhaust the care provider and ultimately lead to rejection (Stuart and Noyes 1999). This further solidifies the insecurely attached individual's belief that adequate care will not be provided, leading to an escalation of demands and further rejection. The insecurely attached individual often does not recognize this pattern or the effect that it has on others, which compounds the problem. IPT helps people to recognize communication patterns and to make modifications, with a threefold benefit: 1) more effective problem solving occurs as patients directly address conflicts, 2) social support improves as patients ask for help in a way that others can respond to more effectively, and 3) these improvements in communication and social support help resolve both interpersonal crises and symptoms (Stuart and Robertson 2003).

Summary of Theoretical Framework

In summary, IPT hypothesizes that psychiatric and interpersonal difficulties result from a combination of interpersonal and biological factors, following the biopsychosocial model of psychiatric illness (Stuart and Robertson 2003). Individuals with a genetic predisposition or biological diathesis will be more likely to become ill when stressed interpersonally. On this foundation rest the individual's temperament, personality traits, and early life experiences, which are reflected in a particular attachment style. This attachment style affects the person's current social support network and the ability to enlist the support of significant others. Finally, interpersonal functioning is determined by the severity of current stressors in the context of this social support (Stuart and Robertson 2003).

The framework and interventions used in IPT are directly linked to attachment and communication theory. IPT is therefore designed to treat psychiatric symptoms by focusing specifically on patients' primary interpersonal relationships, particularly in the problem areas of grief, interpersonal disputes, role transitions, and interpersonal sensitivity (detailed later in this chapter; see "Problem Areas"). The therapist is also concerned with the communication style that the patient uses in initiating, maintaining, and disengaging from relationships. This occurs within the time-limited format of IPT and focuses on here-and-now resolution of symptoms rather than on the transference relationship that develops in therapy. Although fundamental change in either personality or attachment style is unlikely during short-term treatment, symptom resolution is possible when patients repair their disrupted interpersonal relationships and learn new ways to communicate their need for emotional support.

Treatment

IPT can be succinctly divided into assessment, initial sessions, intermediate sessions, and treatment conclusion. During each phase, the clinician has a well-defined set of tasks to accomplish, each of which is designed to foster the therapeutic goals of the patient. The stance taken by the therapist supports the therapeutic tasks and techniques. Clinicians must be active during the course of IPT, maintaining the focus of therapy and keeping the patient on task. The therapist also should be supportive; the "blank screen" approach should be abandoned in favor of a stance that is empathic and strongly encouraging. The therapist also should make every effort to convey a sense of hope to patients and reinforce their gains. There is no need to be concerned about being neutral in order to create an untainted transference reaction; in fact, the therapist can control the transference reaction to a large degree by assuming the role of a "benevolent expert" and facilitating a positive working alliance throughout the treatment.

Assessment

An assessment is conducted to determine when IPT should be used and to whom it should be applied. The therapist should be guided by several factors, including the available empirical evidence of efficacy, the attachment and communication style of the patient, and the patient's motivation and insight (Stuart and Robertson 2003). A DSM-IV-TR diagnosis should be made because IPT appears to be well suited to patients with mood (empirically validated) and anxiety disorders.

Special attention should be paid to patients with personality disorders. Those with Cluster A disorders, such as paranoid, schizoid, or schizotypal personality disorder, may be unable to form effective alliances with their therapists in short-term therapy, whereas those with severe Cluster B disorders, such as narcissistic, histrionic, borderline, or antisocial personality disorder, may require more intensive therapy than can be provided in an IPT format. However, many patients with depression or anxiety superimposed on a personality disorder may benefit from short-term IPT if the focus is on depression or anxiety rather than on personality change.

IPT should not, however, be restricted to patients with DSM Axis I diagnoses (Stuart and Robertson 2003). It is quite suitable for patients with a variety of interpersonal problems such as work conflicts or marital issues. In fact, patients without major psychiatric illness often have greater interpersonal resources and better social support networks. They present with circumscribed and specific interpersonal problems, and they are frequently superb candidates for IPT.

The assessment should include an evaluation of the patient's attachment style (Stuart and Robertson 2003), consisting of the patient's perception of his or her style of relating to others, and an evaluation of the patient's past and current relationships. Questions about what the patient does when stressed, ill, or otherwise in need of care are particularly helpful. The patient also should be queried about his or her typical responses when asked to assist others. The therapist is essentially developing hypotheses regarding the patient's model of relationships—that is, whether the patient tends to see the world as full of people who can generally be trusted, who should be avoided, or who are needed but tend to be unreliable.

The patient's attachment style has direct effects on his or her ability to develop a therapeutic alliance with the therapist and the likelihood that treatment will be beneficial. Unfortunately, in IPT, as in other psychotherapies, the old saying about "the rich getting richer" holds true. Those patients with more secure attachment styles are usually able to form a working relationship with the therapist and, because of their relatively healthy relationships outside of therapy, are also more likely to be able to draw on their social support system effectively. Individuals with more anxious ambivalent attachments usually can quickly form relationships with their clinicians but often have great difficulty with the conclusion of treatment—a particular problem in time-limited therapy. Those with anxious avoidant styles of attachment may have difficulty trusting or relating to the therapist. Consequently, the therapist may need to spend several of the initial sessions working on developing a productive therapeutic alliance, before moving into more formal IPT work.

The therapist should use the assessment to forecast and plan for problems that may arise during therapy. For example, because patients with anxious ambivalent attachment styles may have difficulty in ending relationships, the astute therapist may modify his or her approach by emphasizing the time-limited nature of the treatment and by discussing the conclusion process earlier. Significant others also may be included in sessions more frequently, to ensure that dependency on the therapist does not become problematic. When working with avoidant patients, the therapist should plan to spend several sessions completing an assessment, taking great care to convey a sense of understanding and empathy to the patient. Soliciting feedback from the patient about the intensity of treatment, particularly considering less frequent appointments, is another tactic that may improve the therapeutic alliance with avoidant individuals.

The therapist should assess the patient's communication style. The way in which patients communicate their needs to others has profound implications for the therapeutic process, as well as for the likelihood that the patient will improve. The therapist should directly ask the patient for examples or vignettes in which a conflict with a significant other occurred. Patients who are able to relate a coherent and detailed story are likely to be able to provide the narrative information necessary to work productively in IPT. Insight also can be judged by noting the way in which the patient describes an interaction and the degree to which he or she presents a balanced picture, particularly with regard to being able to accurately represent the other person's point of view.

Finally, the therapist should assess the match between himself or herself and the patient. The old adage "know thyself" cannot be overemphasized, for therapists, like patients, also have idiosyncratic styles of attachment and communication. Therapists who are overly directive may have difficulty with avoidant patients, for example. Therapists who find it difficult to terminate treatment may encounter problems with dependent patients (Stuart and Robertson 2003).

In general, patients who have characteristics that render them good candidates for any of the time-limited therapies will be good candidates for IPT. These include motivation, good insight, average or better intelligence, and high-level defense mechanisms in the context of sufficient ego functioning. Other desirable characteristics for IPT include 1) a specific interpersonal focus, such as a loss, social transition, or interpersonal conflict; 2) a relatively secure attachment style; 3) the ability to relate a coherent narrative, along with the ability to relate specific dialogue from interpersonal interactions; and 4) a good social support system. The selection of patients can best be understood to be on a spectrum, with highly suitable patients on one end and those who may be less suitable on the other. There are no formal contraindications to IPT, but there are clearly patients who might benefit more from treatments other than IPT.

In summary, the initial assessment, which often takes several sessions to complete, should determine the patient's suitability for IPT. The patient's psychiatric status, attachment style, and communication patterns should be assessed. The assessment should assist the therapist in anticipating problems in therapy, such as resistance or dependency, and should direct the therapist to modify his or her therapeutic approach so that these problems are minimized. Only after the assessment, and the determination that the patient is suitable, should IPT formally begin.

Initial Sessions

During the initial sessions of IPT (usually the first one or two meetings following the general assessment), the therapist has four specific tasks:

1) to conduct an interpersonal inventory, 2) to work collaboratively with the patient to determine which problem areas will be the focus of treatment, 3) to present to the patient a rationale for the use of IPT, and 4) to develop a treatment contract with the patient.

The interpersonal inventory (Klerman et al. 1984) consists of a brief description of the important people in the patient's life and for each individual includes information about the amount and quality of contact, problems in the relationship, and the expectations that the patient has about the relationship. These descriptions are not intended to be exhaustive; the relationships that are noted to be problematic and subsequently become treatment foci will be revisited in detail later. The inventory helps the patient (and therapist) determine which relationships are appropriate to work on. It also aids the therapist in gathering further information about the patient's attachment and communication patterns (Stuart and Robertson 2003).

Once the inventory is complete, the patient and clinician should mutually identify one or two problem relationships on which to focus. The therapist should frame the patient's problem as interpersonal and should give specific examples of the way in which the problem fits into one of the four problem areas: grief or loss, interpersonal disputes, role transitions, and interpersonal sensitivity.

The therapist also should explain the rationale for IPT in concrete terms. Attention should be drawn to the interpersonal orientation of the therapy, and the patient should be instructed that he or she will be expected to discuss interpersonal relationships. Furthermore, the patient should be explicitly told that the goal of therapy is to modify communication patterns and/or expectations about relationships and that as these changes occur, symptomatic relief is expected to follow.

As in all psychotherapies, establishing a therapeutic framework—a contract—for the treatment is an essential part of IPT. In fact, because IPT is time limited, and because the IPT practitioner avoids directly addressing the transferential elements of therapy, the contract is particularly important as a point of reference for both patient and therapist. The time limit must be specifically negotiated with the patient, and other issues that might lead to problems in the therapy should also be tackled in the initial stages of treatment.

The contract should specifically address

- The number (generally 12–20), frequency, and duration of sessions
- The clinical foci of treatment: the problem areas that have been agreed on by the patient and therapist

- The roles of the patient and therapist, particularly the need for the patient to take responsibility for working on his or her communication between sessions
- Contingency planning: addressing issues such as missed sessions, lateness, or illness
- Acceptable conduct in the sessions, contact out of hours, emergencies, and behavioral expectations such as those in regard to substance use and aggressive or inappropriate behavior

Despite the establishment of an explicit contract, "violations" may occur. These may vary from simple matters such as lateness or delayed fee payments to more significant problems such as inappropriate behavior in the sessions or other disruptive interactions. It is important that the IPT therapist initially view these problems as interpersonal communications because they provide valuable information about both the patient's experience of the therapeutic relationship and his or her communication problems outside of therapy. In IPT, rather than addressing the transferential implications of such behaviors, the therapist can use them to examine similar problems outside of the treatment. For example, if a patient delays attempting changes in communication, the therapist can hypothesize that the same behavior also occurs in the patient's relationships outside of therapy. The therapist would then ask the patient about similar difficulties he or she might have with others. As we have seen, this is in direct contrast to traditional transference-based therapy, in which the therapist examines the behavior in the context of the therapeutic relationship.

Because of the injunction in IPT against discussing the transference relationship directly, the contract must serve as a rock-solid reference for both patient and therapist. When contract violations occur, the therapist can note to the patient that both had initially agreed on certain guidelines for therapy (such as meeting at the scheduled time rather than 15 minutes later) and that the patient, by failing to meet his or her responsibility, is in essence keeping himself or herself from benefiting maximally from the treatment. The therapist would then proceed to ask questions about similar behavior outside of the therapeutic relationship.

Intermediate Sessions

During the intermediate sessions of IPT, the patient and therapist work together to address the interpersonal problems identified during the assessment. In general, work on these issues proceeds in the following order: 1) identification of a specific interpersonal problem; 2) detailed exploration of the patient's perception of the problem, including whether it is a problem in communication in the relationship or a matter of unrealistic expectations about the relationship; 3) collaborative brainstorming to identify possible solutions to the problem or to identify ways in which the patient may be able to change his or her communication with significant others; 4) implementation of the proposed solution (typically between sessions); and 5) review of the patient's attempted solution and its results, with positive encouragement for the changes made and discussion of refinements to the solution to be carried out by the patient (Stuart and Robertson 2003). The last phase of the problem-solving approach is that the therapist and patient monitor the consequences of the attempted solution and make modifications as needed.

Various solutions can be considered for the problems with which patients present. For instance, a change in communication to a style that is more direct may be of help with a patient who is experiencing a dispute. A change in circumstances, such as a change in location or in employment, may be of benefit for a patient moving through a role transition. A change in expectations, with a movement toward other social support, is also a viable option. In IPT, however, the end point of therapy is not simply insight; it is change in communication, behavior, and social support that leads to symptom resolution.

Case Example of Change in Communication: Ms. M

Ms. M, a 31-year-old woman, presented with complaints of fatigue at 4 months postpartum. She described a lack of energy, poor sleep, low self-esteem, and a feeling of being overwhelmed. She was irritable and had a short temper, which she felt was due in large part to conflicts with her husband, who she felt had not been helping with the care of their baby. She had no psychiatric history, and because she was breast-feeding, she had no desire to take medications.

After obtaining information about her general social support, Ms. M and her therapist agreed to work on her relationship with her husband. When she was asked to describe specific interactions and her communication in detail, it became clear that Ms. M was actually being quite critical of her husband; when he made attempts to help, she often felt it was not adequate and berated him for his efforts. As a result, he had largely quit helping. She narrated a specific example: Ms. M had come home late from work to find her husband giving their son a bath. Rather than seeing this as his attempt to be helpful and giving him positive feedback, she was quite critical of him for not being as careful and thorough as she thought he should have been.

After discussing several such instances, Ms. M was able to see that her style of communication was not encouraging her husband to help her. In fact, it was discouraging him from doing so and was leading her to feel increasingly frustrated. Once she recognized this pattern, she was able to make some changes and was more appreciative of his help. Her husband, who was invited to several of the later sessions, indicated that he felt more appreciated and began to do more of the child care and housework. Both reported an improvement in their relationship, and Ms. M also reported that her fatigue and irritability were greatly improved.

Case Example of Change in Expectations: Mr. N

Mr. N, a 28-year-old man, had recently graduated from medical school. He was seeking help for feelings of fatigue and disappointment. He reported that although he intellectually recognized that he had accomplished a great deal and had a bright future, he felt neither pleasure about his graduation nor any sense that he had accomplished much in his life.

Mr. N reported several good relationships, including a supportive one with his fiancée, and some close relationships with medical school colleagues. The interpersonal inventory, however, showed a very conflicted relationship with his father. Mr. N described him as very demanding and noted that his father rarely appreciated any of his accomplishments. Mr. N's father was a prominent lawyer and had expressed a great deal of disappointment that Mr. N had gone to medical school. His father had refused to attend the graduation and commented to Mr. N that "at least you can go to law school now that you've finished medicine."

Mr. N and the therapist spent a great deal of time discussing Mr. N's anger at his father, with the goal of helping him to communicate this anger more directly and to be more direct in asking for the support he wanted. After several sessions, Mr. N talked with his father about his disappointment that he had not attended the graduation and his wish that his father would recognize what Mr. N had accomplished. Despite several valiant attempts on the part of Mr. N at communicating his feelings, Mr. N's father seemed incapable of responding to his son's requests and continued to be somewhat distant and critical.

As a result, therapy shifted to a discussion about Mr. N's expectations of his father. Given the history and consistency of his father's interactions with him, Mr. N began to recognize that it was quite likely that his father would never be able to respond in the way in which he wanted and was likely to continue to be distant despite Mr. N's improved communication with him. Time was spent helping Mr. N to literally grieve the loss of the father he wished to have.

Mr. N also recognized that because of his interactions with his father, he was likely to be self-critical and downplay his achievements. Nonetheless, he liked and needed more positive feedback from others. In contrast to his father, Mr. N's fiancée and several of his close friends were able to discuss this with him and were very supportive. Mr. N reported that he felt better after revealing the conflictual relationship with his father to others for the first time and that it helped a great deal that they had been sympathetic and responsive. His fiancée had even thrown him a belated graduation party, which he enjoyed.

When concluding treatment, the therapist pointed out that even though Mr. N had made a great deal of improvement, he might encounter other difficult life transitions. Getting married, having his own children, and attaining other life goals might be times when Mr. N's feelings about his father might resurface. Furthermore, the death of his father at some point might be very difficult. Both Mr. N and his therapist agreed that should such problems arise in the future, Mr. N would be welcome to return for another course of therapy.

Dealing With Resistances

Although this approach sounds rather simple, it is in fact often difficult. It is useful for clinicians to remind themselves that most patients have already had their fill of "good advice" by the time they arrive at the therapist's office. The issue is rarely that the patient does not know or has not been told what to do to solve the problem but rather that the patient has not been able to accept or implement the proposed solution. It is rare that patients will improve with nothing more than good advice from the therapist.

Consequently, in addition to the various techniques described later in this chapter, much of the therapist's work in the intermediate sessions of IPT involves dealing with the patient's resistance to the therapeutic process and his or her ambivalence regarding change. Resistances can be divided into two categories for the purposes of IPT interventions: 1) those that are contractual, such as missed appointments or being late for appointments; and 2) those that involve implementation of changes, such as the patient being unwilling to attempt agreed-on solutions or "forgetting" to take steps to change his or her relationships (Stuart and Robertson 2003).

Within the IPT model, contractual problems should first be dealt with directly by stating to the patient that he or she will not get the full benefit of therapy if he or she misses some appointments or misses some of the time allocated to each session. Because the therapist has already negotiated a detailed treatment contract with the patient, he or she can refer to the agreement reached in the first sessions of IPT (e.g., that the patient has agreed to treatment lasting 12 weeks). The therapist should note that each missed appointment reduces the time available for treatment and reduces the patient's chances for recovery.

Implementation difficulties may be dealt with similarly in a direct fashion when they first appear. The therapist should remind the patient that a time limit to therapy exists and that the benefit of therapy will be maximized if changes are attempted. Second, the therapist should assist the patient in exploring what made the implementation difficult. It is also often useful if the therapist highlights the consequences of not changing and directly addresses the patient's ambivalence.

Many patients will respond to these direct interventions, particularly if they are conveyed with a sense of understanding by the therapist. Occasionally, however, patients persist in their resistance despite these active steps by the therapist. In these cases, it is often helpful to ask the patient what kind of response he or she is expecting from the therapist and others in the face of this unwillingness to change. Addressing the issue in this way often helps the patient appreciate the ways in which his or her pattern of communication provokes unproductive responses in others. Rather than dwell on the patient–therapist relationship, however, the IPT practitioner should then move to other problematic relationships to help the patient appreciate similar communication styles and the responses he or she may be provoking from others.

Completion of Acute Treatment

The best clinical practice in IPT is usually to extend the interval between sessions once the patient is in the recovery stage of acute treatment (Stuart and Robertson 2003). After having met weekly for most of treatment, the patient and therapist may choose to meet biweekly or even monthly toward the end of treatment. For more highly functioning patients, six to eight weekly sessions may be sufficient to resolve their acute problems, but they often derive additional benefit from extending session intervals to biweekly or monthly once their functioning has improved. This gives them the opportunity to further practice communication skills, reinforce the changes that they have made, and develop more self-confidence while remaining in a supportive relationship, all of which facilitate better and more stable functioning. Therefore, it is helpful to negotiate the number of therapy sessions rather than a specified number of weeks of therapy.

Several specific techniques may facilitate the conclusion of therapy. Because the primary goal of IPT is symptom relief and improvement in interpersonal functioning, the specific aim at the time of treatment conclusion is to foster the patient's independent functioning and sense of competence. The idea is to help the patient appreciate that he or she has resources and skills to manage problems and to squarely attribute therapeutic gain to the patient. As acute treatment ends, the therapist should make clear that the patient has improved, has made changes, and has the capability to function independently. The therapist is still available in the background should a future emergency arise, but the expectation is that the patient will function independently and do so quite capably.

It is important to acknowledge a sense of loss that a patient may experience. The therapist may be one of the first people who has taken an interest in the patient, and therapists often underestimate the effect of concluding therapy. After all, therapists have many patients, whereas patients have only one therapist. The therapist should reassure the patient that it is normal to feel a sense of loss. It signifies the effort that the patient has put into the work and into building a relationship with the therapist. Also, it is normal for patients to fear that they will not be able to maintain their gains without the therapist's ongoing support.

The success of therapy is also dependent on the patient's belief that the therapist is absolutely committed to helping the patient. Consequently, if extending the therapy beyond the number of sessions initially agreed on is clearly in the patient's best interest, then it should be extended. The conflict between maintaining the therapeutic contract and extending sessions can be resolved simply by renegotiating a new contract with the patient (Stuart and Robertson 2003).

Maintenance Treatment

Acute treatment with IPT comes to an end as specified by the therapeutic contract. Unlike the end of treatment under the traditional psychoanalytic model, in which "termination" constitutes a complete severing of the therapeutic relationship, the conclusion of acute treatment with IPT does not signify the end of the therapeutic relationship (Stuart and Robertson 2003). In fact, in IPT it is often agreed that the patient and therapist will have therapeutic contacts in the future, and provision is specifically made for these. Not only are many of the major psychiatric disorders (such as depression and anxiety disorders) relapsing and remitting in nature, but also clear evidence indicates that provision of IPT as a maintenance treatment after recovery from depression is helpful in preventing relapse (E. Frank et al. 1990). The IPT practitioner should always discuss maintenance treatment with his or her patient (Stuart and Robertson 2003).

Several alternatives exist for the provision of this maintenance treatment. A specific contract should be established with the patient for whichever option is chosen. Options include specifically scheduling maintenance sessions at monthly or greater intervals, concluding acute treatment with the understanding that the patient will contact the therapist should problems recur, or planning to have the patient contact another provider in the future if the therapist is not available. Decisions about how to structure future treatment must rely on clinical judgment.

Although providing intermittent maintenance treatment with IPT may potentially lead to transference problems, the development of problematic transference and the drive to focus on it as a necessary element of therapy is a function of three things (Stuart and Robertson 2003). The first is the patient himself or herself: the more maladaptive the patient's attachment style and communications, the more likely transference will become problematic and need to be addressed. Second, the intensity of treatment is positively correlated with the intensity of the transference: as therapy sessions are held more frequently (e.g., weekly vs. five times per week), transference becomes a greater therapeutic issue. Third, the duration of treatment is correlated with the development of problematic transference: the longer treatment continues, the more likely transference is to become a focus of therapy. Monthly or bimonthly follow-up sessions consequently confer little risk of precipitating transference problems, while giving great benefit to the patient (Stuart and Robertson 2003).

Clinical experience, theory, and empirical evidence all make clear that IPT should be conceptualized as a two-phase treatment, in which a more intense acute phase of treatment focuses on resolution of immediate symptoms and a subsequent maintenance phase follows with the intent of preventing relapse and maintaining productive interpersonal functioning (Stuart and Robertson 2003). In essence, IPT can be understood as following a "family practice" or "general practitioner" model of care, in which short-term treatment for an acute problem or stressor is provided until the problem is resolved (Stuart and Robertson 2003). Once this occurs, however, the therapeutic relationship is not terminated; like a general practitioner, the therapist makes himself or herself available to the patient should another crisis occur, at which time another time-limited course of treatment is undertaken. In the interim, the therapist may choose, in the same fashion as the general practitioner, to provide "health maintenance" sessions periodically.

Techniques and the Therapeutic Process

Although several techniques (described later in this section) are specific to IPT, it is the focus on extratherapeutic interpersonal relationships rather than any particular intervention that characterizes the therapy. Not surprisingly, given its psychodynamic roots, IPT incorporates several traditional psychotherapeutic methods, such as exploration, clarification, and even some directive techniques. Indeed, no techniques are actually forbidden in IPT. All of them are used, however, in the service of helping the patient to modify his or her interpersonal relationships.

More important than any techniques, however, is the establishment of a productive therapeutic alliance. Warmth, empathy, genuineness, and conveying unconditional positive regard, although not *sufficient* for change in IPT, are all *necessary* for change in IPT (J. Frank 1971; Rogers 1957). Specific techniques are of no benefit if the patient is not present in the therapy. Without a productive alliance, the patient will flee therapy, an obstacle that no amount of technical expertise can overcome.

The primary goal of the IPT practitioner should be to understand the patient. If the patient does not perceive that the therapist is truly committed to doing this, the patient will not disclose information as readily, will not feel valued as an individual, and will not develop a meaningful relationship with the therapist. Working to understand the patient should always take precedence over any technical interventions. Furthermore, all IPT interventions should be therapeutic—the ultimate value of an intervention is the degree to which it helps the patient. Techniques should not be used simply because they are included in a manualized protocol; the benefit to the patient should guide the interventions used in treatment.

Nonspecific Techniques

Nonspecific techniques are those that are common to most psychotherapies. Examples are the use of open-ended questions and clarifications and the expression of empathy by the therapist. These techniques play a crucial role in IPT because they serve to help the therapist understand the patient's experience, convey that understanding to the patient, and provide information about the genesis of the patient's problems and potential solutions to them. Techniques such as brainstorming with the patient, giving directives, and assigning homework can be used judiciously as well in the service of facilitating change. In IPT, all of the techniques that are used should focus primarily on the patient's interpersonal relationships and also should facilitate the therapeutic alliance.

Communication Analysis and Interpersonal Incidents

The analysis of the patient's communication patterns is one of the primary techniques used in IPT. The therapist's task is to help the patient to communicate more clearly what he or she wants from significant others and to convey his or her needs more effectively. Patients often assume that their communication is clear, when in fact it may not be understood at all by the people to whom it is directed.

Communication analysis requires that the therapist elicit information from the patient about important interpersonal incidents (Stuart and Robertson 2003). Interpersonal incidents are descriptions by the patient of specific interactions with his or her significant other. If the identified dispute results in a pattern of fighting between spouses, the therapist might ask the patient to "describe the last time you and your spouse got into a fight" or to "describe one of the more recent big fights you had with your spouse." The therapist should direct the patient to describe the communication in detail, re-creating the dialogue as accurately as possible. The patient should be directed to describe his or her affective reactions and both verbal and nonverbal responses and to describe observations of his or her spouse's nonverbal behavior. The purpose of discussing an interpersonal incident is twofold: 1) to provide information about the miscommunication that is occurring between the parties and 2) to provide insight to the patient about the unrealistic view that the problem is intractable.

A typical patient will describe an interaction with a significant other in very general terms, leaving the therapist with little information about the specific communication that occurred. For instance, a patient may say that her husband "never listens to her." General statements such as "My husband never listens to me," although containing a grain of truth, almost always represent only one side of the story. What is more likely is that the patient's husband may indeed be insensitive, but some of his nonresponsiveness is a result of the reciprocal communication style of the couple. The patient may, although she is intending otherwise, come across as critical or uncaring or may simply be trying to communicate at a time when her words will not be well received. She may, as may her husband, also be unwittingly ignoring important communications. The problem is framed as a communication difficulty within the relationship rather than blaming either individual.

Therefore, the therapist's goal in eliciting interpersonal incidents is to have the patient re-create, in as much detail as possible, a specific interaction between herself and her husband. Because this is not usually how patients spontaneously present information about their conflicts, the therapist must actively direct the patient to produce this material. The therapy proceeds from a general problem statement on the part of the patient to a specific re-creation of the dialogue between the patient and her spouse. The therapist should ask about not only the verbal interactions but also the nonverbal communications that occurred, such as using silence in a hostile fashion, slamming doors, and leaving the situation in the middle of an interaction. The re-creation should include a detailed description of what the patient said to begin the interaction, how her husband responded, what she understood him to say, how she responded in turn, and so forth. Special note should be made of the end of the interaction because many conflicts may carry over to the next day or may be brought up again in subsequent disagreements. The goal is to use this step-by-step report to understand the way in which the patient conveys her attachment needs, acting on the hypothesis that she is communicating in a way that is being misunderstood, and she is therefore not being responded to as she would like.

Case Example: Ms. O

Ms. O, a 36-year-old woman, complained of depression that she attributed to constant conflicts with her husband of 10 years. She described him as uninterested in her and stated that he "never appreciates all the work that I do." She described that despite her full-time job, her husband expected her to do all of the housework and never offered to be of any help. Her depressive symptoms and decrease in functioning apparently had gotten his attention, however, because she reported that they had recently had a big fight over the fact that the housework was left undone. The following dialogue is from session 3:

> Ms. O: Last week was the same as always—he ignored me all week. I don't think he'll ever change. (Note the implication from Ms. O that the conflict between her and her husband is intractable.)
>
> Therapist: The way you describe the problem with your husband, it sounds as if you don't think there will ever be any improvement. Let's take a closer look at one of your fights. Tell me about the last time you and your husband got into a fight because you felt he ignored you.
>
> Ms. O: Last night was typical. After supper, he went into the living room and turned on the TV. I was feeling depressed and angry, so I turned off the TV so he'd pay attention to me.
>
> Therapist: What happened after that?
>
> Ms. O: He looked at me for a minute, then ignored me again by picking up the newspaper.
>
> Therapist: How did you respond to that?
>
> Ms. O: Like anyone would! I said, "If you're going to treat me like that, I'm leaving!"
>
> Therapist: You seem really angry right now as you're talking about that incident.
>
> Ms. O: I'm furious! He always does that to me!
>
> Therapist: It sounds like you certainly conveyed your feelings to him through your actions. I wonder, though, if your husband understood that your original intent was to get him to pay attention to you: to acknowledge that you are important to him. How does he usually respond to you when you're angry?
>
> Ms. O: Well, he usually just withdraws. He grew up in a family that didn't communicate much, and he doesn't like conflict.
>
> Therapist: So when you express anger to him, especially through your actions, he usually withdraws or ignores you. It seems

as if communicating with him angrily is not a very effective way to get him to listen to you.

Ms. O and her therapist went on to discuss the likely effect of her communications to her husband. Mr. O acknowledged his withdrawal response during a conjoint session several weeks later. As Ms. O made attempts to communicate her needs more directly to her husband, and especially as she stopped her threatening comments, she found that he was more willing to be supportive both emotionally and physically.

Use of Affect

The more the patient is affectively involved in therapy, the more likely the patient will be motivated to change his or her behavior or communication style. Consequently, one of the most important tasks for the IPT practitioner is to attend to the patient's affective state. Of particular importance are those moments in which the patient's observed affective state and his or her subjectively reported affect are incongruent. Examining this inconsistency in affect can often lead to breakthroughs in therapy.

Affect can be divided into that experienced during therapy (process affect) and that reported by the patient to have occurred at some time in the past (content affect) (Stuart and Robertson 2003). *Content affect* is the predominant affect experienced at the time of the event. For instance, a patient might describe feeling "numb" at the time of the death and funeral of a significant other. *Process affect*, on the other hand, is the affect experienced by the patient as he or she is describing to the therapist the events surrounding the loss. The same patient, for example, might describe a "numb" feeling at the time of the funeral but while describing the event to the therapist might be in tears and feeling sadness, or perhaps anger. When met with this incongruence in affect, the therapist can focus directly on the discrepancy between content and process affect.

Case Example: Mr. P

Mr. P, a 35-year-old man, presented with symptoms of depression 6 months after the death of his father, who had died unexpectedly from pancreatic cancer. Mr. P's father had been a salesman who was frequently away on business trips and appeared to the therapist to be someone who prioritized his work over his family. Nonetheless, during the first few sessions, Mr. P consistently described his father as loving, caring, and an excellent father. Mr. P described having no feelings of sadness about his father's death and felt very guilty that he had none of what he considered to be "socially appropriate" feelings. The following dialogue occurred in the fourth session:

Therapist: Tell me more about your experiences at your father's funeral.

Mr. P: It was a warm, pleasant day—I remember thinking that I would rather be outside working in the yard than going to the funeral. I just...I just felt numb—nothing, the whole time.

Therapist *[noting the patient's sad affect]:* Tell me what you *feel right now* as you're describing the funeral to me. (Note the therapist distinguishing between the process and the content affect.)

Mr. P *[becoming tearful]:* I'm not sure....I guess I feel sad but not quite like I expected. I guess I also feel rather angry at my dad. You know, he wasn't really around all that much. I remember when I was about 14 years old and had a big baseball game, and I begged him to come....He said that he was too busy, and I remember being angry with him all day after the game.

Mr. P went on to describe several other incidents with his father. During therapy, he developed a much more balanced and realistic picture of his father, including both his positive attributes and his shortcomings.

Use of Transference

Given the interpersonal and psychodynamic foundation on which IPT rests, transference can and does play an extremely important role in the therapy. By observing the developing transference, the therapist can begin to develop hypotheses about the way that the patient interacts with others outside of the therapeutic relationship, because the way in which a patient relates to the therapist is a reflection of the way he or she relates to others. Thus, the transference recognized by the clinician provides a means of understanding other relationships in the patient's interpersonal sphere.

Case Example: Mr. Q

Mr. Q, a 40-year-old man, had been referred by the human relations officer at his company for continuing conflicts with supervisors. Although his sales work was excellent, the human relations officer reported that Mr. Q often got into arguments with his supervisors and peers and was on the verge of losing his job as a result.

Mr. Q reported that the problem was with the company, which "obviously doesn't appreciate that good salesmen need to be encouraged to operate independently and not be constantly interfered with." He was quite clear that he did not see himself as the problem; it was the attitude of others that was at issue. He had agreed to come to treatment only because he realized that if he did not comply, he might lose his job.

Recognizing that the therapeutic alliance was tenuous, the therapist spent the first several sessions listening patiently to Mr. Q's side of the story, expressing empathy about the difficult situation that Mr. Q was in. Furthermore, the therapist assured Mr. Q that he was working only for Mr. Q's benefit, not for the company, and that confidentiality would be completely maintained.

As Mr. Q began to develop more trust in the therapist, he began to reveal more about how difficult it had been at work. Although he had done well with sales, he did not feel that he had any close friends and felt that he had little support. He stated that he wanted to have colleagues at work with whom he could talk about the stress of his job and to whom he could go for new ideas or advice. He did recognize that he had trouble asking for help, largely because he did not trust others and because he believed that they would have little to offer.

A turning point in therapy came at session 6, for which the therapist was about 15 minutes late. After entering the therapist's office, Mr. Q began berating the therapist about his lack of respect because of his lateness. Mr. Q said that he "had lots of important things to do, and the therapist obviously didn't realize that Mr. Q's time was valuable: time was money."

Rather than deal with the transferential elements directly, the therapist responded by doing two things. First, he chose to honestly tell Mr. Q why he had been late: he had been called to his child's school earlier in the morning because his son's arm had been broken, and his son had been admitted to the emergency department. This revelation would have been contraindicated in a more transferentially based therapy, but in IPT, it had the effect of allowing the therapist to give direct feedback to Mr. Q about the therapist's reaction to Mr. Q's angry statements.

Second, the therapist stated directly that Mr. Q's immediate assumption that he had been wronged had initially made the therapist quite angry. The therapist stated that he had wanted to ask Mr. Q to leave and simply stop seeing him for therapy. However, the therapist went on to state that after thinking about it further, he realized that his reaction had helped him to understand how others at Mr. Q's workplace might be feeling when Mr. Q got angry with them.

Mr. Q somewhat sheepishly apologized for his angry statements, which the therapist graciously acknowledged. The therapist, using the patient–therapist interaction that had occurred as a basis for his next set of questions, began to ask Mr. Q in more detail about work interactions in which he had gotten angry and during which others had gotten angry in return. The in-session interaction both informed the questions that were asked about Mr. Q's extratherapy relationships and provided the impetus for Mr. Q to begin to develop a different perspective on how others perceived him. Over the next several sessions, Mr. Q and the therapist developed the hypothesis that Mr. Q's expressions of anger, although at times warranted, usually had the effect of causing others to respond by getting angry in return. His impulsive anger was keeping him from developing the close relationships with others that he desired.

By the end of therapy, Mr. Q reported that he was getting along better with others at work. His supervisor also endorsed these changes. Mr. Q continued to have some difficulty with his anger, but in contrast to his behavior pretherapy, he usually felt able to "control" his anger on most occasions by stopping to think about the reaction that he was likely to get from others.

Problem Areas

IPT focuses on four specific problem areas that reflect the interpersonal nature of the treatment: grief, interpersonal disputes, role transitions, and interpersonal sensitivity. Psychosocial stressors from any of the problem areas, when combined with an attachment disruption in the context of poor social support, can lead to interpersonal problems or psychiatric syndromes (Stuart and Robertson 2003).

Grief and Loss

It is useful to formulate many types of losses as grief issues. In addition to the death of a significant other, loss of physical health, divorce, and loss of employment are examples of interpersonal stressors that might be experienced by the patient as grief (Stuart and Robertson 2003). In general, it is usually best for the therapist to place the patient's problems within the problem area that makes the most intuitive sense to the patient. Moreover, grief need not be considered as "normal" or "abnormal", it is the task of the IPT practitioner to attempt to understand the patient's experience, not pathologize it.

Once a grief issue is established as a focus of treatment, the therapist's tasks are to facilitate the patient's mourning process and to assist the patient in developing new interpersonal relationships or in modifying his or her existing relationships so as to obtain increased social support. New or existing relationships cannot replace the lost relationship, but the patient can reallocate his or her energies and interpersonal resources over time.

Several strategies are useful in dealing with grief issues. Primary among these is the elicitation of feelings from the patient, which may be facilitated by discussing the loss and the circumstances surrounding it, both of which serve to help the patient to realistically reconstruct the relationship. The use of process and content affect may be quite useful during this type of discussion. Grief issues commonly involve layers of conflicted feelings surrounding the lost person, and assisting the patient to develop a three-dimensional picture of the lost person, including a realistic assessment of the person's good and bad characteristics, is a necessary process in the resolution of the grief. Often the patient will initially describe the lost person as "all good" or "all bad" and be unaware that this idealization (or devaluation) covers other contradictory feelings that may be difficult for the patient to accept. The development of a balanced view of the lost individual greatly facilitates the mourning process.

This same process can be used for other losses as well: the loss of a job, a divorce, or loss of physical functioning. In such instances, the patient also will need to grieve the loss and to move toward establishing new social supports. Encouraging patients to develop a more realistic view of their loss may be of help as well.

Interpersonal Disputes

The first step in dealing with interpersonal disputes is to identify the stage of the conflict and to determine whether both parties are actively working to solve the problem, have reached an impasse, or have reached a point at which dissolution of the relationship is inevitable (Klerman et al. 1984). It is important to keep in mind that successful treatment does not necessarily require that the relationship be repaired. The important point is that the patient makes an active and informed decision about the relationship.

One of the primary goals with interpersonal disputes is to help patients to modify their patterns of communication. Particularly in relationships of longer duration, patients often become locked into patterns of communication with their significant others that result in misunderstanding or in cycles of escalating affect. The therapist can show the patient how to communicate his or her needs more clearly and in a way that is more likely to gain what the patient is requesting rather than provoke hostile responses. The therapist should model direct communication to the patient and may engage the patient in role-playing to reinforce the new communication. Although IPT is generally an individual therapy, inviting a significant other to therapy for several conjoint sessions can be invaluable because the therapist can observe the communication in vivo and can begin to help the couple to make changes in the way in which they interact.

Role Transitions

The problem area of role transitions encompasses a huge number of possible life changes. Included are life-cycle changes such as adolescence, childbirth, and a decline in physical functioning and social transitions such as marriage, divorce, change in job status, and retirement. Typical problems include sadness at the loss of an old familiar role, as well as poor adaptation to or rejection of the new role. Role transitions often include loss of important social supports and attachments and may include a demand for new social or other skills. A diminishment of self-esteem and depression may result.

The therapist should assist the patient in giving up his or her old role, which includes helping the patient to experience grief over the loss, often using some of the techniques described for dealing with grief issues. It is crucial to help the patient to develop a realistic and balanced view of his or her old role, including both positive and negative aspects. Assisting the patient to develop new social supports and skills is also an essential part of the therapy.

Interpersonal Sensitivity

Some patients may have problems with poor interpersonal functioning because of personality traits, avoidant attachment styles, or other factors. Interpersonal sensitivity (Stuart and Robertson 2003) refers specifically to a patient's difficulty in establishing and maintaining interpersonal relationships. Consequently, patients with interpersonal sensitivities often require a somewhat different approach than is used with patients who have better social skills.

Patients with interpersonal sensitivities may have few, if any, interpersonal relationships to discuss in therapy. Relationships with family members, even though they may be quite disrupted, may be some of the only relationships the patient has. The therapy relationship also may take on greater importance with these patients because it, too, may be one of the only relationships in which the patient is engaged. The therapist should be prepared to give feedback to the patient about the way he or she communicates in therapy and should be prepared to use role-playing as a means of practicing skills with the patient. In addition, the therapist often must be active in assisting the patient in getting involved in appropriate social groups or activities in the community. Above all, the therapist and patient must keep in mind that the therapy is not designed to "correct" the social difficulties but rather to teach the patient some skills with which he or she can continue to build new relationships and to relieve his or her acute distress.

Summary of Interpersonal Problem Areas

These categories are very helpful as a means of focusing the patient on specific interpersonal problems, but it is important to be flexible when using them. Rather than "diagnosing" a specific category, the therapist should use the problem areas primarily to maintain focus on one or two interpersonal problems, particularly because the time available in IPT is, by definition, limited. In general, the patient's view of the nature of the problem should be accepted. For example, if the patient feels that his or her recent divorce is a grief issue rather than a role transition, then the grief area should be used. The therapeutic alliance should not be sacrificed for the sake of a "correct diagnosis" of the problem area.

The interpersonal problems experienced by patients are similar in that they all derive from an acute interpersonal stressor combined with a social support system that does not sufficiently sustain the patient. In addition to addressing the specific problem, effort always should be directed toward improving the patient's social supports (Stuart and Robertson 2003).

Interpersonal Psychotherapy and Medication

The use of medication is perfectly compatible with IPT—in fact, the original studies of IPT reported that combination treatment was more successful and better accepted by patients than either medication or psychotherapy alone (Weissman et al. 1979). Given the biopsychosocial diathesis stress model of illness that is used in IPT (Stuart and Robertson 2003), the use of medication is theoretically defensible as well. Although more empirical data are needed, it is common practice for IPT and medication to be used together to treat psychiatric illnesses.

Summary Case Illustration: Mrs. R

Mrs. R, a 27-year-old woman, was 3 months postpartum. She had been married 4 years to a "relatively" supportive husband. They had moved within the last year, so that he could begin his residency training in internal medicine at the local hospital, and in the process had moved some distance from family and friends. Mrs. R described that her pregnancy was planned but reported that she and her husband had decided to have a baby largely because their medical costs would be covered while Mr. R was in training.

Her current complaints included trouble sleeping, low energy, and a poor appetite. She reported that she felt depressed at times, but her primary mood was irritability. This was particularly evident in her relationship with Mr. R. She denied any thoughts of self-harm and also denied any thoughts of harm toward her baby. When asked about such thoughts, she responded that her only satisfying relationship was with her baby daughter.

Mrs. R denied any previous psychiatric problems. She also noted no medical problems and reported that her pregnancy and postpartum course to date were unremarkable. The only complicating factor was that she was breast-feeding and wanted to continue doing so for at least a year and did not want to consider any medication because she did not want to expose her baby to potentially harmful drugs. She was not taking any oral contraceptives and laughingly stated that "at the moment, birth control isn't a problem because I don't even want my husband to touch me, much less do anything else!"

She denied any formal family psychiatric history but did note that her mother had remarked on several occasions that she might have had postpartum depression, although she was never treated. Mrs. R had an older sister with two children, and her sister had experienced no difficulty with either child. She denied any use of substances other than occasional alcohol and stated that she had only recently had her first glass of wine in more than a year, having forsworn any alcohol during the pregnancy.

Her early childhood and development were unremarkable. She did report that her parents highly valued education and were fairly demanding about her academics but not to a degree she considered to be outside of the norm. Both were professors at a university distant from her current residence. Mrs. R had completed a master's degree in psychology and had started her doctoral work, but she and Mr. R decided that she would put her work on hold both to accommodate the move to another city and to allow her to care for the baby. She did have plans to resume her education, but it was not clear when that would occur.

Mrs. R described herself as hardworking, honest, and conflict-avoidant. She had been quite successful in school and impressed the therapist with her intellect and insight. She had several good friends in the city in which she had lived previously, and although she frequently talked on the telephone with them, she found that it was not the same as getting support in person. Furthermore, she noted that she had not made any close friends after the most recent move. She attributed this to the time needed to get established and the subsequent need to stay at home with the baby.

After the therapist conducted an interpersonal inventory, the therapist and Mrs. R mutually identified two primary problems. The first was a role transition in which she was faced with being a new mother, a role that was both unfamiliar and about which she had some ambivalent feelings. The second was a conflict with her husband. She was clear that he was not emotionally supportive and that he was not meeting her expectations regarding help with child care. The therapist also felt strongly that in addition to these problems, Mrs. R would benefit greatly from increased social contact and support. They agreed to meet for 12 sessions during the next several months.

Over the next several sessions, the therapist elicited several detailed interactions between Mr. and Mrs. R. As Mrs. R described these, she began to realize that her communication was not clear and that she at times expected her husband to literally "anticipate" her need for help without her having to ask him for specific help. She tended to interpret this failure on his part as a lack of emotional support. One particular incident highlighted this communication style:

Therapist: Mrs. R, tell me about one of the more recent conflicts you and Mr. R have had about child-care duties.
Mrs. R: Two nights ago was typical. My husband got home around 8:00 P.M., and I was upset because he had not called to let

me know that he was going to be late. I had waited for him for dinner, and I was even more irritated about that....He's so inconsiderate.

Therapist: Tell me more about what exactly was said.

Mrs. R: I said, "Late again, I see—you could have called to let me know."

Therapist: And what did Mr. R say in response?

Mrs. R: He didn't say anything; he just walked in, sat down on the couch, and turned on the TV.

Therapist: And then?

Mrs. R: I took Jennifer over to the table with me and started eating. My husband eventually came over, and we pretty much sat there in silence the whole meal.

Therapist: So, how did the interaction end?

Mrs. R: It didn't really—he went to bed early and then left for the hospital early in the morning. *[Somewhat sheepishly]* I found out the next day that he had been in surgery most of the evening and couldn't get out of the operating room to call me.

Therapist: It sounds to me that there was a lot of nonverbal communication in that interaction. What was it exactly that you were trying to communicate to Mr. R?

Mrs. R: Well, that I was feeling frustrated and that I needed some help and some adult interaction after being cooped up all day with Jennifer. I don't think he realizes how much work is involved. Also, he has a lot of interaction with other people, and I'm pretty desperate for someone to talk to at the end of the day.

Therapist: How well do you think he understood that from your communication, especially the nonverbal communication and silence that you used in the incident you described?

Mrs. R: I doubt he got any of it. I just wish he would recognize what I need.

Therapist: It sounds to me that you have a mismatch in needs when he arrives home from work. He probably needs a break from people, and you really need some interaction. The net result seems to be that you both get angry and withdraw, and neither of you gets what you want and need.

Mrs. R: I hadn't thought of it in that way....

Therapist: What ways can you think of that you can address this more directly?

Mrs. R: Well, this weekend he has some time off from his clinical responsibilities, so maybe we could spend some time talking. I don't really want to do it, but it seems pretty clear that if I don't address this with him directly, and let him know what I need from him, things aren't going to get any better.

Over the next several weeks, Mrs. R had several lengthy discussions with Mr. R about her need for time with him, communication with him, and physical help with child care. To her surprise, he was quite receptive to her requests, and although she continued to feel that she bore the weight of the responsibilities because of his work schedule, she was clear that he was making an effort and wanted to help. Before therapy concluded, they had arranged for a babysitter on two occasions and had gone out together without the baby.

In addition, the therapist suggested to Mrs. R that she begin making some additional efforts to enlarge her social network. To accomplish this, he specifically suggested that she try out a support group for the spouses of residents employed at the hospital. She was initially resistant because she was concerned that the women there "would only be interested in being moms and wouldn't understand my interest in education and other intellectual things." After session 4, she reluctantly attended a group and found instead that there were many women in very similar situations, many of whom had small children and had moved from other places. She even arranged to meet with two of the other women for coffee the next week. Over the course of therapy, she established friendships with several other women with small children. She found these to be extremely helpful both because the women were able to understand and empathize with her situation and because they fulfilled much of her need for adult social contact.

In addition to these two issues, therapy also focused on the role transition in which she was engaged. Mrs. R was quite insightful and readily described mixed feelings about her daughter. She clearly felt very attached to Jennifer and loved her dearly but also was aware that she had put plans for further schooling on hold and that she had given up a great deal of spontaneity as well. She reported that giving voice to these ambivalent feelings, as well as talking about them with other women in similar circumstances, was of great help. She also discussed with her husband her desire to return to school part-time within the next 2 years.

Over the course of therapy, Mrs. R had discovered that Mr. R was stressed out as well, and to maintain their relationship, the two of them needed to schedule time together. The greater time and spontaneity that they had enjoyed previously simply was not available anymore but could be compensated for by scheduling time. In addition, the friendships that she was developing had also met many of her social needs and provided empathic support.

At session 10, Mrs. R and the therapist reviewed her progress and discussed her understanding of what had led to her difficulties. Mrs. R described that the stress of having a baby, coupled with Mr. R's diminished availability because of his residency schedule and the move they had made, which took them away from familiar social supports, had made it much more difficult to cope with things. She felt that even though there continued to be stressors, she was coping with them much better. She also emphasized that her relationship with Mr. R had improved greatly and that she was "enjoying life again."

The last two sessions were spaced over a 2-month period. Mrs. R continued to do well and at the end of therapy agreed to contact the therapist should problems arise in the future.

Summary

IPT is characterized by three essential elements: a focus on interpersonal relationships, a contract that specifies a time limit for therapy, and a focus on relationships outside of therapy rather than on the transference relationship. Attachment theory supports the approach used in IPT, and the attachment style of the patient should instruct the therapist about the patient's suitability for treatment, prognosis, and potential problems that may arise in therapy. Furthermore, the patient's attachment style should inform the therapist about the ways in which the therapy can be modified to be more effective for patients with less secure attachment styles.

Interpersonal problems and psychiatric symptoms are conceptualized as developing within a biopsychosocial context. An acute interpersonal crisis, such as a loss, an interpersonal dispute, or a difficult life transition, creates problems for people for two reasons: 1) their interpersonal communication skills within their significant relationships are not adaptive, and 2) their social support network is not sufficient to sustain them through the interpersonal crisis. IPT helps patients to communicate more effectively to meet their attachment needs, to realistically assess their expectations of others, and to improve their social support in general. In essence, the goal of IPT is to assist the patient in getting his or her attachment needs met more effectively given his or her attachment style. This should help resolve interpersonal problems and reduce suffering.

IPT is best suited to patients who are more securely attached and who present with more specific interpersonal problems. Both clinical experience and research evidence make clear, however, that IPT also works well for patients with various DSM-IV-TR diagnoses and that even patients with personality problems may benefit from treatment. Research is under way to investigate more applications of the treatment.

Finally, IPT must be based on a three-point foundation. First, the practice of IPT should rest on the empirical research that supports its use. Second, the practice of IPT should reflect clinical experience with its use. Third, and most important, the practice of IPT should include the use of clinical judgment: the therapist must recognize the unique nature of his or her relationship with each patient and must always place the needs of the patient above strict adherence to a manual. Given these foundational supports, IPT is an efficacious, effective, and extremely useful clinical approach to interpersonal problems.

References

American Psychiatric Association: Diagnostic and Statistical Manual of Mental Disorders, 4th Edition, Text Revision. Washington, DC, American Psychiatric Association, 2000

Beck AT, Rush AJ, Shaw BF, et al: Cognitive Therapy of Depression. New York, Guilford, 1979

Bowlby J: Developmental psychiatry comes of age. Am J Psychiatry 145:1–10, 1988

Elkin I, Shea MT, Watkins JT, et al: National Institute of Mental Health Treatment of Depression Collaborative Research Program: general effectiveness of treatments. Arch Gen Psychiatry 46:971–982, 1989

Frank E, Spanier C: Interpersonal psychotherapy for depression: overview, clinical efficacy, and future directions. Clinical Psychology: Science and Practice 2:349–369, 1995

Frank E, Kupfer DJ, Perel JM: Three-year outcomes for maintenance therapies in recurrent depression. Arch Gen Psychiatry 47:1093–1099, 1990

Frank J: Therapeutic factors in psychotherapy. Am J Psychother 25:350–361, 1971

Kiesler DJ, Watkins LM: Interpersonal complementarity and the therapeutic alliance: a study of the relationship in psychotherapy. Psychotherapy 26:183–194, 1989

Klerman GL, Weissman MM, Rounsaville BJ, et al: Interpersonal Psychotherapy of Depression. New York, Basic Books, 1984

Kupfer DJ, Frank E, Perel JM: Five year outcomes for maintenance therapies in recurrent depression. Arch Gen Psychiatry 49:769–773, 1992

O'Hara MW, Stuart S, Gorman L, et al: Efficacy of interpersonal psychotherapy for postpartum depression. Arch Gen Psychiatry 57:1039–1045, 2000

Rogers CR: The necessary and sufficient conditions of therapeutic personality change. J Consult Psychol 21:95–103, 1957

Stuart S, Noyes R: Attachment and interpersonal communication in somatization disorder. Psychosomatics 40:34–43, 1999

Stuart S, Robertson M: Interpersonal Psychotherapy: A Clinician's Guide. London, Edward Arnold, 2003

Weissman MM, Prusoff BA, Dimascio A, et al: The efficacy of drugs and psychotherapy in the treatment of acute depressive episodes. Am J Psychiatry 136:555–558, 1979

Weissman MM, Markowitz JW, Klerman GL: Comprehensive Guide to Interpersonal Psychotherapy. New York, Basic Books, 2000

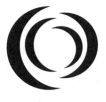

Time-Limited Dynamic Psychotherapy

Formulation and Intervention

Hanna Levenson, Ph.D.

"We don't say 'cure.' We say you had a 'corrective emotional experience.'"

Therapist [Billy Crystal] to gangster/patient [Robert DeNiro] in the movie Analyze This

Some material in this chapter is from *Time-Limited Psychotherapy: A Guide to Clinical Practice* (copyright © 1995 by Hanna Levenson, reprinted by permission of Basic Books, a member of Perseus Books, LLC) and from "Time-Limited Dynamic Psychotherapy: An Integrationist Approach," *Journal of Psychotherapy Integration* 13:300–333, 2003.

Time-limited dynamic psychotherapy (TLDP) is an interpersonal, time-sensitive approach for patients with chronic, pervasive, dysfunctional ways of relating to others. Its premises and techniques are broadly applicable regardless of time limits. However, its method of formulating and intervening makes it particularly well suited for the so-called difficult patient seen in a brief or time-limited therapy. The brevity of the treatment promotes therapist pragmatism, flexibility, and accountability (Levenson et al. 2002b). Furthermore, time pressures help keep the therapist attuned to circumscribed goals with an active, directive stance (Levenson et al. 2002a). The focus is not on the reduction of symptoms per se (although such improvements are expected to occur) but rather on changing ingrained patterns of interpersonal relatedness or personality style. TLDP makes use of the relationship that develops between therapist and patient to kindle fundamental changes in the way a person interacts with others and himself or herself. In this chapter, I review theory, research, and training relevant to TLDP and illustrate its practice with a case study.

Overview

TLDP was first formalized in a treatment manual constructed for a research program investigating briefer ways of intervening with challenging patients. This manual eventually was reproduced in book form: *Psychotherapy in a New Key: A Guide to Time-Limited Dynamic Psychotherapy* (Strupp and Binder 1984). In a more recently published clinical casebook, *Time-Limited Dynamic Psychotherapy: A Guide to Clinical Practice*, Levenson (1995) translated TLDP principles and strategies into pragmatically useful ways of thinking and intervening for the practitioner. The Levenson text places more emphasis on behavioral changes through experiential learning than on insight through interpretation. TLDP maintains continuity with psychoanalytic modalities, however, by emphasizing the role of the therapeutic relationship in evoking and resolving past problem patterns.

Historically, TLDP is rooted in an object relations framework. According to object relations theory, images of the self and others evolve out of human interactions rather than out of biologically derived tensions. The search for and maintenance of human relatedness are considered to be major motivating forces within all human beings. Specifically, the self is seen as an internalization of interactions with significant others. This relational view sharply contrasts with that of classical psychoanalysis, which emphasizes the role of innate mental structures in mediating conflicts between instinctual impulses and societal constraints. Indeed, the

TLDP interpersonal perspective reflects a larger paradigm shift occurring within psychoanalytic theory and practice from a one-person to a two-person psychology (Messer and Warren 1995).

TLDP embraces an interpersonal perspective, as exemplified by the early work of Sullivan (1953), and is consistent with the views of modern interpersonal theorists. Strupp and Binder (1984) made clear that their "purpose is neither to construct a new theory of personality development nor to attempt a systematic integration of existing theories. Rather, we have chosen interpersonal conceptions as a framework for the proposed form of psychotherapy because of their hypothesized relevance and utility" (p. 28). The relational view of TLDP focuses on transactional patterns in which the therapist is embedded in the therapeutic relationship as a participant observer. Transference (the repetition of past conflicts within the therapeutic relationship) is not considered a distortion but rather a patient's plausible perceptions of the therapist's behavior and intent. Similarly, countertransference (the emergence of a therapist's emotional patterns within the therapy) does not indicate a failure on the part of the therapist. Rather, it represents his or her natural reactions to the pushes and pulls from interacting with patients.

Interestingly, other theories of psychotherapy are also incorporating interpersonal perspectives in their conceptualizations and practice. This can be seen in cognitive therapy, behavior therapy, and gestalt therapy. Data from child development research (e.g., Stern 1985) point to how one's world is essentially interpersonal. Recent information from the field of neurobiology suggests that "relationships early in life may shape the *very structures* that create representations of experience and allow a coherent view of the world. Interpersonal experiences directly influence how we mentally construct reality" (emphasis added, Siegel 1999, p. 4). This growing recognition of the import of interpersonal relatedness promotes compatibility across a variety of theoretical and strategic viewpoints, allowing for meaningful psychotherapy integration (see Greenberg, Chapter 8, in this volume).

Essential Assumptions

The TLDP model makes five basic assumptions that greatly affect treatment:

1. *Maladaptive relationship patterns are learned in the past*—Disturbances in adult interpersonal relatedness typically stem from faulty relationships with early caregivers—usually in the parental home. Bowlby

(1973) elaborated that early experiences with parental figures result in mental representations of these relationships or working models of one's interpersonal world. These models, or schemas, inform one about the nature of human relatedness and what is generally necessary to sustain and maintain emotional connectedness to others. Children filter the world through the lenses of these schemas, which allows them to interpret the present, understand the past, and anticipate the future.

2. *Such maladaptive patterns are maintained in the present*—This emphasis on early childhood experiences is consistent with much of psychoanalytic thinking. From a TLDP framework, however, the individual's personality is seen not as fixed at a certain point but rather as continually changing as it interacts with others. Data from neurobiology research appear to confirm that although relationships play a crucial role in the early years, this "shaping process occurs throughout life" (Siegel 1999, p. 4). Although one's dysfunctional interactive style is learned early in life, this style must be supported in the person's current adult life for the interpersonal difficulties to continue. For example, if a child has learned to be placating and deferential because he or she grew up in a home with authoritarian parents, that child will unwittingly and inadvertently attempt to maintain this role as an adult by encouraging others to act harshly toward him or her.

   This focus is consistent with a systems-oriented approach, which stresses the context of a situation and the circular processes surrounding it. "Pathology" does not reside within an individual but rather is created by all the components within the (pathological) system. Maladaptive patterns are maintained through their enactment in the current social system, as others unwittingly replicate familiar responses from one's troubled past.

3. *Dysfunctional relationship patterns are reenacted in vivo in the therapy*—A third assumption is that the patient interacts with the therapist in the same dysfunctional way that characterizes his or her interactions with significant others (i.e., transference) and tries to enlist the therapist into playing a complementary role. This reenactment is an ideal therapeutic opportunity because it permits the therapist to observe the playing out of the maladaptive interactional pattern and to experience what it is like to try to relate to that individual. Because dysfunctional interactions are presumably sustained in the present, including the current patient–therapist relationship, the therapist can concentrate on the present to alter the patient's dysfunctional interactive style. Working in the present allows change to happen more quickly because there is no assumption that one needs to work through child-

hood conflicts and discover historical truths. This emphasis on the present has tremendous implications for treating interpersonal difficulties in a brief time frame.

4. *The therapeutic relationship has a dyadic quality*—A corollary assumption to the TLDP concept of transference is that the therapist also enters into the relationship and becomes a part of the reenactment of the dysfunctional interpersonal interaction. In Sullivan's (1953) terms, the therapist becomes a participant observer. The relational-interactionist position of TLDP holds that the therapist cannot help but react to the patient—that is, the therapist inevitably will be pushed and pulled by the patient's dysfunctional style and will respond accordingly. This transactional type of reciprocity and complementarity (what I call *interactional countertransference*) does not indicate a failure on the part of the therapist but rather represents his or her "role responsiveness" or "interpersonal empathy" (Strupp and Binder 1984). The therapist inevitably becomes "hooked" into acting out the corresponding response to the patient's inflexible, maladaptive pattern, or in Wachtel's (1987) terms, patients induce therapists to act as "accomplices."

That the therapist is invited repeatedly by the patient (unconsciously) to become a partner in a well-rehearsed, maladaptive two-step has its parallels in the recursive aspect of mental development. For example, children who have experienced serious family dysfunction are thought to have disorganized internal mental structures and processes as a result. These disorganized processes impair the child's behavior with others, which causes others not to respond to the child in empathic ways, thereby disorganizing the development of the mind further.

To get "unhooked," the therapist must realize how he or she is fostering a replication of the dysfunctional pattern. The TLDP practitioner uses this information to attempt to change the nature of the interaction in a positive way, thereby engaging the patient in a healthier mode of relating. In addition, the therapist can collaboratively invite the patient to look at what is happening between them (i.e., metacommunicate), either highlighting the dysfunctional reenactment while it is occurring or solidifying new experiential learning following a more functionally adaptive interactive process.

5. *The TLDP focus is on the chief problematic relationship pattern*—Although patients may have a repertoire of different interpersonal patterns, the emphasis in TLDP is on discerning a patient's most pervasive and problematic style of relating (which may need to incorporate several divergent views of self and other). This is not to say that

other relationship patterns may not be important. However, focusing on the most frequently troublesome type of interaction should have ramifications for other less central interpersonal schemas and is pragmatically essential when time is of the essence. The presence of a clear interpersonal focus is an important element distinguishing time-limited psychoanalytic therapy from longer-term efforts at personality reconstruction.

Goals

The TLDP therapist seeks two overriding goals with patients: *new experiences* and *new understandings*.

New Experiences

The first and major goal in conducting TLDP is offering the patient a new relational experience. *New* is meant in the sense of being different and more functional (i.e., healthier) than the maladaptive pattern to which the person has become accustomed. And *experience* emphasizes the affective-action component of change—behaving differently and emotionally appreciating the different behavior. From a TLDP perspective, behaviors are encouraged that signify a new manner of interacting (e.g., more flexibly, more independently) rather than specific, content-based behaviors (e.g., going to a movie alone). The new experience is actually composed of a set of focused experiences throughout the therapy in which the patient gains a different appreciation of self, of the therapist, and of their interaction. These new experiences provide the patient with experiential learning so that old patterns may be relinquished and new patterns may evolve.

The focus of these new experiences centers on those that are particularly helpful to a patient based on the therapist's formulation of the case (see "Time-Limited Dynamic Psychotherapy Formulation" later in this chapter). The therapist identifies what he or she could say or do (within the therapeutic role) that would most likely subvert or interrupt the patient's maladaptive interactive style. The therapist's behavior gives the patient the opportunity to disconfirm his or her interpersonal schemas. The patient can actively try out (consciously or unconsciously) new behaviors in the therapy, see how they feel, and notice how the therapist responds. This information then informs the patient's internal representations of what can be expected from self and others. This in vivo learning is a critical component in the practice of TLDP.

These experiential forays into what for the patient has been frightening territory make for heightened affective learning. A tension is created when the familiar (but detrimental) responses to the patient's presentation are not provided. Out of this tension, new learning takes place. Such an emotionally intense, here-and-now process is thought to "heat up" the therapeutic process and permit progress to be made more quickly than in therapies that depend solely on more abstract learning (usually through interpretation and clarification). I believe this experiential learning is important for doing brief therapy and becomes critical when working with a patient who has difficulty establishing a therapeutic alliance or exploring relational issues in the here and now. As Frieda Fromm-Reichmann is credited with saying, "What the patient needs is an experience, not an explanation."

There are definite parallels between the goal of a new experience and procedures used in some behavioral techniques (e.g., exposure therapy), in which clients are exposed to feared stimuli without the expected negative consequences. Modern cognitive theorists voice analogous perspectives when they talk about interpersonal processes that lead to experiential disconfirmation. Similarities can also be found in the plan formulation method (Sampson and Weiss 1986), in which opportunities for change occur when patients test their pathogenic beliefs in the context of the therapeutic relationship.

The concept of a *corrective emotional experience* described more than 50 years ago is also applicable (Alexander and French 1946). In their classic book, *Psychoanalytic Therapy: Principles and Applications*, Alexander and French challenged the then-prevalent assumption concerning the therapeutic importance of exposing repressed memories and providing a genetic reconstruction. By focusing on the importance of experiential learning, they suggested that change could take place even without the patient's insight into the etiology of his or her problems.

Decades of clinical and empirical data within psychology clearly support this conclusion (Fisher and Greenberg 1997). Now, neurobiological data appear to indicate that most learning is done without conscious awareness (Siegel 1999). This view has major implications for the techniques one uses. It questions the pursuit of insight as a necessary goal and thereby challenges the use of interpretation as the cornerstone of psychodynamic technique. From an empirical standpoint, Henry and colleagues (1994) presented data indicating that transference interpretations in particular may not be effective and may even be countertherapeutic.

Alexander and French's (1946) concept of the corrective emotional experience has been criticized for promoting manipulation of the transference by suggesting that the therapist should respond in a way diametrically opposite to that expected by the patient. For example, if the patient was raised by an intrusive mother, then the therapist should maintain a more restrained stance. The TLDP concept of the *new relational experience* does not involve a direct manipulation of the transference and is not solely accomplished by the offering of a "good enough" therapeutic relationship. Specifically, a therapist can help provide a new experience by selectively choosing—from all of the helpful, mature, and respectful ways of being present in a session—those particular aspects that would most effectively undermine a specific patient's dysfunctional style. A warm stance that supports a patient's independence, for example, may counter expectations of intrusiveness as readily as a stance of restraint would.

New Understandings

The second goal, providing a new understanding, focuses more specifically on cognitive changes than the first goal just discussed, which emphasizes the affective-behavioral arena. The patient's new understanding usually involves an identification and comprehension of his or her dysfunctional patterns. To facilitate such a new understanding, the TLDP therapist can point out repetitive patterns that have originated in experiences with past significant others, with current significant others, and in the here and now with the therapist. Therapists' judicious disclosing of their own reactions to patients' behaviors also can be beneficial. If undertaken in a constructive and sensitive manner, such disclosure allows patients to recognize similar relationship patterns with different people in their lives. This new perspective enables them to examine their active role in perpetuating dysfunctional interactions.

Differentiating between the idea of a new experience and a new understanding helps the clinician attend to aspects of the change process that would be most helpful in formulating and intervening as efficiently and effectively as possible. In addition, because psychodynamically trained therapists are so ready to intervene with an interpretation, placing the new experience in the foreground helps them regroup and focus on the "big picture"—how not to reenact a dysfunctional scenario with the patient. This emphasis on the new experience is a departure from the central role of understanding through interpretation in the original TLDP model (Strupp and Binder 1984). It is my current thinking that experiential learning broadens the range of patients who can benefit from brief therapies, leads to more generalization to the outside world, and permits therapists to incorporate a variety of techniques and strategies that might be helpful.

Inclusion and Exclusion Criteria

TLDP was developed to help therapists deal with patients who have trouble forming working alliances because of their lifelong dysfunctional interpersonal difficulties. However, it could be applicable for anyone who is having difficulties (e.g., depression, anxiety, emptiness) that affect their relatedness to self and other. Previously, I (Levenson 1995) endorsed the TLDP selection criteria as outlined by Strupp and Binder (1984). My current thinking is that TLDP may be helpful to patients even when they do not quite meet these criteria, as long as adequate descriptions of their interpersonal transactions can be elicited.

The following five major selection criteria are used to determine a patient's appropriateness for TLDP:

1. Patients must *be in emotional discomfort* so that they are motivated to endure the often challenging and painful change process and to make sacrifices of time, effort, and money as required by therapy.
2. Patients must *come for appointments and engage with the therapist*—or at least talk. Initially, such an attitude may be fostered by hope or faith in a positive outcome. Later, it might stem from actual experiences of the therapist as a helpful partner.
3. Patients must *be willing to consider how their relationships have contributed* to distressing symptoms, negative attitudes, and/or behavioral difficulties. The operative word here is *willing*. Suitable patients do not actually have to walk in the door indicating that they have made this connection. Rather, in the give-and-take of the therapeutic encounters, they show signs of being willing to entertain the possibility. Note that they do not have to understand the nature of interpersonal difficulties or admit responsibility for them to meet this selection criterion.
4. Patients must *be willing to examine feelings* that may hinder more successful relationships and may foster more dysfunctional ones. Also, Strupp and Binder (1984) elaborated that the patient needs to possess "sufficient capacity to emotionally distance from these feelings so that the patient and therapist can jointly examine them" (p. 57). Because of my emphasis on the experiential goal, the strength of the patient's ability to step back from feelings and metacommunicate what is going on is less important than in the original model.
5. Patients should *be capable of having a meaningful relationship* with the therapist. Again, it is not expected that the patient initially relate in a collaborative manner. But the potential for establishing such a relationship should exist. Patients cannot be out of touch with reality or

be so impaired that they have difficulty appreciating that their therapists are separate people.

Formulation

Cyclical Maladaptive Pattern

In the past, psychodynamic brief therapists used their intuition, insight, and clinical savvy to devise formulations of cases. These methods may work wonderfully for the gifted or experienced therapist, but they are impossible to teach explicitly. One remedy for this situation was the development of a procedure for deriving a dynamic, interpersonal focus—the *cyclical maladaptive pattern* (Binder and Strupp 1991).

Briefly, the cyclical maladaptive pattern outlines the idiosyncratic vicious cycle (Wachtel 1997) of maladaptive interactions that a particular patient manifests with others. These cycles or patterns involve inflexible, self-defeating expectations and behaviors and negative self-appraisals that lead to dysfunctional and maladaptive interactions with others.

Development and use of the cyclical maladaptive pattern in treatment is essential to TLDP (Levenson and Strupp 1997). It is not necessarily shared with the patient but may well be, depending on the patient's abilities to deal with the material. For some patients with minimal capacity for introspection and abstraction, the problematic interpersonal scenario may never be stated per se. Rather, the content may remain very close to the presenting problems and concerns of the patient. Other patients enter therapy with a fairly good understanding of their self-perpetuating interpersonal patterns. In these cases, the therapist and patient can jointly articulate the parameters that foster such behavior, generalize to other situations as applicable, and readily recognize the behavior's occurrence in the therapy.

In either case, the cyclical maladaptive pattern plays a key role in guiding the clinician in formulating a treatment plan. It provides an organizational framework that makes a large mass of data comprehensible and leads to fruitful hypotheses. A cyclical maladaptive pattern should not be seen as an encapsulated version of truth but rather as a plausible narrative, incorporating major components of a person's current and historical interactive world. It is a map of the territory—not the territory itself (Strupp and Binder 1984). A successful TLDP formulation should provide a blueprint for the therapy. It describes the nature of the problem, leads to the delineation of goals, serves as a guide for interventions, and enables the therapist to anticipate reenactments within the context of the therapeutic interaction. The cyclical maladaptive pattern also provides a way to assess whether the therapy is on the right track, in terms of both outcome at termination and in-session mini-outcomes. The focus provided by the cyclical maladaptive pattern permits the therapist to intervene in ways that have the greatest likelihood of being therapeutic. Thus, there are possibilities for the therapy to be briefer and more effective.

Constructing the Cyclical Maladaptive Pattern

To derive a TLDP formulation, the therapist lets the patient tell his or her own story (step 1) in the initial sessions rather than relying on the traditional psychiatric interview that structures the patient's responses into categories of information (e.g., developmental history, education). By listening to how the patient tells his or her story (e.g., deferentially, cautiously, dramatically) as well as to the content, the therapist can learn much about the patient's interpersonal style. The therapist then explores the interpersonal context of the patient's symptoms or problems (step 2). When did the problems begin? What else was going on in the patient's life at that time, especially of an interpersonal nature?

The clinician obtains data that will be used to construct a cyclical maladaptive pattern (step 3). This process is facilitated by using four categories to gather, organize, and probe for clinical information:

1. *Acts of the self*—These acts include the thoughts, feelings, motives, perceptions, and behaviors of the patient of an interpersonal nature. For example, "When I meet strangers, I think they wouldn't want to have anything to do with me" (thought). "I am afraid to take the promotion" (feeling). "I wish I were the life of the party" (motive). Sometimes these acts are conscious, as those above are, and sometimes they are outside awareness, as in the case of the woman who does not realize how jealous she is of her sister's accomplishments.
2. *Expectations of others' reactions*—This category pertains to all the statements having to do with how the patient imagines others will react to him or her in response to some interpersonal behavior (act of the self). "My boss will fire me if I make a mistake." "If I go to the dance, no one will ask me to dance."
3. *Acts of others toward the self*—This third grouping consists of the actual behaviors of other people, as observed (or assumed) and interpreted by the patient. "When I made a mistake at work, my boss shunned me for the rest of the day." "When I went to the dance, guys asked me to dance but only because they felt sorry for me."
4. *Acts of the self toward the self (introjection)*—In this category belong all of the patient's behaviors or attitudes toward the self—when the self

is the object of the interpersonal pattern. How does the patient treat himself or herself? "When I made the mistake, I berated myself so much that I had difficulty sleeping that night." "When no one asked me to dance, I told myself that it is because I'm fat, ugly, and unlovable."

For the fourth step, the therapist then listens for themes in the emerging material by being sensitive to commonalities and redundancies in the patient's transactional patterns over person, time, and place. As part of interacting with the patient, the therapist will be pulled into responding in a complementary fashion, re-creating a dysfunctional dance with the patient. By examining the patterns of the here-and-now interaction, and by using the "expectations of others' reactions" and the "acts of others toward the self" components of the cyclical maladaptive pattern, the therapist becomes more aware of his or her countertransferential reenactments (step 5).

One's reactions to the patient should make sense given the patient's interpersonal pattern. Of course, each therapist has a unique personality that might contribute to the particular shading of the reaction that is elicited by the patient. The TLDP perspective, however, is that the therapist's behavior is predominantly shaped by the patient's evoking patterns (i.e., the influence of the therapist's personal conflicts is not so paramount as to undermine the therapy).

By using the four categories of the cyclical maladaptive pattern and the therapist's own reactions to the developing transactional relationship with the patient, a cyclical maladaptive pattern narrative is developed that describes the patient's predominant dysfunctional interactive pattern (step 6). The cyclical maladaptive pattern can be used to foresee likely transference-countertransference reenactments that might inhibit treatment progress. By anticipating patient resistances, ruptures in the therapeutic alliance, and so on, the therapist is able to plan appropriately. Thus, when therapeutic impasses occur, the therapist is not caught off guard but rather is prepared to capitalize on the situation and maximize its clinical effect—a necessity when time is of the essence.

From the cyclical maladaptive pattern formulation, the therapist then discerns the goals for treatment. The first goal involves determining the nature of the new experience (step 7). This new experience should contain specific transference-countertransference interactions that disconfirm existing negative expectations. After determining the nature of the new experience, the therapist can use the cyclical maladaptive pattern formulation to determine the second goal for treatment, the new understanding (step 8) of the client's dysfunctional pattern as it occurs in relationships.

The last step (9) in the formulation process involves the continuous refinement of the cyclical maladaptive pattern throughout the therapy. In a brief therapy, the therapist cannot wait to have all the "facts" before formulating the case and intervening. As the therapy proceeds, new content and interactional data become available that might strengthen, modify, or negate the working formulation. These steps should not be thought of as separate techniques applied in a linear, rigid fashion but rather as guidelines for the therapist to be used in a fluid and interactive manner.

Other Formulation Methods

The cyclical maladaptive pattern is only one of the formal ways relationally oriented therapists can represent patterned, repetitive interpersonal transactions. Some others include the core conflictual relationship theme (Luborsky 1984), plan diagnosis method (Weiss and Sampson 1986), structural analysis of social behavior (Schacht and Henry 1995), and role-relationship models configuration (Horowitz 1987). This focus on patterned, recursive, interpersonal processes provides meaningful opportunities for therapeutic integration at the formulation and intervention levels.

Therapeutic Strategies

Implementation of TLDP does not rely on a set of techniques. Rather, it depends on therapeutic *strategies* that are useful only to the extent that they are *embedded in a larger interpersonal relationship*. Because the focus is on experiential interpersonal learning, theoretically any intervention that facilitates this goal could be used. However, it is critical for the therapist to understand how the meaning and effect of such interventions taken out of their original context might shift when they are incorporated within TLDP. Moreover, any intervention (even psychodynamic standbys such as clarification and interpretation) must be assessed with regard to how much it might alter the interpersonal interchange in an undesirable direction or reenact the patient's cyclical maladaptive pattern. Also, in brief therapies, therapists are more directive and active. They are more willing and (hopefully) able to incorporate a variety of potentially useful strategies as a way of working, and patients come to expect this more pragmatic attitude.

Here, I would like to focus on one treatment strategy that incorporates behavioral, experiential, and interpersonal elements.[1] Specifically, the

---

[1]For information on more traditional TLDP interventions, the reader is referred to the Vanderbilt Strategies Scale (Levenson 1995, Appendix).

therapist needs to provide opportunities for the patient to have new experiences of himself or herself and/or the therapist that are designed to help disrupt, revise, and improve the patient's cyclical maladaptive pattern. The following examples illustrate how to intervene with two patients with seemingly similar behaviors but differing experiential goals.

> Ms. S's maladaptive interpersonal pattern suggested that she had the deeply ingrained belief that she could not be appreciated unless she maintained the role of the charming, effervescent ingenue. When she attempted to joke throughout most of the fifth session, her therapist directed her attention to the contrast between her joking and her anxiously twisting her handkerchief. (New experience: The therapist introduces to Ms. S the possibility that he can be interested in her even if she is anxious and not entertaining.)

> Ms. T's lifelong dysfunctional pattern, in contrast, was a meek stance fostered by repeated ridicule from her alcoholic father. She also attempted to joke in the fifth session, nervously twisting her handkerchief. Ms. T's therapist listened with engaged interest to the jokes and did not interrupt. (New experience: The therapist can appreciate her taking center stage and not humiliate her when she is so vulnerable.)

In both cases, the therapist's interventions (observing nonverbal behavior; listening) were well within the psychodynamic therapist's acceptable repertoire. There was no need to do anything feigned (e.g., laugh uproariously at Ms. T's joke), nor was there a demand to respond with a similar therapeutic stance to both presentations.

In these cases, the therapists' behavior gave the patients a new interpersonal experience—an opportunity to disconfirm their own interpersonal schemas. With sufficient quality and quantity of these experiences, patients can develop different internalized working models of relationships. In this way, TLDP is thought to promote change by altering the basic infrastructure of the patient's transactional world, which then reverberates to influence the concept of self.

Termination

Because TLDP is based on an interpersonal model, with roots in attachment theory and object relations theory, issues of loss are interwoven through the therapy and do not solely appear in the termination phase. Toward the end of therapy, the best advice for the TLDP therapist is to maintain the dynamic focus and the goals for treatment, while examining how these patterns appear when loss and separation issues are most salient.

How does the TLDP therapist know when the patient has had "enough" therapy? In doing TLDP, I use five sets of questions to help the therapist judge when termination is appropriate.

1. Has the patient had interactional changes with significant others in his or her life? Does the patient report more rewarding transactions?
2. Has the patient had a new experience (or a series of new experiences) of himself or herself and the therapist within the therapy?
3. Has there been a change in the level on which the therapist and patient are relating (from parent–child to adult–adult)?
4. Has the therapist's countertransferential reaction to the patient shifted (usually from negative to positive)?
5. Does the patient manifest some understanding about his or her dynamics and the role he or she was playing to maintain them?

If the answer is "no" to more than one of these questions, then the therapist should seriously consider whether the patient has had an adequate course of therapy. The therapist should reflect why this has been the case and weigh the possible benefits of alternative therapies, another course of TLDP, a different therapist, nonprofessional alternatives, and so forth.

As with most brief therapies, TLDP is not considered to be the final or definitive intervention. At some point in the future, the patient may feel the need to obtain more therapy for similar or different issues. Such additional therapy would not be viewed as evidence of a TLDP treatment failure. In fact, it is hoped that patients will view their TLDP as helpful and as a resource to which they could return over time. This view of the availability of multiple short-term therapies over the individual's life span is consistent with the position of the therapist as family practitioner.

Training

In the Brief Psychotherapy Program at the California Pacific Medical Center in San Francisco, clinical service is combined with a comprehensive, structured training program for psychiatry residents and psychology interns. Brief Psychotherapy Program training consists of a 1-hour didactic seminar and a 2-hour group supervision per week for five to seven trainees at a time over a 6-month training rotation. The didactic portion of the training covers the theoretical and clinical aspects of TLDP. Videotapes of actual therapy sessions (conducted by the supervisor as well as by beginning students) are used to illustrate important basic principles, strategies, and common therapeutic dilemmas. Commercially available instructional videotapes are also used.[2]

As trainees watch videotapes of sessions in a stop-frame approach, they are asked to describe what is going on in the vignettes and to distinguish between relevant and irrelevant material. They propose interventions, think aloud about the reasons for their choices, disclose how they are reacting to the material, and anticipate the moment-to-moment behavior of the patients and therapists. Each trainee is assigned to videotape one patient for an entire therapy (up to 20 sessions) with the TLDP model. The average number of actual sessions is approximately 14 (because of vacations, illnesses, holidays, and cancellations). Trainees write up their cyclical maladaptive patterns and goals at the beginning of therapy and share these with the others in the class. In this way, the driving force of the therapy is made explicitly salient, and supervision focuses on how to devise strategies designed to further the goals consistent with the formulation.

Each trainee privately reviews his or her entire videotape of that week's session and selects portions to show in the group supervision. This format allows trainees to receive peer and supervisory comments on their technique as well as to observe the process of a brief therapy with other patient–therapist dyads. In this way, trainees learn how the model must be adapted to address the particular dynamics of each case. They also learn what is generalizable about TLDP across patients.

In both instruction and supervision, I strongly believe that videotape is an essential part of TLDP training because it provides a vivid account of what actually occurs in therapy, permitting an examination of the nuances of the therapeutic relationship. In addition, the realistic context provided by videotape can be used to facilitate an active wrestling with relevant material, which counteracts the negative effects of inert knowledge. Most important is the focus on specific therapist–patient interactions, by using very brief segments of tape to illustrate interactional sequences. (See Levenson and Strupp 1999 for specific recommendations concerning training in brief dynamic psychotherapy.)

---

[2]For instructional TLDP videotapes, contact Levenson Institute for Training, 2323 Sacramento Street, Second Floor, San Francisco, CA 94115 (510-666-0076); American Psychological Association, 750 First Street NE, Washington, DC 20002 (800-374-2721); Psychological and Educational Films, 3334 E Coast Highway #252, Corona del Mar, CA 92625 (888-750-4029).

Research

Several research programs investigating TLDP have been undertaken since the 1970s, yielding a steadily growing body of empirical findings pertaining to the process and outcome dimensions of this short-term treatment approach.

From the standpoint of psychotherapy process, a series of studies at Vanderbilt University in the 1970s (Vanderbilt I) suggested that therapists become entrapped into reacting with negativity, hostility, and disrespect and, in general, antitherapeutically when patients are negative and hostile. Moreover, the nature of therapists' and patients' behavior in relation to one another has been shown to be associated with the quality of therapeutic outcome. Quintana and Meara (1990) reported that patients' intrapsychic activity became similar to the way in which they perceived their therapists treated them in short-term therapy. Similarly, Harrist and colleagues (1994) found that patients internalized both their own and their therapists' contributions to the therapeutic interaction and that these internalizations were associated with better outcomes. A recent study examining relational change (Travis et al. 2001) found that patients significantly shifted their attachment styles (from insecure to secure) and significantly increased the number of their secure attachment themes following TLDP.

The VA Short-Term Psychotherapy Research Project—the VAST Project—examined TLDP process and outcome in a population with personality disorders (Levenson and Bein 1993). It found that approximately 60% of the 89 male patients achieved positive interpersonal or symptomatic outcomes following TLDP (average of 14 sessions). At termination, 71% of the patients felt that their problems had lessened. One-fifth of the patients moved into the normal range of scores on a measure of interpersonal problems.

In the VAST Project long-term follow-up study (Bein et al. 1994), patients were reassessed a mean of 3 years after TLDP. Findings indicated that patient gains from treatment (measured by symptom and interpersonal inventories) were maintained and slightly bolstered. In addition, at the time of follow-up, 80% of the patients thought that their therapies had helped them deal more effectively with their problems. Other analyses indicated that patients were more likely to value their therapies the more they perceived that sessions focused on TLDP-congruent strategies (i.e., trying to understand their typical patterns of relating to people, exploring childhood relationships, and trying to relate in a new and better way with their therapists).

With the VAST Project data, Hartmann and Levenson (1995) discovered important associations between patients' cyclical maladaptive patterns and facets of clinical process and outcome. Specifically, their data indicated that a statistically significant relationship was found between the interpersonal problems raters felt should have been discussed in the therapy (based solely on the patients' cyclical maladaptive patterns) and those topics the therapists said actually were discussed. Perhaps most meaningful is the finding that better outcomes were achieved when these therapies maintained a focus relevant to the patients' cyclical maladaptive patterns. Thus, these preliminary findings indicate that the TLDP case formulations convey reliable interpersonal information to clinicians who are otherwise unfamiliar with the case, guide the issues that are discussed in the therapy, and lead to better outcomes when therapists can adhere to them.

Summary Case Illustration: Mr. U

Mr. U, a 74-year-old man, was about to be discharged from an inpatient psychiatry unit. I knew very little about him prior to our first session. I had been told that he had been given a diagnosis of major depression and was a retired widower with four grown children. Mr. U had cooperated with treatment during his 1-month inpatient treatment, which consisted of individual sessions with a psychiatrist, antidepressant medications, and milieu therapy.

Much of Mr. U's background emerged in a piecemeal fashion as the therapeutic alliance strengthened and Mr. U became more aware of the relevance of his personal history. I eventually learned that Mr. U's father had had alcoholism and that his mother had been "a saint." Mr. U said that he felt love for his father until he saw him beat his mother when he was about 10 years old. Mr. U lived his early adult years as a loner, obtained a college degree in education, and became a teacher. Following this, he married a woman who was referred to in the inpatient records as "a domineering alcoholic." The couple had continual marital stress, and at one point, when they came close to divorcing, Mr. U was hospitalized in a psychiatric unit. When Mrs. U suddenly died of cancer, Mr. U was left to raise four children, the youngest of whom was his 10-year-old daughter, Sue Ellen. His older daughter left to get married, and his teenage sons ran away to work on a fishing boat.

Mr. U lived with Sue Ellen in an interdependent relationship for 12 years, until they were evicted from their house. Sue Ellen left to find a place of her own. Mr. U then moved into an apartment with his younger son and his son's girlfriend. About a year later, Mr. U was again hospitalized and was subsequently referred to me for outpatient treatment. His goal was to "not be depressed."

Formulation

Because of space constraints, I cannot fully articulate here how I derived the data for Mr. U's rudimentary cyclical maladaptive pattern.[3] Suffice it to say that I was looking for repetitive themes built around the four categories of the cyclical maladaptive pattern. In addition, I was mindful of my own countertransference. To obtain a narrative of Mr. U's interactive themes, I strung together the components of the cyclical maladaptive pattern combined with my own reactions to tell a story of his pattern of role relationships. Those themes that occurred over time, across situations, and with several different persons gained preeminence.

In the first session, Mr. U presented as the proverbial cork floating on the sea of life. He was an isolated, depressed, dependent man who expected that others knew best what he should do, so he waited for them to assume responsibility for his life. Others did step in and direct him because they initially felt sorry for him, they were worn down by his complaining, or they felt guilty for not wanting to do more. However, eventually they became frustrated and irritated by his defeatist attitude and sometimes became angry and/or rejected him. Although Mr. U may have initially complied with others' directives and demands, he ended up feeling not helped but rather rejected, unloved, and worthless. Unable to feel effective and nurtured, he became more helpless and hopeless. This led to his increased isolation and depression, completing the cycle. Consistent with the behavior from others, I also was aware of having negative feelings toward Mr. U. As he told his story, I found myself becoming somewhat bored, irritated, and emotionally disconnected. I also had some feelings of pity for his plight as an elderly man who felt abandoned by his children.

From this initial cyclical maladaptive pattern, I considered what *new experience* of our interaction would provide a healthy disruption in Mr. U's usual pattern. I reasoned that a more empowered, active sense of himself leading to more confident behaviors with me might help jog him out of the familiar rut of his dependency and despondency. And the experience of not being rescued from his helplessness nor punished for decisiveness and independence might further encourage him to begin to internalize a new relationship model.

In terms of a *new understanding*, I assessed that Mr. U's recognition that his feelings were important (especially the more energizing ones) would be helpful to him in directing his own life. In addition, I hoped that he could

---

[3]For more specifics on developing a cyclical maladaptive pattern, including more elaboration on Mr. U's cyclical maladaptive pattern, see Levenson 1995.

see that he was already making decisions and taking actions that affected people. I wanted him to have some awareness that if he changed his customary passive pattern, he would not necessarily be deserted—in fact, in many ways, he was his own worst enemy. Finally, it would be critical for Mr. U to appreciate his strengths and capabilities and have some compassion for how and why he might have needed to develop such a style of relating.

I concluded that Mr. U met the five basic selection criteria, but his concrete thinking style, impoverished descriptions of his relationships, and limited ability to reflect on his own behavior would call for a correspondingly more didactic and directive version of TLDP. At the conclusion of the first session, I offered Mr. U a 20-session brief therapy and suggested that we could focus on ways to help him feel less hopeless and depressed. Despite his lack of psychological-mindedness and a depression severe enough to warrant hospitalization, I was encouraged by the relative clarity of his interactive pattern. Given his dependency needs and difficulties with losses, a specific time limit would be expected to raise the saliency of these issues and thereby facilitate the work.

When I proposed the focus and time frame, Mr. U was characteristically compliant and resigned ("Whatever you say, doctor. Whatever you say."). I wondered if I had already fallen into a countertransferential reenactment of taking too much control and direction, thereby colluding with his helpless stance. I thought it likely, given Mr. U's cyclical maladaptive pattern, that I could become hooked into reenacting several scenarios with him, such as becoming impatient or angry with his passivity, directive in response to his submission, and as hopeless as he was.

By the end of the first session, I had a rudimentary blueprint of the therapy, consisting of the case formulation, goals, and anticipated stuck spots in the treatment. In the second session, Mr. U explained that he felt responsible for his daughter's moving out of the apartment they had shared for 21 years.

Course of Treatment

> Therapist: So this is what has been gnawing away at you, Sue Ellen's leaving and the role you might have played in it?
>
> Mr. U: Yeah. And then our being used by real estate people over and over again. We've had to move. Not over and over again, but we've had to move. We're stranded out there. Now Sue Ellen pays too high rent for her salary because she doesn't have anything left. And it's...I don't know. We did have enough money and a pretty happy life. But all of a sudden we're up against it like all the street people almost.
>
> Therapist: Do you think Sue Ellen's sorry she moved?

Mr. U: I don't know. *[plaintively]* She still calls me Daddy. But then when she's gone, you know she's with her friends. I guess she's forgetting me, and it hurts. *[emphatically]* It hurts. I don't see her. She says, "Oh, Dad, I have other things to do." I ask her to come over—I say, "Let's meet and have an afternoon." *[mimicking daughter]* She says, "I have other things I have to do." One of her friends has a boat in College View. They go out on the bay—*[pejoratively]* baying it. And I just feel left out.

Therapist: *[matter-of-factly]* Well, you are.

Mr. U: I am. *[lamenting]* Yeah, I'm really left out. So, I don't know...*[resigned tone, voice becomes plaintive and trails off]*

Therapist: The least she could do after you went to all the trouble of raising her and giving her things was to stick around for the rest of your life.

Mr. U: Anyway, I guess these are the things, the...

Therapist: *[interrupting]* How do you feel about what I just said?

Mr. U: What did you say? *[pause]* At least she could have stuck around? *[pause]* I'm not that possessive. Really, I'm not that possessive to want her to stick around. I just want her in the same household. That's what I really want.

Therapist: *[nodding]* Yeah. How do you feel about the fact that I said the least she could do is not move out?

Mr. U: I don't know. If I answer that, it would seem like a selfish answer. If I just said, "Well, I feel that she's unjust or she's unfair," it would be a selfish answer on my part. Because I know kids have to grow up and go their own way.

Therapist: Well, you know that in your head, but I'm really asking how your gut feels.

Mr. U: *[begins crying]* I don't want her to go! I want to be with her. She's my little kid. *[pause]* Oh, Christ. You know, my wife and I fought quite a bit, and she always won. And she was able to domineer me completely. And we just withdrew from each other. So when she died, I turned all my love that I would normally have toward a wife toward this little kid who didn't leave me. My two sons left me, and my older daughter left me. I never would have sold the house if they had all stuck together, but they started giving me all kinds of trouble. And I think I had all these frustrated feelings toward my wife because she was—she insisted on being boss. And it really bothered me. I was angry inside all the time with her. I turned on to this young girl all the feelings. So what it amounts to is that I love Sue Ellen. I want her to be around. It's a fatherly love, but it's a real close attachment. And I don't want it broken. *[pause]* If Sue Ellen goes, I don't really have anybody. *[pause]* Well, I'm feeling sorry for myself, but that's the truth of the matter. *[sighs]* Anger at myself for making, *[pause]* you know, for getting rid of a house that could have kept us all together.

At the beginning of the hour, I wondered whether Mr. U was angry with his daughter for not being with him in his time of need, especially given that he was there for her as a child. My statement ("The least she could do…was to stick around for the rest of your life.") was intended to be an empathic connection with what I sensed was his longing for his daughter and anger toward her that she was not living up to her part of the implicit quid pro quo. My hunch was confirmed a few seconds later when Mr. U stated that he only "wanted her in the same household." My intervention was designed to state "out loud the thought that can't be spoken, [and thereby] increase the likelihood that the patient will begin to be exposed to the therapeutically relevant cues" (Wachtel and McKinney 1992, p. 340). However, despite my conscious intentions to be empathic, my voice had a sarcastic tone, and the phrasing of my words seemed condescending.

Based on my working understanding of Mr. U's cyclical maladaptive pattern, I judged that my provocative statement was a countertransferential reenactment showing my irritation and frustration with his self-pity. From a TLDP perspective, the goal is not to avoid becoming ensnared in an interactive web with the patient but rather to make use of this entanglement to further the therapeutic process. Fortunately, I was aware of this reenactment as soon as the words left my mouth (the "observing participant"). In addition, Mr. U's changing the subject ("Anyway…") was another clue that something significant had just transpired. I surmised that Mr. U probably was having some internal reaction to my provocative statement about his daughter's obligation to him. Thus, I asked him how he felt about what I had just said to him.

Could Mr. U avail himself of the opportunity to express his anger (either toward me or about his daughter) and then determine whether there were dire consequences? My stepping back and inviting Mr. U to examine what had transpired between us was an opportunity for him to have a new interpersonal experience—specifically, to be more assertive in expressing his negative feelings. In addition, I was concerned that my harsh comment might have ruptured the developing working relationship between us. One of the ways to try to repair a rupture in the therapeutic alliance is to address the patient's problematic feelings about what is transpiring between therapist and patient. In a brief therapy, in particular, it is critical to discuss in the here and now of the therapy anything that might contribute to a negative transference. However, in his characteristic style, Mr. U did not tell me directly how he was feeling. At this point, I was hypothesizing that this entire interchange—his passive and martyr-like presentation precipitating my frustration and insensitivity, possibly causing him to feel criticized and to withdraw—was a mini-reenactment of what transpires outside of therapy.

I see such a rupture in the therapeutic alliance as consistent with what Safran and Segal (1990), writing on interpersonal processes in cognitive therapy, called a "useful window into the patient's subjective world" (p. 89). From a TLDP perspective, it affords the therapist an opportunity to understand more fully the schemas behind a patient's cyclical maladaptive pattern because the nature of the patient's underlying characteristic construal of self and others is thereby implied. With this information, the therapist can learn how to provide the patient with a mini–new experience in the service of modifying the maladaptive schemas sustaining his or her cyclical maladaptive pattern.

Following this interchange, Mr. U described what happened when he and his wife had argued—"She always won. And she was able to domineer me completely. And we just withdrew from each other." Perhaps I had fallen into an interactional pattern like the one he had had with his wife. Rather than tell me directly that I was too overbearing, Mr. U alluded to how he was dominated by his wife. Interactional psychoanalytic theorists refer to this behavior as an "allusion to the transference." In this way, Mr. U may have unconsciously (and more safely, indirectly) communicated to me his views about our current interaction. The TLDP therapist should be alert to the possibility that comments about other people are disguised communications about how the patient experiences the therapeutic relationship and what the consequences might be. Would he keep his anger "inside all the time" and "withdraw" from our therapeutic work if I continued to respond to his passivity in a "domineering" fashion?

Mr. U came to the third session hungry (he had not eaten breakfast) and having soiled his pants (caused by a stool softener). He was almost saying in an infantile fashion, "Feed me. Change me. Take care of me." I was increasingly more confident in my formulation—Mr. U's indirect and childlike stance was preferable to taking the risk of stating his needs and showing his anger, because he feared that the more direct route would result in physical or emotional abandonment. Later in the session, Mr. U said that he felt sad about having been left alone for 3 days by his family. However, I hypothesized that he might also have felt angry at being abandoned yet again. Repeatedly, I saw the same theme of his feeling sad and blaming himself rather than feeling anger and confronting others. Given his early childhood experiences with a violent, alcoholic father, such an interpersonal pattern is quite understandable. Whenever I attempted to engage Mr. U in a discussion of his feelings about being left alone, he switched to complaining that he could not concentrate because he had not had anything to eat that morning.

Mr. U: *[half-hearted laugh] [pause]* There isn't a place in here where I could get a tomato juice or anything?
Therapist: No, not here.

Mr. U: *[distressed]* Oh, boy.

Therapist: Mr. U, you are saying two different things. You're saying that you would have trouble sitting here continuing with our session because you haven't had breakfast; then you say that it's more than that. You would have trouble sitting here talking because you're upset about the things that have gone on this week, and it would make this session hard anyway.

Mr. U: Well, they decided to go up to Oregon to visit some people, and they just left, and I've been alone for 3 days in the house, and I haven't been going out.

Therapist: But right here, sitting here now, do you feel that talking with me is difficult because we'll be talking about some upsetting things, or do you think that sitting here talking with me is difficult because you didn't have breakfast this morning?

Mr. U: I think it's because I didn't have breakfast.

In my training classes, I like to show the videotape of this session and stop the tape here. I ask the trainees what they would say or do at this point. Most of the time, if they have been trained in long-term psychodynamic psychotherapy, they volunteer various interpretations (e.g., "I was wondering if you might be feeling angry because your family abandoned you"; "It seems like you want to avoid talking about upsetting things"; "Does this remind you of how you interact with your family?"). After I hear these various interventions, I ask the students to evaluate whether such communications would help Mr. U take a step toward feeling more activated and empowered (i.e., the experiential goal emanating from the formulation of the case). Usually, the trainees have no difficulty seeing that their (accurate) interpretations would only serve to make the patient feel worse because they so easily can be heard as blaming indictments, a conclusion reached by interpersonal researchers.

Because my goal for the therapy was to have Mr. U feel more empowered and show more assertive behaviors instead of feeling so dependent and being so compliant, I let that goal guide my intervention. I, therefore, asked him to clarify whether being hungry or knowing that we would be talking about some upsetting things was making it difficult to be in the session. When he replied that it was because he was hungry, I did not interpret his response as an indication of resistance. Rather, I took his response seriously (which does not mean that I automatically believed him) and simply asked him what would keep him from getting something in his stomach right then. I was trying to afford Mr. U the opportunity to make a decision on his own behalf—to take care of what he saw as *his* needs.

Resistance from the perspective of TLDP is viewed within the interpersonal sphere as one of many transactions between therapist and patient. The patient is attempting to retain personal integrity and ingrained perceptions of himself or herself and others. The patient's perceptions support his or her understanding of what is required to maintain interpersonal connectedness and safety. Resistance in this light is the patient's attempt to do the best he or she can with how he or she construes the world.

> Mr. U: If I just got something in my stomach, I would feel better.
>
> Therapist: Uh-huh. And what keeps you from getting something in your stomach right now?
>
> Mr. U: I'd have to go over to the cafeteria over there.
>
> Therapist: That's right.
>
> Mr. U: *[sigh]*
>
> Therapist: And what would keep you from deciding to do that?
>
> Mr. U: *[sigh]* Well, the fact that we're having a session, and I don't want to be rude.
>
> Therapist: So, rather than be rude, you'll sit there and be uncomfortable for an hour.
>
> Mr. U: Well, I don't know. I guess so. Unless you'd let me go.
>
> Therapist: Unless *I'd* let you go?
>
> Mr. U: *[taken aback]* Well, I feel obligated to come and see you because you're helping me.
>
> Therapist: *[pause]* Mr. U, it seems you're faced with a dilemma. Right here, right now, with me in this room. And the dilemma is—can you concentrate and really make use of the time, or do you need some food in you to be able to do that? Your dilemma is whether to take care of *you* or to take care of *me*.

After this segment, Mr. U tried to avoid making an active decision in the room by simply continuing to talk. After listening to him for a couple of minutes, I interrupted him and said that I was not clear as to what his decision was—whether he had decided to stay or to get something to eat. Mr. U said that he was feeling better and could stay.

I would have felt more secure in Mr. U's truly having had a new experience if he had chosen to leave the session and chance my displeasure. This would have clearly been the riskier choice and a significant break with his familiar pattern. Nonetheless, he voiced his decision, and our interaction around the breakfast issue had raised the salience of his customary way of denying his own needs in favor of what he thinks others want.

In the process of exploring why Mr. U did not decide to get something to eat, I pointed out one level of the interpersonal dynamic that was occurring between us in the here and now: "Your dilemma is whether to take care of you or to take care of me." Exploring patterns that constitute dysfunctional transactions between patient and therapist is a critical step in accomplishing the second goal of helping the patient have a new understanding.

In the fourth session, Mr. U talked about loaning money to his younger daughter. This money allowed her to live separately from him—something I knew from the second session that he did not want ("I just want her in the same household."). This afforded me the opportunity to ask Mr. U how he felt about loaning her money, with the intent of determining whether he could express some of his more negative feelings as a way for him to feel more empowered and entitled.

Not unexpectedly, Mr. U had considerable difficulty expressing his anger. Although I was still interested in Mr. U's feelings, I became more interested in his manner of interacting with me—in this case, how he subverted showing anger.

After attempting to reveal Mr. U's affect directly several times without success, I commented on the process ("Seems like this is a difficult question."). This led Mr. U to claim that his feelings were unknown to him. With more probing, he was able to say that his feelings were hidden. I then asked him if there might be a good reason to keep the feelings hidden from his point of view (i.e., allying with the resistance). I decided to raise the issue of a "good reason" because I suspected, based on Mr. U's cyclical maladaptive pattern, that he feared that I would be displeased, condemning, or incited to delve deeper by his withholding.

My next intervention was psychoeducational; I explained why people might keep feelings hidden, even from themselves. I was inviting Mr. U to explore the reasons he might go through life not acknowledging what he felt. However, he was not willing to engage with me on this level and became flustered. As a way to help him tune into what he did feel, I asked him to concentrate on his bodily sensations. Given that he often somaticized his emotional pain, I asked him to communicate in a way that was familiar to him. His response ("I'm so constipated.") was relevant on two levels—literally (I am physiologically blocked) and symbolically (I am psychologically blocked). In response, I interpreted that he was more comfortable talking about his physical feelings than his emotional ones.

Later in the session, I shared an observation with Mr. U: "I notice that when I ask you these kinds of questions, you tear up and your voice gets a little quivery. Do you notice that too?" By keeping my process comment at a basic descriptive level, I hoped to avert his hypersensitivity to being blamed. I then asked him what he was feeling at those moments. My goal here was to help him become curious about his own behaviors as markers for understanding his feelings and the effect he had on others. In response, Mr. U replied in a stuttering voice that he wanted to keep his feelings hidden and not talk about them. In keeping with the goal of wanting to promote his taking risks in letting people know his wants and needs directly, I did not chastise him (e.g., interpret his withholding). Instead,

I underscored what he had said ("I think you are saying something very important, Mr. U. You're saying that you want to keep the feelings hidden."). Following this interchange, I conveyed to him I would be open to changing the subject if he wished.

Toward the end of this session, Mr. U again complained that he was constipated. He mentioned that he had a stool softener in his car and said that he would like to leave the session early to take it. From a physiological standpoint, it would not have made much difference if he took the stool softener immediately or when our session ended. However, subjectively, this seemed like a big step for Mr. U—to put forth his needs despite his expectation that they might conflict with my desire to have him remain in the session.

In the previous session, Mr. U had decided not to leave to get something to eat. In this session, his saying that he wanted to leave early appeared to be an unconscious test to see if I really would "let him go." I was encouraged by Mr. U's direct statement of what he wanted to do. Here was another opportunity in the therapy for him to have a different experience of himself and me. Rather than interpreting what I thought was going on, I simply told him that I would look forward to seeing him at our usual time next week.

Throughout the rest of the therapy, I remained focused on the goals for the treatment. I felt free to use various interventions that might facilitate his feeling more assertive and empowered and less passive. For example, I used behavioral rehearsal (for him to feel what it might be like to assert his needs in an anticipated new living situation) and the gestalt empty-chair technique (for him to talk to himself as a boy), allowing him to be more compassionate with himself for his "failure" to protect his mother. In this particular case, the use of such techniques did not appear to jar Mr. U. Given the brevity of the therapy, Mr. U was accustomed to my using a variety of pragmatically designed strategies. Furthermore, because the interventions were all designed to achieve one major goal, they had a common theme, lending to their coherence (i.e., phenomenologically they made sense).

However, it is important to note that because of Mr. U's dependency needs and his comfort with my taking control, I broached the possibility of using these techniques in a low-key, collaborative way. I was also ready to process their use should Mr. U's reaction be untoward or result in a reenactment of his cyclical maladaptive pattern. However, it is not just the introduction of techniques from other schools that requires such careful monitoring. The TLDP therapist needs to attend to the current relational context for judging the appropriateness as well as the effectiveness of any intervention. The critical question is whether the intervention has potential for promoting the idiosyncratically defined new experience.

Glickhauf-Hughes et al. (1996) described a gestalt technique of encouraging the client to "say no." They indicated that "it is important to help clients truly know that they can choose to say 'no,' even to suggestions by the therapist" (p. 50). As an example of this technique, they indicated that the therapist should state to a client who was saying no indirectly, "My hunch is that you really didn't want to answer that question. Can you say to me, 'No. I don't want to answer that question right now?'" (p. 51). However, for Mr. U, the use of such an intervention would have been counterproductive; he might have submissively followed my instructions to say no or learned that such "assertive behaviors" would please me. In either case, Mr. U would not have had to risk my disapproval if he said no and therefore would not have had the full experience of confronting me. The opportunity for disconfirming his own pathogenic beliefs would have been lost (Weiss and Sampson 1986).

Termination

Mr. U began our last session by relating how his children were visiting more and inviting him to do things. His improved relationships with them illustrate the chief principle whereby TLDP is thought to generalize. Ideally, patients' experiences in brief therapy help disconfirm their ingrained dysfunctional interpersonal expectations and alter their internalized views of self and others. This encourages them to try out new, but shaky, behaviors with other people. In Mr. U's case, he took risks to be more assertive with me in the therapy. His increased confidence in his abilities to get his own needs met led him to be less anxious, placating, and resentful. As a result, his children experienced him as more delightful to be around and consequently involved him more in their lives. This was what Mr. U wanted in the first place, so he was happier and further encouraged to be more independent in his life. In this way, Mr. U would be expected to be able to continue his therapeutic work in his naturalistic environment, even though the sessions with me would be coming to a close. Such continued therapeutic work is at the crux of TLDP because a brief treatment usually only helps the patient to start moving in the desired direction and does not take him or her to the final destination.[4]

---

[4]For a session-by-session commentary, including a videotaped portrayal of this case and information on Mr. U's 1-year and 6-year follow-up, see Levenson 1998.

Summary

In this chapter, I presented an overview of TLDP, which stems from traditional psychoanalytic theory and therapy roots but has an effective approach with a different emphasis than that of classical psychoanalysis. The approach stresses the importance of the therapy relationship as a vital factor in eliciting and changing maladaptive interpersonal modes of behavior and personality patterns. Basic assumptions of the TLDP model were reviewed, followed by a discussion of the treatment's goals (which focus on new experiences and new understandings). Finally, I discussed criteria for patient selection along with case formulation guidelines, strategies for treatment interventions, and an illustrative case. The approach shows that meaningful changes can be obtained with a relatively brief treatment format based on a psychodynamic framework.

References

Alexander F, French TM: Psychoanalytic Therapy: Principles and Applications. New York, Ronald Press, 1946

Bein E, Levenson H, Overstreet D: Outcome and follow-up data from the VAST Project. Paper presented at the annual international meeting of the Society for Psychotherapy Research, York, England, June 1994

Binder JL, Strupp HH: The Vanderbilt approach to time-limited dynamic psychotherapy, in Handbook of Short-Term Dynamic Psychotherapy. Edited by Crits-Christoph P, Barber JP. New York, Basic Books, 1991, pp 137–165

Bowlby J: Attachment and Loss, Vol 2: Separation, Anxiety, and Anger. New York, Basic Books, 1973

Fisher S, Greenberg RP: Freud Scientifically Reappraised: Testing the Theories and Therapy. New York, Wiley, 1997

Glickhauf-Hughes C, Reviere SL, Clance PR, et al: An integration of object relations theory with gestalt techniques to promote structuralization of the self. Journal of Psychotherapy Integration 6:39–59, 1996

Harrist RS, Quintana SM, Strupp HH, et al: Internalization of interpersonal process in time-limited dynamic psychotherapy. Psychotherapy 31:49–57, 1994

Hartmann K, Levenson H: Case formulation in TLDP. Presentation at the annual international meeting of the Society for Psychotherapy Research, Vancouver, BC, Canada, June 1995

Henry WP, Strupp HH, Gaston L: Psychodynamic approaches, in Handbook of Psychotherapy and Behavior Change. Edited by Bergin AE, Garfield SL. New York, Wiley, 1994, pp 467–508

Horowitz M: States of Mind: Analysis of Change in Psychotherapy, 2nd Edition. New York, Plenum, 1987

Levenson H: Time-Limited Dynamic Psychotherapy: A Guide to Clinical Practice. New York, Basic Books, 1995

Levenson H: Time-Limited Dynamic Psychotherapy: Making Every Session Count: Video and Viewer's Manual. San Francisco, CA, Levenson Institute for Training, 1998

Levenson H, Bein E: VA Short-Term Psychotherapy Research Project: outcome. Paper presented at the annual international meeting of the Society for Psychotherapy Research, Pittsburgh, PA, June 1993

Levenson H, Strupp HH: Cyclical maladaptive patterns in time-limited dynamic psychotherapy, in Handbook of Psychotherapy Case Formulation. Edited by Eells TD. New York, Guilford, 1997, pp 84–115

Levenson H, Strupp HH: Recommendations for the future of training in brief dynamic psychotherapy. J Clin Psychol 55:385–391, 1999

Levenson H, Butler SF, Bein E, et al: Brief dynamic individual psychotherapy, in The American Psychiatric Publishing Textbook of Clinical Psychiatry, 4th Edition. Edited by Hales RE, Yudofsky SC. Washington, DC, American Psychiatric Publishing, 2002a, pp 1151–1176

Levenson H, Butler SF, Powers T, et al: Concise Guide to Brief Dynamic and Interpersonal Psychotherapy. Washington, DC, American Psychiatric Publishing, 2002b, pp 1151–1176

Luborsky L: Principles of Psychoanalytic Psychotherapy: A Manual for Supportive-Expressive Treatment. New York, Basic Books, 1984

Messer SB, Warren CS: Models of Brief Psychodynamic Therapy: A Comparative Approach. New York, Guilford, 1995

Quintana SM, Meara NM: Internalization of the therapeutic relationship in short term psychotherapy. J Couns Psychol 37:123–130, 1990

Safran P, Segal ZV: Interpersonal Process in Cognitive Therapy. New York, Basic Books, 1990

Sampson H, Weiss J: Testing hypotheses: the approach of the Mount Zion Psychotherapy Research Group, in The Psychotherapeutic Process: A Research Handbook. Edited by Greenberg LS, Pinsof NM. New York, Guilford, 1986, pp 591–614

Schacht TE, Henry WP: Modeling recurrent relationship patterns with structural analysis of social behavior: the SASB-CMP. Psychotherapy Research 4:208–221, 1995

Siegel DJ: The Developing Mind: Toward a Neurobiology of Interpersonal Experience. New York, Guilford, 1999

Stern D: The Interpersonal World of the Infant. New York, Basic Books, 1985

Strupp HH, Binder JL: Psychotherapy in a New Key: A Guide to Time-Limited Dynamic Psychotherapy. New York, Basic Books, 1984

Sullivan HS: The Interpersonal Theory of Psychiatry. New York, WW Norton, 1953

Travis LA, Binder JL, Bliwise NG, et al: Changes in clients' attachment styles over the course of time-limited dynamic psychotherapy. Psychotherapy 38:149–159, 2001

Wachtel PL: Action and Insight. New York, Guilford, 1987

Wachtel PL: Psychoanalysis, Behavior Therapy, and the Relational World. Washington, DC, American Psychological Association, 1997

Wachtel PL, McKinney MK: Cyclical psychodynamics and integrative psychodynamic therapy, in Handbook of Psychotherapy Integration. Edited by Norcross JC, Goldfried MR. New York, Basic Books, 1992, pp 335–372

Weiss J, Sampson H: The Psychoanalytic Process: Theory, Clinical Observation and Empirical Research. New York, Guilford, 1986

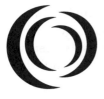

7

Brief Couple Therapy

Donald H. Baucom, Ph.D.
Norman B. Epstein, Ph.D.
Laura J. Sullivan, M.A.

Several different theoretical approaches use a brief therapy format to assist couples who are experiencing relationship distress. Three of these approaches—cognitive-behavioral couple therapy (Epstein and Baucom 2002), emotion-focused couple therapy (Johnson and Greenberg 1995), and insight-oriented couple therapy (Snyder and Wills 1989)—have empirical support indicating their efficacy in working with maritally distressed couples.[1] A fourth approach—integrative behavioral couple therapy (Christensen et al. 1995)—appears to be equally efficacious, although the empirical findings for this approach are still being analyzed

---

[1] Although almost all of the empirical treatment research has been conducted with married couples, in this chapter, the term *couple therapy* is used to recognize that many couples who are not legally married have problems and are assisted by these intervention strategies.

(see Baucom et al. 1998 for a detailed description of the empirical status of various forms of couple therapy). Cognitive-behavioral couple therapy, the focus of this chapter, has documented evidence of its effectiveness, which dates back to the 1970s, in approximately 20 controlled investigations on several different continents (Baucom et al. 2003).

Theoretical Background

Behaviors, Cognitions, and Emotions

Cognitive-behavioral couple therapy has evolved over several decades and owes its origins to more strictly behavioral approaches to understanding relationship distress. Several principles characterize the theoretical and treatment strategies used in the early forms of behavioral couple therapy. A traditional behavioral model assumes that the behavior of both partners is shaped, strengthened, weakened, and modified by environmental events, particularly those events involving the other partner. In addition, influential events outside the relationship (e.g., meeting another very appealing person) affect the partner's tendency to remain in the relationship as well as his or her subjective feelings of satisfaction (Jacobson and Margolin 1979). As a result, marital satisfaction is viewed as a function of the ratio of rewards derived to costs incurred from being in the marriage. A great deal of research and clinical experience confirm that distressed couples typically express much more negative behavior and much less positive behavior than do nondistressed couples (Epstein and Baucom 2002).

Behavioral couple therapy also is based on an assumption that couples are distressed, in part, because they have not developed or maintained the skills necessary to meet the demands of an ongoing relationship. These include skills for making decisions, as well as skills necessary to make behavioral changes and communicate constructively. Difficulties with such skills are presumed to result from a "skills deficit" or a "performance deficit," the latter implying that a couple who has a dysfunctional interaction pattern has the ability to perform more constructive skills but fails to do so for some reason, such as a choice to behave negatively in order to retaliate for a partner's negative actions. In traditional behavioral couple therapy, heavy emphasis was placed on teaching couples the skills necessary for the performance of relationship roles and functions.

Although learning skills is beneficial to many distressed couples, improvements in relationship adjustment across a broad range of couples cannot be accounted for by improvement in communication skills alone (Halford et al. 1993; Iverson and Baucom 1990). In addition, comparisons of behavioral couple therapy with other treatment approaches that do not emphasize behavioral skills training have found these other treatment approaches to be equally efficacious in alleviating distress, indicating that skills training may not be necessary or sufficient for positive treatment outcomes (Baucom et al. 1998, 2000).

The combination of these findings suggests that a behavioral skills deficit model is too narrow to explain or treat couple distress and highlights the need to attend not only to partners' behavior but also individuals' *interpretations* and *evaluations* of their own and each other's behavior (Baucom and Epstein 1990). As cognitive models of individual psychopathology brought attention to the important role of cognitive factors in clinical phenomena (Beck et al. 1979), marital researchers focused on cognitive variables as a critical element in understanding the relationship between couple behavior and marital distress (Baucom et al. 1995).

Thus, cognitive-behavioral couple therapy evolved from the gradual expansion of behavioral couple therapy and its treatment strategies to include a focus on cognitive factors in the onset and treatment of couple distress. A major premise of this approach is that some partners' dysfunctional emotional and behavioral responses to relationship events are influenced by inappropriate information processing, whereby cognitive appraisals of the events are either distorted or extreme (e.g., "You went to the football game with your friends and stayed out late because you don't really love me. Football, your friends, and everything else in life are more important to you than I am.") or are evaluated according to extreme or unreasonable standards of what a relationship should be (e.g., "If you really loved me, you'd want to spend all your free time with me, not with your friends. That's what a marriage should be."). Often partners fail to recognize that their thinking has become distorted or extreme and, instead, trust their own subjective, stream-of-consciousness thoughts or automatic cognitions as absolute truth. Because these distorted thoughts are almost always skewed in the negative direction in distressed relationships, the partners' thinking maintains and exacerbates the relationship distress. Consequently, a major task of the cognitive-behavioral couple therapist is to help couples become more active observers and evaluators of their own automatic cognitions (e.g., attributions) and their longstanding assumptions and standards about their relationship. Cognitive-behavioral approaches assume that altering the information processing and cognitions in partners who have notable distorted or extreme cognitions subsequently will lead to positive changes in emotions and behaviors (Epstein and Baucom 2002).

Although altering the ways that partners behave toward each other and think about their relationship can at times change significantly their feelings toward each other, in some important instances, one or both partners' emotions are of central importance and serve as the focus for intervention. At one end of the continuum, some individuals have difficulty accessing, experiencing, and/or expressing emotions. This could include problems in being aware of emotions, differentiating among emotions, experiencing certain emotions as dangerous or unacceptable, relating emotional experience to internal and external events, and having skills to express these emotions to one's partner. The partners of these individuals who struggle in the emotional realm often experience them as intellectual, unemotional, and/or distant. At the other end of the continuum, some individuals have difficulty containing their emotions and express them in an unmodulated, destructive manner. Often, they experience emotional dysregulation, in which their emotions are easily aroused, are experienced at a high level, and are slow to return to a more reasonable level (Linehan 1993). This emotional dysregulation can lead to destructive behaviors that are focused on the individual himself or herself or are directed at the partner. Partners of such individuals often report that they must "walk on eggshells" so as not to upset the person. Cognitive-behavioral couple therapists must attend to important emotional factors at both ends of the continuum to be of assistance to a broad range of couples.

The Individual, the Couple, and the Environment

A healthy relationship is one in which the relationship contributes to the growth and well-being of both partners as individuals, the two partners work well together as a unit or team, and the couple relates to their broader environment in an adaptive fashion—contributing to their social and physical environment and using environmental resources for the well-being of the couple. Relationship distress can result from difficulties in any or all of these domains.

The negative behaviors, cognitions, and emotions typical of distressed couples can be explained partially as a skills or performance deficit, but this explanation is too narrow as a way to understand the numerous factors that contribute to relationship discord. Epstein and Baucom (2002) proposed that relationship difficulties can result from factors at three different levels: the individual, the relationship, and the environment.

Individual Factors

On an individual level, even two psychologically healthy, well-adjusted partners can experience relationship distress if what they want or need from their relationship differs. Epstein and Baucom enumerated the important needs and motives that often become problematic in couples' relationships. These include important relationship-focused needs, such as 1) the need to affiliate or be part of various groups, including a couple relationship; 2) the need for intimacy or closeness with one's partner; 3) the desire to be altruistic or give to one's partner; and 4) the need to be attended to by one's partner. For example, when two partners differ in the amount of closeness and intimacy they desire or the ways in which that intimacy is to be expressed, this often leads to relationship distress. The individual who seeks more closeness often will approach the partner, who, desiring more distance, then withdraws. This withdrawal then leads to greater attempts at closeness from the first partner, with corresponding greater withdrawal from the second partner; over time, this pattern can evolve into a demand/withdraw pattern that characterizes many distressed relationships.

Partners also have individually focused needs that can serve as a source of relationship distress. That is, partners can differ in their needs for autonomy, control, and achievement, and these differences can spell problems for many couples. For example, one partner with a high need for control might want to keep the home environment well organized and engage in detailed planning on a regular basis. If this individual is married to someone who is more relaxed, spontaneous, and less planful, the two partners can experience daily frustrations in their attempts to reconcile their different tendencies and live harmoniously as a couple.

In both of the examples above, partners who differ in their desire for intimacy or in their personal preferences for control, organization, and planning might respond to their frustrations by becoming emotionally upset, distorting their interpretations of the partner's behavior, and behaving negatively toward each other as they attempt to get their needs met. Elsewhere (Epstein and Baucom 2002), we differentiated between *primary distress* associated with partners' experiences of unresolved differences and unmet needs and *secondary distress* associated with partners' dysfunctional ways of interacting in response to those unresolved issues. That is, when people do not get their important needs and desires met in their relationship, this can be the primary basis of their dissatisfaction with the relationship. In addition, they often respond in destructive ways to not getting their needs met, a secondary source of distress. For example, getting mired in a demand/withdraw pattern can be a secondary source of distress in response to the partners' differing needs for intimacy. Often, these secondary sources of distress take on a life of their own, and the cognitive-behavioral couple therapist must be responsive to both primary and secondary distress, such as differing desires for intimacy *and* the demand/withdraw pattern that the couple has developed. Thus, helping partners to understand and find ways to negotiate normal, healthy individual differences is an important part of couple therapy. Although it is beyond the scope of the current chapter, the therapeutic context becomes increasingly complex if one or both partners have significant individual psychiatric problems, a personality disorder, or long-term, unresolved individual issues. Elsewhere, we described how to integrate the treatment of relationship distress and individual psychopathology in a couple context (Epstein and Baucom 2002).

Couple Factors

A relationship is more than the sum of the two individuals involved; it takes on a unique character that typifies the relationship itself. Important interactive patterns can contribute to relationship discord and can serve as the focus of cognitive-behavioral couple therapy. These patterns have been noted for many years and have been particularly well documented in the research of Christensen and his colleagues (Christensen and Heavey 1993). First, a couple might show mutual engagement, in which both partners are highly involved in the interaction. If the two partners engage in constructive behaviors and communication while interacting, this can be a highly rewarding interaction pattern. However, in the context of poor communication skills or negative emotions, mutual engagement can involve frequent and destructive arguments and fights. Second, as described earlier, some couples engage in a demand/withdraw pattern in which one partner pushes for engagement and the other partner attempts to distance. This pattern is particularly common among distressed couples, and the most typical pattern is for the woman to assume the demanding role and for the man to assume the withdrawing role, unless the couple is discussing a topic of particular importance to the man. Third, some couples have a mutual avoidance or withdrawal pattern, in which both partners maintain significant distance. Such couples often seek assistance from therapists because of a lack of vitality or sense of disengagement in their relationship. Cognitive-behavioral couple therapy assists couples in recognizing these maladaptive interaction patterns, understanding the basis of these patterns, and helping them develop more constructive ways to interact with each other.

Environmental Factors

Couples do not live in isolation; rather, they exist in a broader social and physical environment that includes their families, communities, broader institutions, and cultures. Often these environmental factors outside of the couple exert demands on the couple to adapt, at times beyond the couple's capabilities. For example, economic downturns can result in partners being unemployed or underemployed, with a wide range of subsequent stresses. Similarly, dealing with in-laws and the partners' families of origin can be a major source of difficulty for partners as they try to navigate different family rituals, expectations, and roles. On the other hand, the environment can provide important resources for the couple, including practical support (e.g., babysitters) and emotional support. Often, both couples and therapists overlook or minimize the role of external stressors, which can interfere significantly with optimal relationship functioning.

Focus of Therapy

In order for a couple to make progress in a brief therapy context, it is important for the therapist and couple to agree on the important foci for treatment and maintain these foci. In most instances, the therapist can identify two or more major themes around which to develop an intervention plan. These themes can be organized into the domains described earlier: individuals, couple interaction, and environment. For example, the therapist might conclude that the couple's major difficulty centers around individual differences in their needs for intimacy or the degree to which they are achievement oriented in approaching careers. In most instances, distressed couples are responding to these individual differences in maladaptive ways. Therefore, the therapist helps the couple recognize these differences, helps them stop their maladaptive ways of interacting around these issues (e.g., demanding and withdrawing), and searches for more adaptive ways to address these individual differences. Similarly, the therapist and couple might conclude that the couple lacks communication skills, which serves as the basis of their maladaptive interaction patterns, leading to communication training as described later in this chapter (see "Skills-Based Interventions"). Or it might be determined that the couple is responding to overwhelming environmental stressors, leading to interventions focused on helping the couple change the environment where possible, support each other through the difficult times, and seek outside support when appropriate.

At times, the beginning therapist can feel overwhelmed by the large number of issues with which a distressed couple presents and not know how to proceed. There is no algorithm for deciding what the major themes are for a couple. Typically, a couple will show their central difficulties multiple times to a therapist, and the major themes are seen in various specific situations. When several themes are present, the therapist must decide what to address first. In doing so, at least two factors are of importance. First, the therapist wants the couple to experience success in their efforts to improve their relationship, particularly given that many distressed couples feel hopeless when they seek treatment. Therefore, treatment should begin with an area in which the couple can be successful and develop an increased sense of their ability to improve their relationship. Second, many studies indicate that negative behaviors between partners prove to be particularly destructive and become the focus of a couple's experiences (for a recent review, see Epstein and Baucom 2002). Therefore, the therapist should work diligently early in therapy to decrease highly aversive interactions between the partners. Increasing positive interactions is important, but it is critical to decrease destructive interactions early in treatment.

Numerous investigations have found that brief cognitive-behavioral couple therapy is efficacious with distressed couples (Baucom et al. 1998). A hallmark of this approach is that it is focused on specific concerns and teaches couples to take control of their own difficulties by using the interventions learned during sessions in their everyday lives.

Assessment of Couple Functioning

To provide brief therapy for couples, the therapist and couple must identify a few major themes that are interfering with couple functioning or that detract from optimal relationship satisfaction. At the same time, a hallmark of cognitive-behavioral couple therapy is its focus on specific behaviors, cognitions, and emotions within the couple's relationship. A careful and thoughtful understanding of these specifics can allow the therapist to organize them into broader themes, which can then be addressed in therapy. As we noted earlier in the chapter, to understand a couple's functioning, it is essential to consider individual factors, couple interactions, and the environmental context within which the couple operates. A detailed consideration of conducting a couple assessment to evaluate these factors is beyond the scope of this chapter. Elsewhere, we wrote at length about how to conduct such an assessment (Epstein and Baucom 2002). A brief description of the basic steps and strategies used in an initial assessment follows.

Conducting a couple assessment involves several steps:

1. The initial identification of presenting problems and the partners' goals in seeking therapy

2. A relationship history and assessment of current relationship functioning, including observation of the couple's interaction patterns
3. An individual history and assessment of current functioning of each partner
4. The therapist's assessment feedback summary to the couple

Typically, the assessment begins with a joint interview with the couple, with a brief description of their current concerns, problems, and reasons for seeking couple therapy. At this point in the assessment, only a brief amount of time is spent defining their concerns, lest couples deteriorate into protracted arguments, blaming each other, and defending themselves.

Once the therapist has an overall understanding of the couple's concerns, it is valuable to place this into a historical context to understand how current concerns have developed. Consequently, the therapist conducts a rather detailed history of the couple's relationship, attending to major themes, periods during which changes occurred in both a positive and a negative direction, and how the couple arrived at the current state of relationship functioning. Throughout the history, the therapist attends to individual, couple, and environmental factors that have contributed to relationship distress. As a couple describes their history, often it is possible to identify significant themes in their relationship that serve as the focus for intervention. These might include long-term interaction patterns, such as partners mutually avoiding each other, one person needing a greater degree of intimacy than the other individual, or the couple not coping well with significant environmental stresses.

Once the couple has completed a relationship history, the assessment returns to a fuller consideration of current relationship functioning, emphasizing both relationship difficulties and relationship strengths. With both people present, each partner is given an opportunity to express his or her concerns, along with that individual's perceptions of relative strengths within the relationship. This detailed description of current concerns and relative strength from each partner can augment the therapist's observations of the relationship history to round out important themes and the specific ways in which they are enacted within the relationship.

Although there are varying perspectives among couple therapists, individual interviews with each partner are often helpful. During these interviews, the therapist can obtain an individual history for each person, obtain additional information about issues that arose during the couple's joint assessment interview, and attempt to develop a positive working relationship with each partner. It is important during these individual interviews not to develop an allegiance with either partner to the detriment of the other member of the relationship; thus, one should not hold secrets or collude with one individual. These individual interviews can provide detailed information about how each partner contributes to relationship functioning.

Next, the assessment involves direct observation of the couple's interaction patterns. Although a certain amount of this interaction has occurred during the previous assessment strategies, the current focus involves asking the couple to engage in a series of conversations with each other to allow the therapist to observe the partners' interacting without the therapist intervening. These conversations include a discussion of positive thoughts and feelings that partners have toward each other, expression of their thoughts and feelings about relationship difficulties, attempts to provide support to one individual when that person expresses concerns not focal to the relationship, and the couple's ability to make decisions or solve problems when significant concerns are present in their relationship.

On the basis of these discussions of the couple's relationship history, their current concerns and strengths, an understanding of each individual's history and current functioning, and behavioral observations of the couple's interactions, the therapist develops an initial formulation and related treatment plan. The final step is to share these observations with the couple, pointing out the individual, couple, and environmental factors that appear to be important; how they developed over time; and how the therapist proposes to help the couple make appropriate changes. This feedback and discussion are important to create a shared understanding of the goals of therapy and the strategies that will be used. During this feedback, each partner provides his or her own perspectives on issues that the therapist has isolated, along with additional areas that need to be addressed within the treatment. Once an agreed-on formulation of the couple's relationship distress and related intervention strategies is reached, treatment begins.

Role of the Therapist

Within the context of the earlier discussion, the cognitive-behavioral couple therapist explores the relevant individual, couple, and environmental factors that contribute to relationship discord, as well as those that serve as resources. In all of these domains, the therapist is attentive to important behavioral, cognitive, and emotional factors that must be addressed. Continuing with an earlier example, if two partners differ in the degree of closeness and intimacy that they want from the relationship, behaviorally they might develop a demand/withdraw pattern. Cognitively, the pursuer in the couple might think that he or she is unloved as the partner seeks greater distance, and emotionally, the pursuer may become angry at being deprived of the closeness that he or she wants.

In assisting the couple, the cognitive-behavioral couple therapist uses a wide variety of cognitive, behavioral, and emotional interventions, as described below (see "Interventions for Modifying Behavior"). A developmental and historical perspective on both individuals and the relationship is taken into account in understanding the couple's current relationship distress, but the primary focus is on the couple's current functioning and ways of responding more adaptively to each other in the future. At times, the therapist assumes the role of educator, providing psychoeducation as needed. For example, if a couple is seeking assistance because they both feel more distant from each other than they would like, the therapist might talk with them about various ways that couples can foster intimacy in their relationships by connecting verbally, physically, and behaviorally and about how these principles might apply to their relationship. This role of educator also might involve helping the couple learn and apply new communication skills as they seek to be more open and disclosing with each other.

The therapist is also a facilitator, creating a safe environment within which the couple can address difficult issues. A safe environment can be created in a variety of ways, ranging from maintaining control over emotional expression for a couple who has strong and frequent emotional outbursts to creating opportunities for caring interactions between partners who have been distant from each other. Cognitive-behavioral couple therapy is predicated on the notion that couples must learn to enact their new ways of behaving, thinking, and feeling outside of therapy sessions, as well as within sessions. Therefore, the therapist helps couples decide on new strategies that they will use between sessions to help their new learning generalize to their everyday lives.

In essence, the role of the cognitive-behavioral couple therapist is similar to that of cognitive-behavioral therapists in other contexts—reviewing the couple's homework since the last therapy session; setting an agenda for the current session; following the agenda with a variety of behavioral, cognitive, and emotional interventions during the session; and guiding the couple in setting up new homework activities to be completed before the next session. Although the length of treatment varies as a function of the characteristics of the particular couple, most treatment outcome studies have reported between 8 and 26 therapy sessions. Recently, Christensen and colleagues (in press) found that couples continue to improve at a linear rate for approximately 26 sessions; that is, gains appear to occur throughout treatment and not only in the early or late stages of intervention.

Interventions for Modifying Behavior

Almost all distressed couples are unhappy with the way that they are behaving toward each other. Within this broader context, their concerns take a variety of forms. Many individuals are focused on the unacceptability of their *partner's* behavior, with complaints such as the partner being too hostile or negative or the partner not engaging in enough constructive or helpful behavior. Other individuals focus on problems of the couple as a *unit;* for example, they cannot communicate well with each other, or they have lost the ability to have fun together. A notable number of others raise concerns about *themselves;* for example, "I can't stand who I have become in this relationship. It brings out the worst in me. I don't like being petty or nasty to another person." In cognitive-behavioral couple therapy, there has always been a strong emphasis on helping members of couples behave in more constructive ways with each other, and this emphasis continues in our current conceptualization. The therapist might use any of the numerous available specific behavioral interventions with the couple, but they fall into two major categories: guided behavior change and skills-based interventions (Epstein and Baucom 2002).

Guided Behavior Change

Guided behavior change involves interventions that focus on changing particular types of behavior without teaching partners specific skills. At times, these interventions have been referred to as *behavior exchange interventions*, but this term can be misleading because these interventions do not involve an explicit exchange of behaviors in a quid pro quo fashion. In fact, often it is helpful for the therapist to discuss with the couple the importance of each person committing to make constructive behavior changes irrespective of the other person's behavior (Halford et al. 1994). Too often, distressed couples operate in a quid pro quo fashion in which each person is only willing to change contingent on the other person's efforts. Asking each person to make appropriate changes and be responsible only for himself or herself helps to alleviate this "Who goes first?" mentality, and it gives each individual a sense of personal control in improving the relationship.

We might introduce interventions of this type as follows:

> What I want each of you to do is to think about how you would behave if you were being the kind of partner that you truly want to be. What does that mean that you would do and not do? If you behave in this manner, it likely will have two very positive consequences. First, your partner is likely to be much happier and to respond to you in a positive manner. Second, you are likely to feel better about yourself. So, I want you to get back to being the kind of person that you enjoy being in this relationship, so that the relationship can bring out the best in you as an individual.

Thus, we rarely attempt to establish rule-governed behavior exchanges (e.g., contracts) that were common in the early days of behavioral couple therapy (Jacobson and Margolin 1979). Instead, we work together with couples to develop a series of decisions about how they want to make changes in their relationship to meet the needs of both people, to help the dyadic relationship function effectively, and to interact positively with their environment.

These types of guided behavior changes can be implemented at two levels of specificity and for different reasons (Epstein and Baucom 2002). First, a couple and therapist might decide that they need to change the overall emotional tone of the relationship, so they choose a broad-based, general guided behavior change strategy. Many couples complain that it simply is no longer pleasant being around each other because the general tone of the relationship has become so dissatisfying; very few positive interactions occur between them, and an excess of negative, hurtful, or critical interactions take place. Various interventions have been developed to shift this overall ratio of positives to negatives. These include "love days" (Weiss et al. 1973) and "caring days" (Stuart 1980). These interventions generally involve having each partner decide to engage in some positive behaviors intended to make the other person happier. The selected behaviors might include small tasks or chores, such as making coffee in the morning, or more direct caring and affectionate behaviors, such as making a telephone call during the week to say hello. Typically, these types of interventions are used when the therapist and couple conclude that the partners have stopped making much effort to behave in caring and loving ways toward each other, have allowed themselves to become preoccupied with other life demands, and have treated their relationship as a low priority.

In essence, these rather broad-based interventions are intended to help couples regain a sense of relating in a respectful, caring, thoughtful manner. One hallmark of courtship is the great amount of time and effort that partners typically put into creating a positive relationship environment and making the other individual happy. Although no attempt is made in therapy to rekindle courtship on a long-term basis, it is reasonable to help couples reestablish an ongoing positive, caring atmosphere. It is important to recognize that these broad-based, general guided behavior changes are intended only to create a shift in atmosphere; they are not intended to address long-term, complex problems in the couple's relationship. Those are addressed through a variety of additional interventions described later in this chapter. In the following example, the therapist uses a guided behavior change with Mr. and Mrs. V to help them create a more positive tone in their relationship.

> Therapist: Mr. and Mrs. V, one of the things that you have mentioned is that you both believe that you have gotten away from really making much of an effort to make each other happy and create a generally positive atmosphere in your home. I believe that is very common among couples, and as you said, as life gets busy, it is easy for everything else to take priority over your relationship. To get things back on track, it might be helpful if you make a special effort to start treating each other in helpful and caring ways again. Let me describe for you a somewhat structured way that many couples have found helpful to get back to a more positive way of interacting with each other. What I would recommend is that every day, each of you does at least one small, caring, or helpful act for the other person that you do not typically do. And I really do want you to keep it small, so that these are the types of things that you could sustain over time. For example, you might prepare breakfast for the other person or run an errand for your partner. Both of you will be doing this, but I want each of you to do it independently, irrespective of whether the other person follows through. As we discussed, it is important for each of you to take personal responsibility to try to make the relationship better. How does that part sound to each of you?
>
> Mr. V: I think it sounds OK, as long as I can remember to do it. I really don't mind trying to be thoughtful to my wife; it's just that we're out of the habit. I don't even think about it. So I'm mainly concerned that she will get upset if in a few days I forget to follow through with this.
>
> Therapist: I can understand, and that does happen. When people are out of the habit of making special efforts, they might have good intentions, but it is hard to follow through. People try various things to remember, so you may need to experiment a bit with things that can serve as a reminder to you. For example, I would like each of you to write down the specific actions that you take each day to behave more positively toward your partner and bring the record with you to our next session, so I can get a picture of what both of you are doing. Writing down what you did might help you keep in mind your goal of increasing positive behavior. Also, some people put up

sticky notes to remind themselves, write reminders in their calendars, or set alarms on their watches. Do you have any ideas of what might work for you?

Mr. V: I hadn't thought about that, but I do have one of these digital organizers, and I could have it pop up a reminder at the beginning of each day. But that's a pretty sad state of affairs when you need a reminder to do something nice for your partner, isn't it?

Therapist: It is in a way, isn't it? And this is not something I'd recommend that you do forever. It really is a way to help you make some changes and break some old habits that you have gotten into. Once most couples begin doing this regularly, they find it rewarding, and they don't need to continue using this much structure. Mrs. V, what are your reactions to what I'm proposing that the two of you do?

Mrs. V: I think it sounds good, and I don't think I'll have any trouble remembering to do nice things for my husband. In my opinion, I do that fairly often already. What is hard for me is that he does not seem to notice it, and then I'm not very motivated to continue doing it.

Therapist: I'm glad you mentioned that. There is actually a second part to what I'm proposing that you do. I call it "Find your partner doing something nice, and thank him or her for it." People do get discouraged and quit trying if they don't believe that their partner notices or appreciates what they are doing. Therefore, it is just as important to acknowledge as it is to give. How do each of you do in terms of expressing appreciation or acknowledging what the other person does?

Guided behavior changes also can be used in a more focal manner. As a result of the initial assessment, the therapist and couple focus on important issues and themes that serve as the basis of the couple's relationship distress. In the following excerpt, the therapist responds to the couple's major complaint that after being married for 23 years, they no longer feel close to each other. They rarely argue, but there is little vitality in their marriage.

Therapist: Mr. and Mrs. W, it is understandable that after 23 years, life can start to feel routine, without much of a sense of closeness or excitement. Let's start to think about what you might do to create a greater sense of closeness with each other. There is no single thing that people do to feel close to each other; it really varies from individual to individual and from couple to couple. Some couples find that they experience a sense of closeness when they talk with each other, sharing their thoughts and feelings about a variety of things. In fact, disclosing inner thoughts and feelings is one of the most effective ways to increase intimacy between two people. But that is not the only way to develop a sense of closeness. Some people feel close to their partners when they are having fun together, joking around and being silly. Other people feel close to each other when they're learning together, taking a class and discussing their perspectives on a variety of issues. I know couples who feel close to each other when they sit quietly together in a room, both reading books. Other people have a sense of closeness when they are out together enjoying nature. Some couples feel close when they are functioning well as a team, perhaps working on a joint task around the house. And other people feel close when they're giving back to others outside of their relationship, working together in a soup kitchen or volunteering for an environmental cause. When you think about the two of you, what are ways that you have interacted with each other in the past that helped you to feel close to each other? Do any of the other ways that I mentioned sound appealing, even if you haven't focused on them previously in your relationship?

Skills-Based Interventions

In contrast to guided behavior changes, skills-based interventions typically involve the therapist's use of didactic discussions and/or media (e.g., self-help books and videotapes) to instruct the couple in the use of particular behavioral skills. This instruction is followed by opportunities for the couple to practice behaving in the new ways. The label *skills-based interventions* suggests that it is assumed that the partners lack the knowledge or skill to communicate constructively and effectively with each other, although this often is not the case. Many couples report that their communication was open and effective at earlier points in their relationship, but as frustrations mounted, they began communicating with each other in destructive ways, or they greatly decreased the amount of communication. Also, many individuals report that they communicate better with other people than with their partners. Regardless of whether this is a skills deficit or a performance deficit, discussing guidelines for constructive communication can be helpful to couples in providing the structure they need to interact in constructive ways. We often differentiate between two major goals of communication between partners: conversations focused on sharing thoughts and feelings and decision-making or problem-solving conversations (Baucom and Epstein 1990; Epstein and Baucom 2002). In conversations for sharing thoughts and feelings, the purpose is for the partners to understand each other and have an opportunity to share their own perspectives. Conversations can be about daily activities or important topics regarding the couple's life goals. In contrast, decision-making conversations are much more goal directed, with the specific goal of making a decision, solving a problem, or resolving a conflict.

Guidelines for these two types of communication are provided in Tables 7–1 and 7–2. These guidelines are presented as recommendations, not as rigid rules. The therapist can emphasize certain points and alter the guidelines, depending on the needs of specific couples. For example, the guidelines for expressiveness emphasize sharing both thoughts and emotions. If the therapist is working with a couple who avoids emotions and addresses issues on a purely intellectual level, then emphasizing the expression of emotion might be of primary importance.

Table 7–1.   Guidelines for couple discussions

Skills for sharing thoughts and emotions

1. State your views *subjectively*, as your *own* feelings and thoughts, not as absolute truths. Also, speak for yourself, what you think and feel, not what your partner thinks and feels.
2. Express your *emotions* or *feelings*, not just your ideas.
3. When talking about your partner, state your feelings about your partner, not just about an event or a situation.
4. When expressing negative emotions or concerns, also include any *positive feelings* you have about the person or situation.
5. Make your statement as *specific* as possible, in terms of both specific emotions and thoughts.
6. Speak in "paragraphs." That is, express one main idea with some elaboration and then allow your partner to respond. Speaking for a long time without a break makes it hard for your partner to listen.
7. Express your feelings and thoughts with *tact* and *timing* so that your partner can listen to what you are saying without becoming defensive.

Skills for listening to your partner

Ways to respond while your partner is speaking

1. Show that you *understand* your partner's statements and accept his or her right to have those thoughts and feelings. Show this *acceptance* through your tone of voice, facial expressions, and posture.
2. Try to put yourself in your *partner's place*, and look at the situation from his or her perspective to determine how the other person feels and thinks about the issue.

Ways to respond after your partner finishes speaking

3. After your partner finishes speaking, *summarize* and restate your partner's most important feelings, desires, conflicts, and thoughts. This is called a *reflection*.
4. While in the listener role, do *not*
    a. Ask questions, except for clarification
    b. Express your own viewpoint or opinion
    c. Interpret or change the meaning of your partner's statements
    d. Offer solutions or attempt to solve a problem if one exists
    e. Make judgments or evaluate what your partner has said

Table 7–2. Guidelines for decision-making conversations

---

1. Clearly and specifically state what the issue is.
   a. Phrase the issue in terms of behaviors that are currently occurring or not occurring or in terms of what needs to be decided.
   b. Break down large, complex problems into several smaller problems, and deal with them one at a time.
   c. Make certain that both people agree on the statement of the problem and are willing to discuss it.
2. Clarify why the issue is important and what your needs are.
   a. Clarify why the issue is important to you, and provide your understanding of the issues involved.
   b. Explain what your needs are that you would like to see taken into account in the solution; do not offer specific solutions at this time.
3. Discuss possible solutions.
   a. Propose concrete, specific solutions that take both people's needs and preferences into account. Do not focus on solutions that meet only your individual needs.
   b. Focus on solutions for the present and the future. Do not dwell on the past or attempt to attribute blame for past difficulties.
   c. If you tend to focus on a single or a limited number of alternatives, consider brainstorming (generating a variety of possible solutions in a creative way).
4. Decide on a solution that is feasible and agreeable to both of you.
   a. If you cannot find a solution that pleases both partners, suggest a compromise solution. If a compromise is not possible, agree to follow one person's preferences.
   b. State your solution in clear, specific, behavioral terms.
   c. After agreeing on a solution, have one partner restate the solution.
   d. Do not accept a solution if you do not intend to follow through with it.
   e. Do not accept a solution that will make you angry or resentful.
5. Select a trial period to implement the solution if the situation will occur more than once.
   a. Allow for several attempts of the new solution.
   b. Review the solution at the end of the trial period.
   c. Revise the solution if needed, taking into account what you have learned thus far.

Similarly, during decision-making conversations, we do not ask routinely that all couples brainstorm a variety of alternative solutions before discussing each one, because some couples easily can identify a mutually acceptable solution. However, if a couple's typical pattern involves each partner presenting his or her own preferred solution, followed by the couple arguing over the two proposals, then brainstorming might help the couple avoid their adversarial approach and each person's premature commitment to a particular solution. Likewise, in the decision-making guidelines, some attention is given to implementing the agreed-on solution. For some couples, reaching a mutually agreed-on solution is the difficult task. Once they have agreed on a solution, they are effective in carrying it out. Other couples reach solutions more readily but they rarely implement their agreements. If a couple has difficulty carrying out what they agree to do, then the therapist can pay more attention to helping them implement their solutions more effectively. In fact, the couple might problem solve strategies to increase the likelihood that a solution will be implemented, discussing possible barriers to following through, as well as ways that both people can be reminded about the actions that they agreed to take during the week. In the following dialogue, the therapist works with Mr. and Mrs. X as they attempt to make decisions about how to spend their holiday time with their families:

Therapist: Good, would you like to spend some time trying to make decisions about how to spend the Thanksgiving holiday this year? And as you work on this, let's try to stay attentive to one of the patterns that we have been picking up in your previous conversations. You both have a tendency to propose the solution that is ideal for you as an individual, and then you lock horns trying to convince each other to accept your own position. As a result, you reach a stalemate. So tonight, let's be particularly aware of the second stage in the decision-making process, when you both share what is important to you about the holiday and spending time with families. Then, when you both understand what is important to each of you, I recommend that you come up with some possible strategies that explicitly take both of your desires and needs into account. If that is OK, I'd like you to start by clarifying the issue that you are facing regarding the holiday.

Mrs. X: I think that the issue is that we have been married for 3 years and still haven't figured out how to spend holidays like Thanksgiving. Both families would want us to spend all our time with them if we could, and obviously, we can't do that because they live in different places. Both my husband and I really enjoy being with our own families, and I think we end up trying to convince each other or make each other feel guilty for wanting to spend time with our own families. So I think the problem is that we do not have a good approach for deciding how to spend the Thanksgiving holiday with our two families.

Therapist: Mrs. X, you stated how you view the concern nicely, without blaming either of you. Mr. X, why don't you continue to focus on the statement of the concern and let Mrs. X know if you see it in the same way, and if not, how you understand the current problem that the two of you are having.

Mr. X: Well, I think that's basically it. I think the problem is that we don't have any good way for making this decision of where to go for

Thanksgiving, and we both end up feeling frustrated and hurt in the process. Honey, I think it is complicated by the fact that you are an only child, and I have three siblings who are married. You seem to feel that we should spend most holidays with your parents, or else they would be alone. My parents always have one or two of my siblings at their home for holidays, even if we're not there. Based on what you have said in the past, you seem to think that we should spend most holidays at your house, and I think it should be 50–50.

Therapist: Mr. X, you also did a nice job of clarifying how you see the problem. You did spend a fair amount of time talking about what Mrs. X thinks and says. In general, be careful when speaking for the other person. I'm not sure if you, Mrs. X, have said these things to Mr. X in the past, or whether you, Mr. X, are making inferences about Mrs. X's emotions and preferences.

Mrs. X: I do think that my husband has a general tendency to try to tell me what I think, and I resent that. I really want to speak for myself. But in this case, we have discussed this many times, and I think that what he is saying is pretty much on target in terms of what I've told him.

Therapist: Fine, if you both feel that you have a common understanding of this concern about how to decide where to spend Thanksgiving, let's move to the next step, in which you both clarify what is important to you and what you prefer. Don't propose specific solutions yet; just share your thoughts and emotions about why this is important to you and what you believe needs to be taken into account in developing a good solution.

Mrs. X: The most critical thing for me is that my parents don't end up feeling unloved or lonely over the holiday. I know that we can't spend all Thanksgivings with them, but it feels horrible talking to them and telling them that there are 20 people gathering at your parents' house for this festive occasion when they will be all alone.

The guidelines for conversations devoted to sharing thoughts and emotions and conversations for decision making both focus primarily on the *process* of communicating, with no particular attention to the *content* of topics that are discussed. However, it also is important for the therapist and couple to develop a joint conceptualization of the content of the primary themes or issues in the couple's concerns. These major themes and issues should be taken into account while the couple engages in both types of conversations. For example, if a lack of intimacy is a major theme in a couple's problem, when the couple has expressive conversations, they might emphasize ways of taking some chances to become more vulnerable with each other, such as discussing more personal feelings with each other.

In essence, during skills training, the therapist should attend to both the process of communication and how the couple addresses important content themes and issues in their relationship. In earlier approaches to cognitive-behavioral couple therapy, therapists commonly restricted their role to being a coach, focusing on the communication process and attending little to the content of what the partners were discussing. We believe that traditional cognitive-behavioral interventions can be used more effectively if the communication process and the important content themes in the couple's relationship are addressed simultaneously. As a result, the therapist might not always be a neutral party when a couple is proposing specific solutions to a problem. If a given solution seems contrary to the changes that are needed to achieve the couple's overall goals, then the therapist might point this out and express concern about the solution. For example, if the members of a couple have expressed that they do not feel respected by each other, the therapist might question their proposal that they "take a break from each other" by spending more leisure time separately with their individual friends. The therapist could note that this solution might temporarily help the couple avoid hurtful confrontations, but it also could increase their sense of hopelessness that they will ever be able to discuss their different preferences in a way that makes them feel validated by each other.

A therapist also can address the content of an issue during a couple's decision-making conversation by providing educational information that will help to guide the couple in devising a solution. Thus, if a couple whose child has challenging behavior problems is discussing parenting issues, the therapist might provide them with information about parenting strategies that are most appropriate for their child's developmental level, which the couple then could take into account in making their decisions. We believe that this is an important shift within cognitive-behavioral approaches, providing a needed balance between addressing the couple's communication and interaction processes and, at the same time, attending to the content of the couple's concerns.

Interventions That Address Cognitions

The ways that people behave toward each other in committed relationships have great subjective meaning for the participants, and these meanings have a capacity to evoke strong positive and negative emotional responses in each person. For example, individuals often have firm standards for how they believe the partners should behave toward each other in a variety of domains. If the standards are not met, the individual is likely to become displeased. For example, Mr. Y grew up in a family where men showed their respect for women by opening car doors for them, pulling up their chairs at a dinner table, and so forth. For him, that is how he believes he should show respect and love for his wife. On the other hand, Mrs. Y grew up in an environment in which such behaviors were seen as demeaning and patronizing to women. For her, people are people and should be treated the same regardless of gender. In addition, as a lawyer, she had to make an extra effort among her male colleagues to be accepted as an equal. When she and Mr. Y were in social gatherings with her colleagues, she did not want him to show traditional gender role behavior toward her that focused on her being a woman. This was a major violation of her standards of egalitarianism and equality. For Mr. Y, Mrs. Y's standard meant that he was not allowed to express his love and respect in a way that he felt that he should, and he interpreted Mrs. Y's behavior as her being ashamed of him in social gatherings. As a result of their different standards for female and male role behavior, they had frequent arguments and finally sought couple therapy.

Similarly, an individual's degree of satisfaction with a partner's behavior can be influenced by the attributions or explanations that the individual makes for the partner's behavior. Thus, a husband might prepare a nice dinner for his wife, but whether she interprets this as something positive or negative is likely to be influenced by her attribution for his behavior. If she views this as his attempt to be thoughtful and loving, she is likely to experience his dinner preparation as positive. However, if she makes an inference that he has done something wrong and has made dinner in order to get in her good graces before telling her about it, she might feel manipulated and experience the same behavior as negative. In essence, partners' behaviors in intimate relationships carry great meaning, and not considering these cognitive factors can limit the effectiveness of treatment. Elsewhere, we have enumerated and described empirical evidence about a variety of cognitive variables that can influence the quality of couples' relationships (Baucom and Epstein 1990; Epstein and Baucom 2002), including

- *Selective attention*—What each person notices about the partner and the relationship
- *Attributions*—Causal and responsibility explanations for relationship events
- *Expectancies*—Predictions of what will occur in the relationship in the future
- *Assumptions*—What each believes people and relationships actually are like
- *Standards*—What each believes people and relationships *should* be like

These types of cognitions are important because they play roles in shaping how each individual experiences the relationship. The therapist does not attempt to have the partners reassess their cognitions simply because they are negative. Instead, the therapist is concerned if one or both partners seem to be processing information in a markedly distorted or unrealistic manner. Thus, an individual might selectively attend to instances when a partner is forgetful, paying little attention to other ways in which the partner accomplishes various tasks successfully. Similarly, this same individual might attribute the partner's failure to accomplish particular tasks as resulting from a lack of respect for the individual's preferences and a clear reflection of a lack of love. Understandably, such cognitions are likely to be related to negative emotions, such as anger, and under such circumstances, the individual is likely to behave negatively toward the partner.

Although distorted or unrealistic cognitions of one or both partners often are the focus of cognitive assessment and intervention, some couples experience relationship distress when both partners have realistic thoughts but they simply interpret or experience the world in different ways. For example, both partners might have very realistic standards for how much time partners should spend together, but if the standards are different, the couple might struggle over their preferences for time together versus time alone.

Therefore, sometimes the focus of therapy will not be on changing behavior but will be on helping the couple reevaluate their cognitions about what is happening in their relationship, so that these events can be viewed in a more reasonable and balanced fashion. A wide variety of "cognitive restructuring" intervention strategies can be used to assist distressed couples:

- Evaluate experiences and logic supporting a cognition.
- Weigh advantages and disadvantages of a cognition.
- Consider worst and best possible outcomes of situations.
- Provide educational mini-lectures, readings, and tapes.
- Use the inductive "downward arrow" method (questions to tap underlying meanings of couple's reactions).
- Identify macro-level patterns from cross-situational responses.
- Identify macro-level patterns in past relationships.
- Increase relationship-schematic thinking by pointing out repetitive cycles in the couple interaction.

Epstein and Baucom (2002) provided a detailed description of each of these intervention strategies. These various cognitive interventions can be categorized into two broad approaches: 1) Socratic questioning and 2) guided discovery.

Socratic Questioning

Cognitive therapy often has been equated with Socratic questioning, which involves a series of questions to help an individual reevaluate the logic of his or her thinking, understand the underlying issues and concerns that are not at first apparent, and so forth. In working with distressed couples, such interventions can be effective but must be used cautiously. The context of individual therapy is quite different from that of couple therapy. In individual therapy, the client participates alone and works with a caring, concerned therapist with whom he or she can be open and honest in reevaluating cognitions. In couple therapy, however, the individual's partner is in the room. Often, the partner has explicitly blamed the individual for the relationship problems, frequently telling the individual that his or her thinking is distorted. Consequently, if a therapist begins to question one person's thinking in the presence of a critical or hostile partner, the individual is more likely to be defensive and unwilling to acknowledge that his or her thinking has been selective or biased to some degree against the other person. If the individual does acknowledge that he or she was thinking in an extreme or distorted way, the partner might use this against the individual in the future. Therefore, Socratic interventions may be more successful when the two partners are less hostile and hurtful toward each other. In the following dialogue, the therapist helps Mrs. Z reevaluate her attribution for Mr. Z's behavior.

> Therapist: Mrs. Z, it sounds like Mr. Z spent more time talking with you in the evenings as you had wanted him to, but it didn't feel very good after all. Is that right?
>
> Mrs. Z: I know that sounds stupid, but that really is how it seems. When he was sitting there and talking to me, I was thinking that he's only doing this because he knows we're going back to therapy next week, and he doesn't want to look bad. It's not that he really wants to talk with me. My husband has always been an excellent "student," and he doesn't want to embarrass himself in front of a therapist. So it really doesn't mean anything when he spends more time talking with me.
>
> Therapist: Given that you interpreted his behavior that way, I can certainly understand why it didn't feel good and didn't make the two of you feel closer as you had hoped it would. If it is OK with you, let's spend a couple of minutes thinking through this a bit more. We have talked about the fact that it is not just what each of you does and doesn't do that influences how you feel about the relationship. When your partner does something or doesn't do something, you interpret it and give it meaning. That meaning often is what determines your satisfaction and feelings at the moment. In this case, you interpreted that Mr. Z talked with you just because

he wanted to impress me and be a good student. Therefore, you didn't feel very good toward him and certainly didn't feel closer to him. Your interpretation certainly could be correct. However, we also talked about the strong tendency you both have to interpret each other's behavior in a negative way and that you often don't give each other the benefit of the doubt. So let's step back and look at Mr. Z's behavior again. Mrs. Z, what are some other possible reasons that Mr. Z spent extra time talking with you this week? I'm not assuming that these will be the actual reasons that he did talk with you, but what are some reasonable possibilities?

Mrs. Z: I guess I can push myself to think of some others, but they certainly didn't go through my mind this week. I suppose he may have suddenly decided that I am an interesting person after all, and he does enjoy talking with me.

Therapist: That is one possibility, but I'm not sure if you are being sarcastic as you say it. Can you see that that is one possibility, even if it is unlikely?

Mrs. Z: I was being sarcastic. It is possible, but why would he suddenly see me as an interesting person after I've begged him to talk with me for years? It seems very unlikely.

Therapist: OK, so it seems unlikely, but it is one possibility. What are some other possibilities for why he might have decided to talk with you more this past week?

Mrs. Z: Well, I guess even if he doesn't find it particularly exciting to talk with me, he might be doing it because he knows it is important to me, and he wants to make our relationship better.

Therapist: Yes, that is another possibility. I don't know if that was what was behind Mr. Z's behavior, but it certainly sounds possible, doesn't it? I think the important thing to realize here is that your interpretation really is very subjective. If things go wrong in your relationship, there really is a tendency to automatically interpret each other's behavior in a negative way. As you said, you didn't even think about any other possibilities for Mr. Z's behavior. To make things better between the two of you, I think it will be important for you to step back and not make these automatic negative interpretations. You will need to check yourself and see if you're being fair to the other person and consider other interpretations. In addition, rather than just interpreting these on your own, often it is helpful to find out from the other person why he or she behaved that way. Why don't we do that? Mr. Z, can you tell Mrs. Z why you spent more time talking with her this past week?

Guided Discovery

Guided discovery involves various interventions in which the therapist creates experiences for a couple so that one or both people may start to question their thinking and develop a different perspective on the partner and/or relationship. For example, if a husband noticed his wife's withdrawal and interpreted it as her not caring about him, the therapist could address this attribution in a variety of ways. First, the therapist could use Socratic techniques, as in the previous case example, such as asking the husband to think of a variety of interpretations for his wife's behavior and asking him to look for evidence either supporting or refuting each of those possible interpretations. In contrast, in guided discovery, the therapist could structure an interaction in which the husband obtained additional information that might alter his attributions. For example, the therapist might ask the couple to have a conversation in which the wife shared what she was thinking and feeling at the time when she withdrew. During the conversation, the man might find out that his partner withdrew because she was feeling hurt and cared about him a great deal. Her vulnerability, rather than a lack of caring, might have been the basis of her withdrawal. This new understanding might alter the man's perspective without the therapist questioning his thinking directly.

Similarly, a woman might develop an expectancy or prediction that her partner does not care about her opinion on a variety of issues. If, however, they agree to start having conversations on a weekly basis and she sees that he is interested in her perspective when she expresses it, her predictions might change. Thus, rather than directly challenging either person's cognitions, the therapist can help the couple arrange interactions that provide additional experiences or information that will challenge each individual's cognitions.

Some cognitions are not addressed best by evaluating their logic, because they are not based on logic. For example, standards involve beliefs about the ways that an individual or the couple should behave; often these involve values of what is right or wrong. It is difficult, if not impossible, to debate the logic or truth of someone's standards and values. Instead, standards for relationships are addressed more appropriately with methods that focus on the advantages and disadvantages of living according to them. In the rest of this subsection, we provide a detailed discussion of addressing relationship standards as one example of cognitive restructuring with couples. These standards might involve an individual's behavior (e.g., whether a partner should have close relationships with members of the opposite sex), the ways that the partners interact with each other (e.g., whether it is acceptable to express disagreement openly with each other), or how to interact with the environment (e.g., how much time one should devote to an ailing parent). In general, in addressing relationship standards, we proceed through the following steps:

1. Clarify each person's existing standards.
2. Discuss advantages and disadvantages of existing standards.

3. If standards need alteration, help revise them to form new acceptable standards.
4. Problem solve on how new standards will be taken into account behaviorally.
5. If a partner's standards continue to differ, discuss the ability to accept differences.

In essence, we discuss how any given standard relevant to the couple usually has some positive and negative consequences. First, it is important to clarify each person's standards in a given domain of the relationship. For example, the couple might differ on their standards for how one should spend free time. A husband might conclude that given that the couple has little free time, they should spend all of it together. However, the wife might believe that partners should spend some free time together but that it is critical to have a significant amount of time away from one's partner as well. Once the partners are able to articulate their standards regarding time together and alone, each is asked to describe the pros and cons of conducting a relationship according to those standards. Thus, the husband would be asked to describe the good things that would result from spending all or almost all of their time together, as well as potential negative consequences. The wife would be invited to add to his perspective. Similarly, the wife would be asked to list the pros and cons of spending some free time together and some free time apart, with the husband adding his perspective. Without intervention, couples often become polarized during this phase, with each person emphasizing the positive consequences of his or her perspective and the other partner noting the negative consequences of the person's point of view. By encouraging each person to share both the positive and the negative consequences of his or her standard, this polarization can be avoided or minimized. A brief excerpt of Mr. and Mrs. A discussing the pros and cons of together time versus time alone follows:

> Therapist: Mr. A, Mrs. A has told you her beliefs about what a relationship should be like relative to spending time together versus having time apart from each other. As we discussed, there's no right and wrong way for a couple to set up their relationship in this area. Any way you do it is likely to have some pros and cons. It sounds like what happens with you and Mrs. A is that you each argue for your own position without trying to understand the other person's perspective. Let's try to change that. Although I know it is not your own perspective, I want you to push yourself to try to see what good things might come from you and Mrs. A spending some time together but also spending some of your free time separately. What good might come from setting up your relationship with Mrs. A in this way?

Mr. A: Well, it would certainly please her, and that would be good. But beyond that, I know that while we are apart, I would look forward to being back with her, so it would lead me to appreciate her. Also, I guess it would mean that we both would have more separate experiences and could bring those back to the relationship and talk about them. Other than when we're at work, we are together almost all the time. So there isn't much new for us to tell each other. I know some good things could come from this, but we have so little free time that it is hard for me to think about spending some of it away from her.

Therapist: Mr. A, thanks. I think you did that in a very sincere way, trying to understand what it is like from Mrs. A's perspective and trying to see good things that could come from spending some time apart from each other. Mrs. A, first let's make sure that you've heard Mr. A correctly. Then, I want you to add to what Mr. A has said. What additional good things do you think could come to the relationship from spending time apart from each other?

After the couple fully discusses their different standards and the pros and cons of each approach, they are asked to think of a moderated standard that would be responsive to both partners' perspectives and that would be acceptable to each person. Individuals typically cling strongly to their standards and values, so rarely is an individual likely to give up his or her standards totally. Much greater success occurs from slight alterations in standards that make them less extreme or more similar to the other person's standards. In the previous example, Mr. and Mrs. A might strive toward some agreed-on standard within which they spend a good deal of couple time together to feel close to each other, along with some time apart from each other to grow as individuals and have unique experiences to bring back to the relationship. This is not an easy task, and it can require several sessions. After the couple agrees on a new standard, they are asked to reach decisions about how this new standard would be implemented in their relationship on a daily basis, in terms of concrete behaviors that each person would perform. Thereby, Mr. and Mrs. A's standard for couple versus individual time would be translated into specific concrete daily activities.

Interventions Focused on Emotions

Whereas many behavioral and cognitive interventions influence an individual's emotional responses in a relationship, at times more explicit attention needs to be paid to addressing emotional factors in the relationship directly. In particular, therapists often work with couples in which one or both partners have either restricted or minimized emotions or excessive emotional responses. Each of these broad domains includes more specific difficulties that individuals have with emotions and particular interventions that are appropriate for them.

Addressing Restricted or Minimized Emotions

Many partners in committed relationships seem to be uncomfortable with emotions in general or with specific emotions. This can take a variety of forms. Some individuals experience and express minimal emotions in general or have problems accessing specific emotions. This can typify the person's experiences in life in general or might be more focal to the current relationship. To a degree, this might reflect an individual's temperament, or it might be the result of being raised in a family or culture in which certain emotions were rarely expressed. Other individuals experience both positive and negative emotions, but their levels of emotional experience are so muted that they do not find their experiences within their relationships very gratifying. Similarly, the partner of such an individual might complain that it is unrewarding to live with someone who has such restricted emotional responses. In addition, some individuals have stronger emotional experiences but have difficulty differentiating among different emotions. They know that they feel good or bad but cannot articulate or differentiate the emotions that they are experiencing. Emotions carry a great deal of meaning, so the ability to make such differentiations can be helpful to both the individual and his or her partner. For example, if an individual can clarify that he or she is feeling sad, this can help both members of the couple understand that the person is experiencing a sense of loss, which then can be addressed. More generally, emotions and cognitions are typically highly related. Sadness usually goes along with some experience of loss; anxiety and fear usually are related to a sense of danger or unpredictability; and anger frequently is associated with an experience of injustice or unfairness. Consequently, knowing the specific emotion that an individual is feeling often gives important clues as to how the person is experiencing the situation cognitively as well.

Although emotions typically are related to thoughts and behaviors, some individuals have difficulty relating their emotions to their internal and external experiences. Thus, a wife might know that she is quite angry but cannot relate this to what she is thinking or to experiences that occurred in an interaction with her husband. This difficulty can make both persons feel that they have little control over the relationship and are at the mercy of the individual's emotions, which appear to occur in an unpredictable manner rather than to be related to specific thoughts or behaviors.

Finally, some individuals avoid what Greenberg and Safran (1987) referred to as primary emotions that are related to important needs and motives. Often, individuals avoid the experience or expression of these emotions because they are seen as dangerous or vulnerable. Greenberg and Safran proposed that people cover these primary emotions with secondary emotions that seem less vulnerable. Consequently, rather than experiencing and expressing fear and anxiety to a partner, an individual might experience negative feelings such as anger and hostility, which help the individual feel less vulnerable.

In some instances, these difficulties in experiencing and expressing emotions might warrant cognitive or behavioral interventions. For example, if one partner believes that it is wrong to experience and express anger, that person might suppress his or her own perception and expression of it and censure the partner for feeling and expressing anger. In this circumstance, the therapist might work with the individual to reevaluate his or her standards regarding the expression of anger. Otherwise, encouraging the person to be aware of and express anger if he or she believes that this is wrong could result in negative consequences.

In addition, a variety of strategies drawn primarily from the emotionally focused therapy developed by Johnson and Greenberg (Johnson 1996; Johnson and Greenberg 1995) can be used to help individuals access and heighten emotional experience. These interventions, which we described in detail elsewhere (Epstein and Baucom 2002), include the following:

- Convey that positive and negative emotional experiences are normal.
- Clarify thoughts and then relate them to emotions.
- Use questions, reflections, and interpretations to draw out primary emotions.
- Describe emotions through metaphors and images.
- Discourage attempts to distract self from experiencing emotion.
- Encourage acceptance of the individual's experience by the partner.

These interventions are based on several broad principles. First, the therapist tries to create a safe atmosphere by emphasizing that the experience and expression of both positive and negative emotions are normal. In addition, the therapist promotes this safe environment by encouraging the partner to respond to the individual in a caring and supportive or, at least, accepting manner when the person expresses various emotions. Even so, the individual might attempt to avoid an emotion or escape once the session is focused on emotions. Therefore, the therapist might need to refocus the individual on an emotional experience and expression if he or she shifts the focus. Of course, this must be done with appropriate timing and moderation to avoid overwhelming an individual with distressing emotions.

Once a safe environment is created, a variety of strategies can be used to heighten emotional experience. These interventions might include asking an individual to recount a particular incident in detail so that the emotional aspect of this experience may be evoked; encouraging the individual to use metaphors and images to express emotions, if directly labeling emotions is difficult or frightening; and using questions, reflections, and interpretations to draw out primary emotions (e.g., "It sounds like when you and your husband start to become intimate sexually, it calls up all those horrible feelings of when you were abused as a teenager. Just being touched is very frightening; is that right?"). The therapist's goal is to help the individual enrich his or her emotional experience and expression in a manner that is helpful to both the individual and the couple, although the experience might be quite painful on a temporary basis.

A decision to focus on this category of interventions should not be based on a therapist's belief that a "healthy" person should have a rich emotional life as well as a full range of emotional expression; instead, the decision to use such interventions should be based on a careful assessment that a restriction in emotional experience and/or expression is interfering with this particular couple's, or the partner's, well-being. In the following example, the therapist is attempting to help Mrs. B reexperience her feelings from a negative interaction with Mr. B. In this instance, the therapist attempts to heighten her emotional experience by having her recount the incident in detail.

Therapist: Mrs. B, it sounds like the interaction that you had with Mr. B last night was pretty upsetting for you, but you're having difficulty clarifying exactly what you were feeling. Mr. B doesn't seem to understand what you were feeling, so I think it might be helpful if we could get more specific about what you were thinking and feeling. One way to do that is to go back and look at that experience in more detail. Would that be OK?

Mrs. B: Sure, I'm willing to do that. It's frustrating; I was so upset, but I couldn't really understand it myself or explain it to my husband, which just makes it that much worse.

Therapist: Fine, let's go back to last night. You mentioned that you were at home and had prepared dinner when Mr. B came in. You mentioned to him that he had a telephone message from his boss, and he made a call right away. Is that right?

Mrs. B: That's right. He called his boss and stayed on the telephone for about 45 minutes. As soon as he got off the telephone, he explained the emergency to me, but by then I already was upset. I felt like I didn't have any reason to be upset, so I just kept it to myself.

Therapist: So you were upset by the time he got off the telephone. What were you thinking about while he was on the telephone?

Mrs. B: Well, I was thinking several different things. First, I was disappointed because I had prepared a nice meal, which was getting cold. What was more upsetting was that he always seems to have something else to do that is more important than I am or our relationship is. Then I feel guilty and stupid for thinking that way. We're dependent on his job, and I know it is not a 9-to-5 job, so he has to respond. Still, it makes me feel very low priority.

Therapist: And when you think that you are unimportant and a low priority to Mr. B, what emotions do you experience? What are the feelings that go along with feeling unimportant and a low priority?

Mrs. B: I guess it's sadness, a real sense of sadness and defeat.

Therapist: Good, I think you're starting to figure it out. Why don't you tell Mr. B directly how you experience it emotionally when he seems to have so many things that take his time?

Containing the Experience and Expression of Emotions

At the other end of the continuum of emotionality, a therapist may work with partners who have difficulty regulating their experience and expression of emotion. Typically, this is of concern to the couple if one or both partners are experiencing and expressing high levels of *negative* emotion or are expressing these emotions in settings that are not appropriate. At the same time, in some couples, one person's extreme exuberance and frequent expression of strong *positive* emotion can become problematic. At times, one person can feel overwhelmed being around another individual who is so excited, upbeat, and happy on an ongoing basis. However, clinicians more often confront couples in which one person has difficulty regulating the experience and expression of negative emotions. The therapist may find such couples quite demanding because their lives appear to revolve around a series of emotional crises, strong arguments, or extreme behaviors (e.g., partner abuse), which result from extreme negative emotions. In addition, the therapy sessions can be very difficult to control because of frequent emotional outbursts as a couple confronts problematic aspects of their relationship.

A variety of strategies can help couples in such circumstances. As noted earlier, behavioral and cognitive interventions often can be of assistance. For example, if an individual frequently is upset and angry because of a partner's displeasing behavior, then the therapist might focus on behavioral interventions to alter the partner's unacceptable behavior. On the other hand, if an individual frequently is upset because he or she holds extreme standards that few partners could satisfy, then focusing on modifying those standards is appropriate. In addition, some interventions are more focal to addressing extreme emotional experiences:

- Schedule times to discuss emotions and related thoughts with the partner.
- Practice "healthy compartmentalization."
- Seek alternative means to communicate feelings and elicit support.
- Tolerate distressing feelings.

One useful strategy is for the couple to schedule times to discuss issues that are upsetting to one or both partners. The goal of this intervention is to restrict or contain the frequency with which and settings in which strong emotions are expressed. If couples have not set aside times to address issues, then an individual with poor affect regulation is more likely to express strong feelings whenever they arise. Some people find that they can resist expressing strong negative feelings if they know that a time has been set aside to address concerns. This intervention can be helpful in making certain that problems and expression of strong negative affect do not intrude into all aspects of the couple's life. In particular, this can be helpful in ensuring that strong negative emotional expression does not occur at times that are likely to lead to increasing frustration for one or both persons. For example, expressing strong anger when one person is leaving the house to go to work, or initiating a conversation with strong negative emotion once the couple has turned off the lights to go to sleep, likely will result in further upset for both people.

Within the context of working with parasuicidal individuals and persons with borderline personality disorder, Linehan (1993) developed a variety of interventions to assist individuals with poor affect regulation. Although her interventions do not focus on addressing strong emotions in an interpersonal context, often they are applicable. One of these interventions involves teaching individuals to tolerate distressing emotions. Some individuals seem to assume that if they are upset, they need to do something immediately to reduce their uncomfortable emotional experience, frequently resulting in strong expressions of emotion to the partner. Helping individuals become comfortable with and accepting of being upset with their partners or their relationship without needing to address every concern immediately can be helpful. Similarly, it can be helpful to coach the individual in focusing on the current moment. Many individuals with poor affect regulation allow their upset in one domain of life to intrude or infiltrate many other aspects of their lives. We explain placing limits on this intrusion to couples as a form of healthy compartmentalization. That is, if one partner is upset about a given aspect of the relationship, it is important for that partner to restrict that sense of upset to that one issue and to allow himself or herself to enjoy other positive and pleasurable aspects of the relationship when they occur.

Poor affect regulation exists on a continuum, and it is influenced by several factors, including the quality of the couple's relationship. Although the previous strategies can be of use to many couples, when individuals have extreme difficulty in regulating their experience and expression of negative emotions, couple therapy alone often is inadequate. In such instances, we typically refer the individual for some form of individual psychotherapy, such as dialectical behavior therapy, which assists the person in developing skills to regulate affect. As the individual becomes more effective in regulating negative affect, it is easier for the therapist to address upsetting aspects of the relationship in a couple therapy context.

Finally, it can be helpful for partners to seek alternative ways to communicate feelings and elicit support, perhaps from individuals other than their partners. Thus, relying on other friends for expressing some concerns, keeping a journal or diary to express emotions, or using other alternatives for releasing tension and strong emotion can be productive for the individual. This approach is not intended as an alternative to addressing an individual's concerns with a partner but as a means of moderating the frequency and intensity with which the person's emotions are expressed to the partner.

Integrating Behavioral, Cognitive, and Emotional Interventions

In working with couples within a brief format, it is imperative that a therapist focus on the most central issues of relevance to a couple. In the current chapter, we have noted a variety of factors that can contribute to relationship functioning, including normal individual differences between the two partners, psychopathology in one or both individuals, couple interactive processes, and the way that the couple relates to their social and physical environment. In considering each of these domains, behavioral, cognitive, and emotional interventions are available to the therapist. Attempting to address all of these factors in a brief therapy format is impossible and would likely be overwhelming to both the therapist and the couple. Furthermore, rarely are all of these factors of central importance to a given couple. Instead, the therapist working collaboratively with the couple identifies the most salient factors to address in couple therapy. Thus, for a given couple, the therapy may focus on how the couple can adapt most effectively to an extraordinary number of external environmental stressors that they are confronting, such as a collection of parenting problems, financial difficulties, and illnesses of aging parents. Other couples may differ in the degree of closeness that they need in order to be satisfied. Yet other couples might lack the ability to express emotions and therefore experience a disengaged relationship. Identifying these most central factors and focusing on them can allow a couple therapist to work in a brief format and make substantial progress with many couples.

In the following example, the therapist focuses on the most central factors in working with Mr. and Mrs. C, a couple in their mid 40s.

Summary Case Illustration: Mr. and Mrs. C

Mr. and Mrs. C had married directly after undergraduate school and were excited to begin their life together. They had dated through most of college and described their early relationship as wonderful. After they graduated, they both began jobs but had decided that Mr. C's career would be the primary one in their relationship. They both wanted children, and once their children were born, they both wanted Mrs. C to stay home and raise the children. They had grown up in what they experienced as wonderful families, and an important part of that was being with their mothers when they were young.

After 24 years of marriage, they sought couple therapy primarily because Mrs. C was unhappy with their relationship and feeling somewhat depressed. As she explained it, there was no room for her in their relationship, and she felt stifled, as if she had stopped growing 20 years ago. She had been the good mother and the good wife, but there had been little for her individually. She almost never did anything for herself and was resentful. She felt caught in a helpless situation. She loved Mr. C and their two children but felt that if she stayed in this marriage any longer, she would "die" emotionally. She had started going out to dinner and movies with some of her female friends, refusing to tell Mr. C and the children where she was going or when she would be back. If they wanted dinner, they could wait until she returned, or they were free to prepare it themselves. Mrs. C had distanced herself from Mr. C; their sexual and affectionate life had come to a halt, and as she expressed it, "Right now, either I as an individual can survive, or our relationship can survive. I've given my whole adult life to our marriage, and now it's time for me."

Mr. C felt totally confused coming into therapy. As he stated it, "I feel like I'm living with a stranger. It looks like my wife, but it's like she got a brain transplant. I don't understand what is happening. I thought everything was fine. We have two wonderful children; we're all healthy; we have enough money, and we have good friends and family. Now she talks about dying if she stays in our marriage. I don't know what to do. It feels like we've been on one life course, and suddenly, she wants to change it. She's going out to dinner, movies, or whatever with her friends at night in the middle of the week without telling us or explaining what is happening. The kids are confused and feel as if they have lost their mother. We really need your help."

After conducting an assessment with the couple, the therapist concluded that they were experiencing difficulty because they had allowed their relationship to become skewed in the following way. In mutual collusion with her husband and with her own full consent, Mrs. C had changed from being a woman with a fulfilling career to being exclusively a wife and mother. In doing so, she undertook in a great deal of self-sacrifice for the well-being of the family overall. From the family's perspective, the arrangement worked quite well. Things functioned smoothly at home, the children made it to their various appointments and sporting events on time, their school projects were always among the best in their class, and Mr. C's career flourished. However, these benefits to the family came at quite a price to Mrs. C personally. She let her personal relationships outside of the family slip, and she spent little time doing things for herself, such as taking additional classes, exercising, or socializing with friends. All couples need to balance individual, family, and couple well-being. Although it was unintended, this couple had allowed their relationship to dominate Mrs. C's individual well-being, and now she was distressed and felt desperate. She was swinging from one extreme approach to another, because the couple had not learned how to integrate a focus on both her individual and their family well-being.

In developing a treatment plan with this couple, the therapist focused on the balance between individual and couple well-being. A central issue of the treatment became whether Mrs. C could experience personal growth within the context of her family. Both Mr. and Mrs. C greatly valued what they had built together during their marriage, and they did not want to lose it. Although Mrs. C was somewhat skeptical that Mr. C and the children could accommodate her individual needs, Mr. and Mrs. C were both eager to try.

First, the therapist focused on helping the couple share their thoughts and feelings about the situation that they were confronting; when they entered therapy, neither partner really knew how the other felt. Mrs. C had learned to keep her feelings to herself and to focus on the family's well-being. As she began to express her concerns, disappointments, and experience of being stifled, Mrs. C found it liberating to see that her husband listened and wanted to understand her. Mr. C found it frightening to hear of Mrs. C's concerns, because he had had no awareness of them. He was quite worried that she might leave their marriage, but with reassurance from the therapist, he came to realize that listening to these feelings would have the greatest likelihood of creating a relationship that was fulfilling to Mrs. C.

After spending considerable time in therapy discussing these concerns and recognizing that they were now in a new developmental stage in their relationship, in which Mrs. C did not have to attend to young children's needs, Mr. and Mrs. C focused their energy on how to rebalance the relative emphases between individual and couple growth and well-being. The couple next spent a considerable amount of time problem solving and decision making regarding these issues. These conversations had several different but related foci. First, the couple spent time talking about what each of them needed as individuals within the marriage to feel fulfilled. The therapist encouraged them to discuss this at two levels: what they needed day to day and what their long-term goals, plans, and dreams were as individuals. As they discussed these issues, Mrs. C was able to clarify both for herself and for Mr. C that she needed time during the week for herself as an individual. She decided to join a health spa and exercise regularly for the first time in 20 years. She also wanted to reestablish some of her female friendships that had lapsed, although this was difficult to do because she had neglected them over the years. She also decided that she wanted to become involved in projects at her local church without Mr. C. She needed a sense of contributing as an individual to her community. From a long-term perspective, Mrs. C wanted to do substantial volunteer work with the animal protection society. As Mr. C heard these various requests from Mrs. C, he was open to incorporating them into their lives. He wanted her to be fulfilled individually but simply had not known what she needed. He acknowledged that it would be difficult, given that they had built their family life in a different way, but he was committed to making these changes. They decided that together they would talk to the children and explain to them some of the changes that they were trying to make in the family for healthy, adaptive reasons.

When the couple discussed Mr. C's needs on a daily basis and his long-term goals, he wanted to change very little for himself personally. They agreed that they had developed their relationship over the years in a way that accommodated his immediate and long-term needs. As Mr. C came to recognize this, he felt somewhat guilty that their relationship had become so skewed. He shared these feelings with Mrs. C, who was supportive of him and pointed out that she willingly had helped to develop their relationship in its current form. They had simply inadvertently gone too far. In discussing these issues, the therapist asked the couple to address their standards for the importance of individual well-being relative to couple and family functioning. They both agreed with the therapist that some balance was necessary, and without focusing on it, they had allowed their family life to drift into a skewed form that ignored Mrs. C's individual needs.

For Mrs. C to place an emphasis on her own growth and well-being, she needed to distance herself somewhat from Mr. C, and he found this difficult to experience. As the couple worked through these issues in therapy, he was able to express to Mrs. C how he sometimes felt rejected and devalued. She was able to explain to him how she had to create some more distance in order to focus on herself because she had such a tendency to give up her own needs for the family. Consequently, during therapy sessions, Mr. C, Mrs. C, and their therapist discussed ways that the couple could maintain their sense of closeness and intimacy while helping Mrs. C develop a healthy sense of autonomy within their relationship. Consequently, they regularly scheduled times to go out together as a couple, continued to have couple conversations during the week, and explored ways to rejuvenate their sexual relationship.

Over a period of approximately 6 months, the therapy was very effective. The therapist used a variety of cognitive, emotional, and behavioral interventions to help the couple address some balance between individual well-being and couple functioning. In part, the couple was successful because both partners were relatively well-adjusted individuals who were committed to their relationship and cared a great deal about each other. Consequently, once they saw the basis for their difficulties, they were able to make changes in a rather rapid fashion, although it was difficult to shift their family patterns that de-emphasized Mrs. C's individual well-being.

Conclusion

Had there been more long-term anger, resentment, disengagement, or insecurity in one or both partners in this case illustration, the treatment likely would have taken longer, or the results likely would have been compromised. Brief couple therapy is not successful with all couples, but the empirical literature is clear in indicating that it is efficacious for many. Often, at the beginning of couple therapy, it is impossible to predict whether a particular couple can make changes in a brief period. Consequently, the therapist should attempt to design interventions in a way that allows and promotes rapid change for a couple, with treatment plans being adapted as the therapy proceeds.

Brief couple therapy is a viable treatment modality when interventions are used that focus on central issues of importance to the couple and when the couple engages in therapeutic strategies in their day-to-day lives outside of the session.

References

Baucom DH, Epstein N: Cognitive-Behavioral Marital Therapy. New York, Brunner/Mazel, 1990

Baucom DH, Epstein N, Rankin LA: Cognitive aspects of cognitive-behavioral marital therapy, in Clinical Handbook of Couple Therapy. Edited by Jacobson NS, Gurman AS. New York, Guilford, 1995, pp 65–90

Baucom DH, Shoham V, Mueser KT, et al: Empirically supported couple and family interventions for marital distress and adult mental health problems. J Consult Clin Psychol 66:53–88, 1998

Baucom DH, Epstein N, Gordon KC: Marital therapy: theory, practice, and empirical status, in Handbook of Psychological Change: Psychotherapy Processes and Practices for the 21st Century. Edited by Snyder CR, Ingram RE. New York, Wiley, 2000, pp 280–308

Baucom DH, Hahlweg K, Kuschel A: Are waiting list control groups needed in future marital therapy outcome research? Behavior Therapy 34:179–188, 2003

Beck AT, Rush AJ, Shaw BF, et al: Cognitive Therapy of Depression. New York, Guilford, 1979

Christensen A, Heavey CL: Gender differences in marital conflict: the demand/ withdraw interaction pattern, in Gender Issues in Contemporary Society: Claremont Symposium on Applied Social Psychology, Vol 6. Edited by Oskamp S, Costanzo M. Newbury Park, CA, Sage, 1993, pp 113–141

Christensen A, Jacobson NS, Babcock JC: Integrative behavioral couple therapy, in Clinical Handbook of Couple Therapy. Edited by Jacobson NS, Gurman AS. New York, Guilford, 1995, pp 31–64

Christensen A, Atkins D, Berns S, et al: Traditional versus integrative behavioral couple therapy for significantly and stably distressed married couples. J Consult Clin Psychol (in press)

Epstein N, Baucom DH: Enhanced Cognitive-Behavioral Therapy for Couples: A Contextual Approach. Washington, DC, American Psychological Association, 2002

Greenberg LS, Safran JD: Emotion in Psychotherapy: Affect, Cognition, and the Process of Change. New York, Guilford, 1987

Halford WK, Sanders MR, Behrens BC: A comparison of the generalization of behavioral marital therapy and enhanced behavioral marital therapy. J Consult Clin Psychol 61:51–60, 1993

Halford WK, Sanders MR, Behrens BC: Self-regulation in behavioral couples' therapy. Behav Ther 25:431–452, 1994

Iverson A, Baucom DH: Behavioral marital therapy outcomes: alternate interpretations of the data. Behav Ther 21:129–138, 1990

Jacobson NS, Margolin G: Marital Therapy: Strategies Based on Social Learning and Behavior Exchange Principles. New York, Brunner/Mazel, 1979

Johnson SM: The Practice of Emotionally Focused Marital Therapy. New York, Brunner/Mazel, 1996

Johnson SM, Greenberg LS: The emotionally focused approach to problems in adult attachment, in Clinical Handbook of Couple Therapy. Edited by Jacobson NS, Gurman AS. New York, Guilford, 1995, pp 121–141

Linehan MM: Cognitive-Behavioral Treatment of Borderline Personality Disorder. New York, Guilford, 1993

Snyder DK, Wills RM: Behavioral versus insight-oriented marital therapy: effects on individual and interspousal functioning. J Consult Clin Psychol 57:39–46, 1989

Stuart RB: Helping Couples Change: A Social Learning Approach to Marital Therapy. New York, Guilford, 1980

Weiss RL, Hops H, Patterson GR: A framework for conceptualizing marital conflict: a technology for altering it, some data evaluating it, in Behavior Change: Methodology, Concepts, and Practice. Edited by Hamerlynck LA, Handy LC, Mash EJ. Champaign, IL, Research Press, 1973, pp 309–342

Part II

Special Topics

Essential Ingredients for Successful Psychotherapy

Effect of Common Factors

Roger P. Greenberg, Ph.D.

Several years ago, I had a psychiatric resident in psychotherapy supervision who dutifully brought audiotapes to each of our supervisory meetings. Each psychotherapy session we reviewed began with minutes of painful silence and a patient made clearly uncomfortable by the soundless process. Finally, after observing the pattern for several weeks, I asked the resident, "Don't you ever greet your patient, say hello, or ask patients how they are doing?"

The resident replied, "You never told me to!"

This vignette presents an extreme example of a novice psychotherapist trying to slavishly adhere to a preconceived notion of how to do psychotherapy while ignoring some of the basic rules of interpersonal sensitivity and human interaction. It is true that psychotherapy sessions have goals and purposes different from those typical of friendships. Yet the ability to help someone open up to threatening thoughts and feelings, as well as be influenced by the interaction, is rooted in a process that establishes a certain amount of safety, security, and respect for the pain of another human being. Therefore, it is important to remember that psychotherapy is enhanced within any particular system when the therapist has good commonsense judgment and hardy interpersonal skills. Not surprisingly, research has clearly supported the idea that there is more to effective psychotherapy than simply picking out a specific psychotherapy model and following the techniques in a robotic manner. In fact, although some research has suggested that it may be useful to learn to do psychotherapy from treatment manuals (which provide a blueprint for applying specific techniques), evidence also indicates that it is possible to go too far in trying to adhere to a manual. Faithfulness to a manual's directives may come at the expense of factors known to have a positive effect on outcome, such as therapist acceptance, flexibility, warmth, and the building of a therapeutic alliance.

Reviews of the psychotherapy empirical outcome literature consistently show that psychotherapeutic treatment produces benefits but also that it is difficult to detect clear differences in the comparative worth of different brands of psychotherapy. The verdict of the dodo bird in *Alice's Adventures in Wonderland* (Carroll 1865/1962)—"Everybody has won, and all must have prizes"—has been used as the subtitle for some classic publications on psychotherapy (Luborsky et al. 1975; Rosenzweig 1936). As the quotation suggests, positive results appear to stem more from a variety of factors common to many forms of treatment than from the application of specific techniques unique to one approach to psychotherapy.

Over the years, the idea that successful psychotherapies have certain things in common has continued to receive research support. The commonalities are of paramount importance, even when therapists feel that they are applying diverse forms of psychotherapy. Seasoned therapists appear to learn this and naturally drift toward similar behaviors as they hone their psychotherapy skills. For example, some well-known studies published more than 50 years ago indicated that there was considerable agreement in descriptions of the ideal therapeutic relationship provided by experienced therapists of varying theoretical persuasions (Fiedler 1950a, 1950b). In fact, senior clinicians espousing different orientations were more similar in their conceptions of ideal therapy relationships than were experienced and novice therapists claiming allegiance to the same theoretical approach!

Common Factors

Attempts to specify those components most needed for successful treatment generally regard techniques unique to particular types of psychotherapy as being less important than some overriding common factors. For instance, notable appraisals of the psychotherapy literature concluded that techniques, such as systematic desensitization or transference interpretations, which are associated with particular models of psychotherapy, account for only about 15% of the improvements that are achieved (Asay and Lambert 1999; Lambert 1992). Three other factors were judged to be more important. These other determinants of outcome are 1) patient variables and extratherapeutic events, 2) relationship factors, and 3) placebo/hope/expectancy effects.

Patient Variables

Some may find it surprising that patient/client variables and the circumstances in an individual's life are considered to play such an important role in outcome. However, a review of the literature led to the conclusion that about 40% of the improvement resulting from psychotherapy can be attributed to these factors. Most prominently mentioned are the patient's ability to relate, degree of psychological-mindedness, severity and number of symptoms, motivation, and capacity to point to a central problem. Also important are life circumstances, such as the level of job stability and the amount of social support or community resources available. Attention to patient factors includes, when needed, educating clients about the role and responsibilities of the psychotherapy patient. This typically requires helping the patient to view psychotherapy as a collaborative effort in which he or she will play an active and important part. It may also mean encouraging the patient to recognize his or her personal assets and the interpersonal support that may be available to him or her. Perhaps most critically, it involves teaching patients that change evolves from their own efforts. Over time, in successful therapies, patients are led to see that things they are doing create either a positive or a negative influence on how situations are likely to turn out. By becoming aware of the effect of their own behaviors, patients learn to repeat those actions that result in beneficial outcomes and to avoid those that turn out to be self-defeating. They also learn that some of the assumptions and expectations they hold about other people's thoughts and judgments are inaccurate.

Another salient point that follows from an appreciation of patient variables is related to trying to create balance between confrontation and support within psychotherapy sessions. All too often, psychotherapy seems to deteriorate into a single-minded exploration of what is going wrong in a patient's life and where his or her particular deficiencies may lie. This can be demoralizing and reinforce already exaggerated negative self-perceptions. It is wise to keep in mind that over time, patients also need to be channeled toward looking at areas of strength and personal assets they may be overlooking. In fact, therapists should routinely mentally catalogue such positive information during the early sessions of treatment so that a balanced picture can be discussed later, when the patient might be more ready to consider it.

Obviously, timing is critical in psychotherapy. The success of interventions is likely to be determined by a blend of therapist experience and artfulness in helping the patient to allow personal material to emerge. Surprisingly, even positive information about a patient can prove threatening if it conflicts with the negative self-portrait the patient has assembled from past experiences with significant figures (such as parents). A therapist may quickly lose credibility and alienate a patient by being too supportive and reassuring. Conflicts between accepting positive information and loyalty to critical parental pronouncements are common and must be handled with sensitivity and patience. This concern is of particular importance in brief psychotherapy because therapists may unwittingly estrange patients in their zeal to intervene swiftly with reassurance and support.

Novice therapists frequently fail to recognize that all patients do not enter treatment with equal commitments to making changes in themselves. Patients are often pressured into treatment by spouses, parents, employers, and even the courts. Therefore, for many patients, attempts to promote active techniques for altering behaviors and emotions can result in resistance and even dropping out of treatment. It is useful to remember that there are stages of change and that therapists need to match their techniques to a patient's degree of readiness to engage in the behavior change process. In the Stages of Change Model as presented by James Prochaska and colleagues (1992, 1995), stages of change unfold over time and involve progression through six levels of patient readiness and involvement: 1) precontemplation, 2) contemplation, 3) preparation, 4) action, 5) maintenance, and 6) termination.

Although I do not review the various stages in detail here, it is important to note that most patients do not present for treatment ready to engage in actions to ameliorate their problems. In fact, the Prochaska group estimated that only about 10%–15% of people are prepared to take action when they enter psychotherapy. Consequently, it becomes the task of the therapist to help patients move from a lack of awareness of their problems (precontemplation), to acceptance of the idea that they have problems (contemplation), to consideration of making changes (preparation), to active attempts to do something to improve the situation (action), and finally to anticipation of future stressors (maintenance). The therapist initially may need to play the role of nurturing parent while helping the patient to examine the reasons for resistance to change and anticipating how he or she might attempt to sabotage the treatment in the future. As patients begin to contemplate making changes, therapists might most appropriately assume the role of the Socratic teacher who facilitates expanded patient self-awareness and insight. When patients start to plan for action, the therapist may take on the role of experienced coach, who, in concert with the patient, helps to develop a game plan for change. During the action phase of brief treatments, psychotherapists behave more as vigorous-change agents and consultants, offering support and advice while patients struggle with the ups and downs of trying to make progress by engaging in new behaviors. Of course, patients' movement through these phases does not proceed uniformly in a straight line, and therapists must learn to regulate their activities to match the patient's level of readiness.

Relationship Factors

Probably the common factor most studied in the research literature is the therapy relationship and the role it plays in determining treatment outcome. Investigators have repeatedly affirmed the importance of a good therapeutic relationship. Even early in treatment, the nature of the relationship—the bond formed between therapist and patient—exerts a powerful influence on how the encounter is likely to turn out. It has been estimated that at least 30% of patient improvement can be attributed to relationship factors (Lambert 1992).

Determining which elements in the relationship are of most importance has been the subject of much speculation and study. Although Freud emphasized the patient's tendency to misread current relationships as reduplications of significant malignant past relationships, he also was aware of the need for patients to identify the therapist with kind, tolerant figures with whom they could develop an interpersonal attachment. This bond of attachment has been labeled the *therapeutic alliance* and is presumed to give the therapist the leverage needed to help the patient face frightening and unacceptable thoughts and emotions. Central to the development of an alliance is the establishment of a collaborative atmosphere in which mutual agreement exists on the goals and tasks of therapy, as well as mutual trust and acceptance. Evidence suggests that the therapist may facilitate this type of atmosphere by showing high levels of empathic understanding, warmth, and unconditional positive regard (factors emphasized in the influential writings of Carl Rogers [1957]). Interestingly, setting up a strong therapeutic alliance seems to be as important for a positive result with psychiatric medications as it is with talk therapy (Greenberg 1999). For example, a positive treatment outcome with antidepressants was found to be more likely when the prescribing clinician was perceived as empathic, caring, open, and sincere.

Other relationship-related findings indicate that treatment gains may stem less from the development of patient insights (as psychoanalysts might expect) than from patients having a "corrective emotional experience." This protherapeutic factor refers to patients perceiving their therapists as treating them in a more constructive and supportive manner than did the significant authority figures in the patient's past. The contrast with the past offered by this more positive relationship might help patients to feel more secure and confident about trying new solutions to old problems.

Several other change-inducing ingredients are common to most forms of psychotherapy. These include catharsis (in which patients release emotional tensions by unburdening themselves of troubling problems), identification (as patients learn to imitate a therapist model), and the development of feelings of mastery (as patients learn some type of framework for making their problems understandable and thereby gain a sense of control).

Incidentally, psychodynamic approaches to therapy sometimes have advocated that unique benefits may arise from focusing interpretations on the relationship between clinician and patient. These *transference interpretations* are designed to show patients that impulses and feelings for the therapist often result from past emotions and thoughts concerning significant others that are then projected (or transferred) onto the therapist. Although the transference concept has proven useful, transference interpretations have a possible downside. Research not only challenges the idea that heavy use of such interpretations is helpful but also actually suggests that use of such interpretations may be harmful, particularly with patients who are interpersonally adept (see review by Fisher and Greenberg 1996). Increased reliance on transference interpretations has been associated with more negative treatment outcomes and more negative effects on the therapist–patient relationship. Such interventions may lead patients to feel criticized and to withdraw. Overly stressing that patients need to examine their relationship with the therapist during psychotherapy sessions tends to lead to perceptions of the therapist as less supportive, less approving, less engaged, and more impatient. All of these qualities operate against the treatment being seen as helpful. In general, if the relationship is to be discussed, the discussion needs to be well timed, handled with great care, and not too frequent. These findings support the brief therapist's stance of downplaying interactions about the transference and emphasizing instead a positive treatment relationship and a well-defined therapeutic focus.

Another relationship-related tip concerning how *not* to conduct psychotherapy involves the concept of *pathogenesis*, which was described in the empirical literature more than 30 years ago. *Pathogenesis* refers to the degree to which therapists (knowingly or without awareness) use others who are dependent on them to satisfy their own needs, no matter what the cost to the dependent individual. A series of studies with very disturbed patients indicated a strong relationship between the level of therapist pathogenesis and negative treatment outcome. This observation seemed particularly striking with novice therapists. It was speculated that as experience increased, therapists either learned to control this aspect of their personalities or actually decreased their levels of pathogenesis. These findings are consistent with other indications that therapists who do not radiate relationship-enhancing characteristics actually might be harmful to those with whom they work. Such practitioners have been labeled *psychonoxious*.

Placebo/Hope/Expectancy Effects

The strength of placebo and expectancy effects in psychotherapy (as well as in all of medicine) has been widely acknowledged. These effects are estimated to be at least as powerful as those attributed to specific techniques and account for a significant portion of the improvement experienced by patients. It is important to realize that even though the term *placebo* is routinely associated with treatments that have no known specific active ingredients, providing a "treatment experience" for patients, no matter what form it might take, is not equivalent to doing nothing. In fact, researchers often have been startled by the improvements observed following a course of treatment presumed to be inert. The mere fact of meeting with a sanctioned caregiver appears to be generally helpful, independent of the specific type of treatment that is being delivered. Although these effects are sometimes demeaned by comments about results being due to *only* nonspecific psychological factors, their consistency and magnitude cannot be ignored. What might account for the ubiquitous power of caregiving encounters? Some important ideas on this topic appear in the classic writings of Jerome Frank (1973; Frank and Frank 1991).

Frank proposed that many individuals enter therapy feeling powerless to change and shaken. They lack confidence in their ability to cope and feel that they will be personally unable to solve problems facing them. He theorized that four factors are inherent in all psychotherapy approaches that help to diffuse these feelings of demoralization and assist the patient in becoming mobilized:

1. Having an emotionally charged relationship through which the therapist can instill hope that change can occur
2. Having a therapeutic setting that reinforces the expectation that others have been helped to change by this particular therapist
3. Having a therapeutic rationale (or "myth") that provides a plausible explanation for problems, compatible with the patient's belief system
4. Having a particular set of procedures or rituals that enhance belief through perception of the therapist as a master of the method

Having these hope-inspiring factors in place increases the likelihood that a patient will engage in the treatment and feel motivated to make changes.

Psychotherapy Integration

There is general consensus among experienced therapists that it is useful to master one or more major approaches to psychotherapy (such as those outlined in this book), but there has also been a growing movement aimed at integrating various approaches to treatment. The desire for integration is fueled by recognition that many approaches have resulted in patient benefits, with no one type of therapy having consistently bested the rest for all patients and most types of problems. Therefore, in the face of expanding numbers of therapy models and acknowledgment that commonalties play a significant role in producing treatment gains, the field has begun to open to the idea of amalgamating theories and techniques from different schools. The idea is to determine which combinations can be expected to produce the best outcomes for which types of problems. The resulting flexibility in case conceptualization and technique application offers a better fit with research evidence than does unwavering allegiance to single-therapy systems. In line with this position is the finding by several surveys that practitioners most often choose the terms *integrationist* or *eclectic* when asked to identify their preferred brand of psychotherapy. Of course, to be skillful as an integrationist, one must develop expertise with several forms of psychotherapy. It is our hope that this book will provide guidance in learning basic strategies associated with several widely accepted forms of psychotherapy.

One obstacle blocking the path to integration is the notion that therapy systems need to compete with one another for superiority. This need not be so. It is perhaps more useful to view diversity as a strength, with different orientations complementing one another. A knowledgeable clinician might then be able to approach problems with a much greater range of therapeutic tools and ways to conceptualize troubling symptom puzzles. In this regard, complementarity often has been suggested as a way to synthesize the strengths of psychodynamic and behavior therapies. For example, Paul Wachtel (1977, 1987) suggested that people are helped when their insights are used to help guide them toward action. Therefore, a psychodynamic approach could be useful in revealing to patients how and why they are unnecessarily defending themselves from certain thoughts, feelings, and behaviors. These insights might then permit the application of behavioral techniques aimed at changing behaviors and altering distorted self-perceptions. Similarly, some have suggested that behavioral techniques might be used at the start of some therapies to provide a degree of initial symptom relief and open the door to patient exploration of some of the dynamic reasons for the turmoil they are experiencing.

The Stages of Change Model (described earlier; Prochaska et al. 1992, 1995) provides another example of how different theories of therapy might be used in a complementary way. For those at the precontemplation stage, unaware or underaware of their problems, a psychodynamic approach may offer some special initial benefits. This is because the approach provides skillful suggestions for how therapists can help patients overcome resistances and increase awareness of the sources of discomfort. When a patient reaches the stage of contemplation, in which he or she has awareness of a problem but no commitment to action, cognitive therapy techniques may prove helpful in focusing the patient on how he or she can move ahead. Once the patient is ready for action, behavioral strategies may be used to particular advantage. By appropriately matching each model to the patient's level of readiness for change, the combination might afford the possibility of moving the patient along to a higher level of benefit than would be attained from any one approach used in isolation.

Conclusion

The purpose of this book is to present a primer on how to conduct treatment with several well-known psychotherapy models. As such, various treatment techniques and rationales are described for the reader. The aim of this chapter has been to briefly outline those factors that cut across virtually all treatment approaches and account for most of the effects obtained with any type of psychotherapy. These factors appear to be necessary ingredients for good outcome, although they alone may not always be sufficient to produce the desired result. In emphasizing common factors, I have highlighted the role played by patient variables, the relationship, and placebo/hope/expectancy effects. Evidence suggests that treatment results are maximized when the therapist can establish an atmosphere of collaboration and trust and an expectation of future well-being. Of special note is the indication that one ultimate goal of effective psychotherapy is to give the patient the confidence and the framework to play an active part in his or her own improvement. It is important, if benefits are to last, that patients be able to attribute gains made to their own efforts.

One of the unexpected findings uncovered by research is that psychotherapy can be for better or for worse. That is, the treatment may be helpful, or it has the power to make patients worse off than they would have been without any treatment at all. Much of the treatment potency for harm (as well as for good) rests in the qualities that the therapist brings to sessions. Investigations indicate that negative outcomes are more likely when the therapist does not listen well, is nonempathic, and is judgmental. Also, as outlined earlier in this chapter, deterioration is most likely when the therapist's needs supersede those of the patient and too much emphasis is placed on analyzing the nature of the treatment relationship. In contrast, the literature offers encouragement through the identification of all the gains that can accrue simply from meeting with a caregiver who presents a reasoned approach to problems, is easy to talk with, and is optimistic that the therapy will be helpful. Clearly, no one approach to therapy has cornered the market on effective ingredients. As specific techniques are matched with the patient's problems and readiness for change, keeping common factors in mind should go a long way toward helping any therapist to optimize treatment effects.

References

Asay TP, Lambert MJ: The empirical case for the common factors in therapy: qualitative findings, in The Heart and Soul of Change: What Works in Therapy. Edited by Hubble MA, Duncan BL, Miller SD. Washington, DC, American Psychological Association, 1999, pp 33–56

Carroll L: Alice's Adventures in Wonderland (1865). Hammondsworth, Middlesex, England, Penguin, 1962

Fiedler FE: A comparison of therapeutic relationships in psychoanalytic, nondirective and Adlerian therapy. J Consult Psychol 14:436–445, 1950a

Fiedler FE: The concept of an ideal therapeutic relationship. J Consult Psychol 14:239–245, 1950b

Fisher S, Greenberg RP: Freud Scientifically Reappraised: Testing the Theories and Therapy. New York, Wiley, 1996

Frank JD: Persuasion and Healing: A Comparative Study of Psychotherapy, Revised Edition. Baltimore, MD, Johns Hopkins University Press, 1973

Frank JD, Frank JB: Persuasion and Healing: A Comparative Study of Psychotherapy, 3rd Edition. Baltimore, MD, Johns Hopkins University Press, 1991

Greenberg RP: Common psychosocial factors in psychiatric drug therapy, in The Heart and Soul of Change: What Works in Therapy. Edited by Hubble MA, Duncan BL, Miller SD. Washington, DC, American Psychological Association, 1999, pp 297–328

Lambert MJ: Implications of outcome research for psychotherapy integration, in Handbook of Psychotherapy Integration. Edited by Norcross JC, Goldstein MR. New York, Basic Books, 1992, pp 94–129

Luborsky L, Singer B, Luborsky E: Comparative studies of psychotherapies: is it true that "Everybody has won and all must have prizes"? Arch Gen Psychiatry 32:995–1008, 1975

Prochaska JO, DiClemente CC, Norcross JC: In search of how people change: applications to the addictive behaviors. Am Psychol 47:1102–1114, 1992

Prochaska JO, Norcross JC, DiClemente CC: Changing for Good. New York, Avon, 1995

Rogers C: The necessary and sufficient conditions of therapeutic personality change. J Consult Psychol 21:95–103, 1957

Rosenzweig S: Some implicit common factors in diverse methods of psychotherapy. Am J Orthopsychiatry 6:412–415, 1936

Wachtel PL: Psychoanalysis and Behavior Therapy: Toward One Integration. New York, Basic Books, 1977

Wachtel PL: Action and Insight. New York, Guilford, 1987

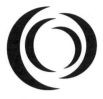

Brief Psychotherapy in a Multicultural Context

Rubén J. Echemendía, Ph.D.
Joël Núñez, Ph.D.

The face of America is rapidly changing. Given the ever-increasing cultural and ethnic diversity in the United States, the need for multicultural awareness and competence among fields providing human services is greater today than ever before. Historically, psychotherapy models have arisen from largely Eurocentric worldviews (Hall and Barongan 1997; Sue and Sue 1999). Although many strides have been made in the advancement of psychotherapy outcome and effectiveness studies, relatively little emphasis has been placed on examining the role of cultural and ethnic differences in current psychotherapeutic approaches. It seems appropriate for the field to engage in a critical self-examination and ask the basic question "Is contemporary psychotherapy an effective means of treating the culturally different?"

Data suggest that many groups that are culturally different from the upper- and middle-class American mainstream significantly underuse mental health services. These seemingly marginalized groups are composed of not only racial and ethnic minorities but also members of divergent religious denominations, sexual orientations, and socioeconomic statuses. At the same time, the data also suggest that many doctoral-level psychotherapists generally perceive themselves as insufficiently trained to work with culturally different clients (Allison et al. 1996; Bernal and Castro 1994). Therefore, there appears to be a cultural chasm between the providers of mental health services and many of those intended to be the users of said services. In this chapter, we attempt to help bridge that chasm by providing a brief introductory overview of issues that are often overlooked in the psychotherapeutic treatment of culturally different peoples, especially in brief psychotherapies, and the contribution of these factors to the underuse and premature termination of mental health services by ethnic minority mental health consumers. We also discuss psychotherapists' lack of training with these populations and the inevitable discomfort this generates when treating individuals from different cultures. Because of space limitations, this chapter is not intended to be a thorough review of the many considerations that should be taken into account in multicultural counseling. It is simply a starting point. Interested readers are encouraged to review comprehensive texts, such as Atkinson et al. (1998), Baruth and Manning (1999), Cuéllar and Paniagua (2000), Ponterotto (2001), and Sue and Sue (1999).

Topics briefly discussed in this chapter include 1) a consideration of the culture-specific context of psychotherapy, 2) the need for awareness and integration of the client's worldview into clinical conceptualizations and treatment planning, 3) the importance of therapist awareness of his or her own worldview and its relationship to that of the client, and 4) multicultural clinical competence as a continual process, not a final state to be achieved.

Cultural Context of Psychotherapy

A fundamental issue that lies at the heart of multicultural clinical competence is the understanding that psychotherapy itself is not a universal phenomenon and that its general tenets, techniques, and expectations as practiced in the United States are not understood and accepted by all. Although this point may appear to be obvious to most clinicians, it is a point worthy of attention.

Many scholars have asserted that traditional forms of psychotherapy were developed within a context in which "normality" was characterized by the beliefs, observations, cognitions, and perspectives of middle- to upper-class heterosexual European and European American men (Lee and Ramirez 2000; Sue and Sue 1999). Subsequently, the criteria of what constitutes normality and the means by which normality is assessed have been set in a culture-specific context. Also, by corollary, significant deviations—including cultural ones—from these norms of character and conduct are, by definition, viewed as abnormal or pathological. For example, homosexuality was categorized as a disorder in DSM-II (American Psychiatric Association 1968) largely because American culture defined homosexual behaviors as aberrant. The subsequent elimination of the diagnosis in DSM-III (American Psychiatric Association 1980) clearly points out the sociocultural aspects of diagnoses. Another powerful example was the nineteenth-century classification by many in the medical community of the ostensibly deviant behavior of runaway African American slaves as a mental disorder (Szasz et al. 1995). By extension, it is not uncommon for Latino individuals to report religious "visions." Do these visions constitute pathological hallucinations or culture-specific expressions of religious beliefs?

These simple examples (of which there are many, many more) should lead clinicians to consider the framework within which psychotherapy operates and to appreciate that for many groups of people, the paradigms, models, methods, and expectations that form the foundation of psychotherapy may be viewed as novel, culturally dissonant, or even alien. In fact, some scholars and researchers have argued that the therapeutic context itself may unwittingly mirror society's cultural power arrangements (Ponterotto 2001). For instance, Americans expect that when a person enters psychotherapy, he or she will divulge highly personal information about himself or herself to a stranger, albeit a professional one, who does not reciprocate by disclosing personal information about himself or herself. This approach may be viewed as inconsistent with the cultural beliefs of many other groups, such as some Asian Americans, Native Americans, or recent Eastern European immigrants. In fact, they may consider it insulting or dehumanizing that the therapist does not respond in a personal manner. The reverse is also true. Some cultures emphasize formality in interpersonal relationships, and a therapist who is gregarious and self-disclosing may be viewed as unprofessional. It is critical, therefore, that the clinician who differs culturally from his or her clients be aware that clients may not share the same suppositions about therapy and its expectations. A lack of clinical awareness at this basic level may lead to misunderstandings, premature termination, and even mistaken assignment of client psychiatric disorders at every level of therapeutic contact, from initial interview to case conceptualization, assessment, and diagnosis (Cuéllar 1998; Harris et al. 2001).

An example may help bring these issues to light. The senior author of this chapter, born in Cuba, began psychotherapy with a Spanish-speaking client during his training. The client was from Puerto Rico. Cuban and Puerto Rican cultures are similar in many regards. One similarity in the culture is that of being *simpático*—encouraging warm, interpersonal relationships between individuals. During the initial interview, the male patient was very much interested in the therapist's background. He asked questions that would otherwise be considered personal and not to be answered within traditional psychoanalytic/psychodynamic perspectives. The therapist's supervisor (an otherwise highly competent United States–born and United States–trained psychologist) indicated that these personal questions should be avoided because they would lead to problems in the transference relationship. The therapist's desire to answer the questions was viewed as a "countertransference issue." However, the therapist replied that a failure to answer the questions would be viewed as disrespectful to the client and neglect to establish the warm relationship that is the basis of Latin cultures. Refusal to answer these questions would create a breach in the therapeutic alliance and likely lead to premature termination. The questions were answered, and the therapy progressed nicely, with the client experiencing significant relief from the issues that led him to seek therapy. Both the therapist and the supervisor also benefited from the experience.

The cultural expectations of clients may particularly clash with basic assumptions underlying the brief therapies. The notion of therapy as a focused, instrumental process, for example, fits far better with traditionally masculine gender roles than feminine ones, which emphasize expressive and relational values (Spence and Helmreich 1978). Also, in their quest for brevity, therapists may be ill prepared to serve as ongoing social supports for culturally different clients who find themselves isolated from the social mainstream. The very notion of time as a scarce commodity to be saved is peculiar to Western cultures (Sue and Sue 1999) and may clash with clients' own expectations of an ongoing bond with a supportive figure.

Awareness of the Client's Worldview

Baruth and Manning (1999) defined *worldview* as the sum of an individual's experiences along with social, religious, and political beliefs and attitudes held in common with other members of the individual's reference group. The reference group may consist of family or community, racial or ethnic group, socioeconomic group, or nation. Baruth and Manning believed that it is imperative that a client's worldview be incorporated into the clinical conceptualization and treatment of clients. They stated that

> a client's worldview is an overriding cognitive frame of reference that in-
> fluences most human perceptions and values. To understand an individ-
> ual's response to a situation and to avoid a communication breakdown,
> the counselor needs to learn the meaning of that response in the client's
> worldview. (Baruth and Manning 1999, p. 9)

A lack of understanding about a client's attitudes, values, lifestyle, and background by therapists has been cited as a factor associated with inad-equate mental health service delivery to multicultural populations, in-cluding racial and ethnic minority groups; lesbian, gay, bisexual, and transgendered groups; and members of nonmainstream religious groups (Baruth and Manning 1999; Patterson 1996).

The dangers of failing to appreciate clients' worldviews, present in any psychotherapy, are magnified in the brief therapies. Because many brief therapies attempt to assess client concerns and achieve a focus for inter-vention within the first session, therapists run the risk of applying "one size fits all" treatments to presenting problems. Indeed, it is difficult to imagine that a therapist could truly enter into a client's unique cultural history and experience in the span of a brief assessment phase of treat-ment. If brief therapies are to be culturally sensitive, they need to ensure that an assessment of the cultural contexts of presenting concerns is a for-mal part of treatment planning (Steenbarger 1993).

Fortunately, the recognition that a client's worldview and sociocultural environment influence behavior has become more acceptable within American psychotherapeutic circles (Cuéllar and Paniagua 2000). With this growing acceptance on the part of psychotherapists and counselors, however, come several new challenges. First, knowledge of and respect for a client's cultural worldview should not imply that universally re-garded pathological behavior such as spousal abuse or child neglect is ac-ceptable under the guise of culturally sanctioned practices (Fontes 1995; Negy 2000). In some instances, an important aspect of treatment with culturally different clients will include the readjustment of client world-views to embrace the social, political, and cultural realities that exist in the United States. For example, a Latino family in treatment may report that a child has missed 3 weeks of school because the child's primary re-sponsibility is to care for an elder who is ill. The clinician may acknowl-edge the Latino cultural tradition that encourages younger family mem-bers to participate in the care of elders but also should inform the family that in the United States, it is not acceptable for minors to be kept from school for such reasons. Perhaps a compromise can be reached that would allow the child to attend school and to assist in the care of the elder in the afternoon. In this manner, accommodation is made and respect accorded to the clients' worldview but not at the cost of the child's welfare or the laws of the land.

Also, awareness of the importance of a client's worldview in treatment implies more than a healthy curiosity about the client's cultural background within sessions. It also requires a serious commitment from the clinician outside of sessions to learn about the cultural groups for which he or she intends to provide services (American Psychological Association 1993; Sue and Sue 1999). It is not the client's responsibility to provide protracted pedagogical instruction for the therapist (Lee and Ramirez 2000).

At the same time, therapists concerned with brevity should be aware of the danger of stereotyping clients as a result of overgeneralizing the cultural information they may have acquired about the group(s) with which the clients identify while ignoring the variability that exists within those groups. There is a potential danger of placing an individual so far within a cultural context that the characteristics and idiosyncrasies of the client in question are lost in cultural stereotypes and overgeneralizations. As a rule, it is safe to assume that there is as much, if not more, variability within a cultural group as between cultural groups. A tenuous balance must constantly be struck between viewing each client as part of the larger group(s) to which he or she belongs and seeing the client as an individual who may sometimes feel, think, and behave in ways that are not consistent with the prevailing knowledge about that group. Although striking the balance may appear to be difficult, it is a crucial element in providing culturally competent mental health services. Careful attention to the maintenance of a collaborative relationship within brief therapy is vital toward assuring that therapists and clients are not operating from opposite sides of a cultural chasm.

The Therapist's Worldview: Acknowledging Differences Within the Therapeutic Relationship

Perhaps one of the most significant, yet most ignored, elements of the therapeutic relationship is the lack of recognition on the part of the therapist of his or her own worldview and how it may differ from, and in some cases even be antagonistic to, the client's worldview. These differences may occur when the client and therapist are from distinctly different cultures (e.g., middle-class Anglo-American therapist and recent

Mexican immigrant) or when the client and therapist are from presumably similar cultures (e.g., Cuban therapist and Puerto Rican client). In both cases, as well as many other permutations, ignorance of the fact that the therapist is an individual embedded within a social, cultural, political, and religious framework that may adversely influence the therapeutic relationship can have devastatingly negative effects on treatment outcome (Cuéllar 1998). The presumption that the therapist can somehow be objective enough to enter into each session being able to bracket out his or her own long-standing perceptions, biases, prejudices, experiences, and attitudes about others in order to impede these from interfering in treatment is, at best, simplistic (Gopaul-McNichol and Brice-Baker 1998; Sue and Sue 1999).

As noted earlier, it is important for therapists to be aware of their worldviews just as it is important for therapy supervisors to be aware of their worldviews. An interesting example of this occurred during training for one of the authors (R.J.E.) in the Midwest. The therapy supervisor and a team of therapists were observing the therapy of a middle-aged Jewish mother through a one-way mirror. The student therapist was from New York City, and the patient was from Long Island, New York. The supervisor was born, lived, and trained in the Midwest. She had limited contact with Jewish people and had little knowledge of Jewish culture. The supervisor had a worldview that valued independence, as an individual and within the family structure.

The patient was describing to the therapist her relationship with her grown children. She expressed concern for them, concern for their career paths, and her desires to help them raise her grandchildren in an "appropriate manner." She found herself often worrying about them. The members of the therapy team who were observing (including the author) felt that the patient was expressing traditional Jewish beliefs about family relationships and the role of the mother within a Jewish family. The supervisor felt that the patient was being "overly intrusive" and pathological in her desires to "control" her family. When it became clear that the woman's children had no objections to the mother's role, the supervisor described the situation as "enmeshed" and pathological. Her approach to treatment would have required the patient to become "independent" and live a life distinctly apart from her children. Those familiar with the culture argued that such a position would lead to culturally inappropriate behavior, increased anxiety, and likely premature termination. The supervisor, to her credit, accepted that she might not be able to fully appreciate the situation because she had little knowledge of the patient's worldview.

This example underscores several important issues. First, issues of culture and worldview are not restricted to the traditional "ethnic minority" categories. Cultural differences exist even within relatively mainstream groups in the United States. Second, therapists, and those who train them, must be aware of their worldviews and examine ways in which their worldviews may interfere with their assessment and treatment of patients. As therapists, we are comfortable recognizing differences when they are readily apparent (e.g., a black Spanish-speaking therapist with a white Southern Baptist client), but we rarely pay attention to differing worldviews when the client and therapist *appear* to be similar. Another example may prove useful. We noted earlier in this chapter that Cuban and Puerto Rican cultures are relatively similar. However, the cultures differ in many ways, particularly if one examines sociocultural status and racial differences within those cultures. Although both Cuban and Puerto Rican people speak Spanish, they differ in several important ways. Differences are found in language, history of colonization, identification with "Spanish" roots, migration patterns, emphasis on education, and so forth. A white Cuban therapist who immigrated to the United States during Castro's revolution may have a very different worldview from that of a dark-skinned Puerto Rican client who came to the United States to improve his family's economic situation. Similarly, a Puerto Rican therapist who was born to a relatively wealthy family in Puerto Rico and who completed her education in the United States may have a very different worldview from that of a mixed-ancestry Cuban refugee who arrived in the United States during the Mariel boat lift.

Studies exploring the construct of cultural encapsulation, or ethnocentrism, have reported that being immersed in and favoring one's own cultural values and beliefs is a normal phase of personality development that one simply does not naturally outgrow (Baruth and Manning 1999; Cross 1991; Gopaul-McNichol and Brice-Baker 1998). Even if people are born with the capacity to be tolerant of differences in others, many people tend to view their own cultural values and beliefs as preferable and/or superior to others. Therefore, these inclinations must be actively discovered and challenged in order to facilitate respect for those of differing cultures and worldviews (Atkinson et al. 1998; Baruth and Manning 1999; Ponterotto 2001). In the absence of this, there is the real danger of consciously or unwittingly viewing the disorders of culturally different clients as being curable only if they were to discard their own culturally maladaptive ways of being and adhere to those of the therapist's culture (Lee and Ramirez 2000). For example, consider an Anglo-American male therapist and his African American female client, who is conflicted about accepting a lucrative job that would require her to leave her family's hometown and move to a distant city. He might believe that this conflict could be eliminated if she ignored her culturally valued stance of familism and collectivism in favor of an individualistic frame of reference that typifies his own culture.

This potential clash between the values and worldviews of therapists and clients is accentuated in brief therapy, in which therapists—in their concern for brevity—may promote symptom relief over goals that are more relevant for culturally different clients. The brief therapist may rapidly diagnose depression and introduce the idea of antidepressant medication, for example, heedless of the cultural implications of such diagnosis and treatment of mental illness. It is not unusual, for example, for international clients to regard the therapist as a wise doctor who can provide advice on life questions. The introduction of emotional exploration and treatments for diagnosed conditions—so basic to the therapist's worldview—may frustrate the legitimate needs of such clients.

At the same time, it should be acknowledged that certain culturally sanctioned beliefs are incompatible with basic assumptions of psychotherapy treatments. These include things such as acceptance of abuse of one individual by another or a requirement that people relinquish the right to have individual identities with unique thoughts and feelings. There are limits, even in psychotherapy, to behaviors and standards that can be unconditionally accepted. It is important to admit that psychotherapy itself does have a cultural component and a worldview, although it may be broad. The worldview encompasses a set of beliefs about the conditions leading to human discomfort and unhappiness. Such beliefs, even though supported by research evidence, may on occasion conflict with the dictates of a particular culture. In the end, clinicians need to decide in each case where to draw the line between being sensitive to cultural practices and offering support for basic human rights.

Instead of ignoring "the elephant in the room"—or worse, becoming convinced that there is no elephant in the room—the divergent worldviews of therapists and clients may be used as a valuable therapeutic tool to elicit and subsequently process potentially beneficial transferential and countertransferential material that may relate to the effects of gender, race or ethnicity, socioeconomic status, religion, sexual orientation, and so on as they impinge on the client's well-being (Cuéllar and Paniagua 2000; Sue and Sue 1999). For example, a male homosexual client with issues surrounding self-acceptance and the lifelong perception of others' condemning his sexuality may benefit greatly from clinical interaction with a heterosexual male therapist who might represent society's institutionalized discrimination against homosexuality. However, this is likely not to be the case if the therapist is unwilling to explore his own ingrained views about his own identity and his beliefs and biases about homosexuality and instead vehemently insists that he perceives his client as "nothing more than a person, just like any other client." The dual problem with this view, of course, is, first, the danger of ignoring what may be an important identity to the client, representing a key determinant of many of his attitudes and behaviors. Second, subtle, inadvertent forms of sexism or insensitive comments and behaviors may occur in therapy as a result of the therapist failing to come to grips with his own identity and experiences that differ from, and may be antagonistic to, the client's (Ponterotto 2001; Sue and Sue 1999). Either or both of these hypothetical circumstances can lead to breakdowns in the therapeutic alliance and thus are counterproductive to clinical change.

Multicultural Clinical Competence at the Graduate and Professional Levels

Failure to recognize the importance of cultural variables and to integrate multicultural perspectives into clinical practice may be directly attributable to the lack of attention paid to these issues in graduate training and continuing education programs despite multiple admonitions to the contrary by many mostly ethnic minority scholars, researchers, and professional organizations (American Psychological Association 1993; Hall and Barongan 1997; Lee and Ramirez 2000). Some have called for the development of multicultural clinical competencies at the graduate and professional levels for psychotherapists. Some training programs have made significant strides in including multicultural training as part of their curricula, yet most have made few changes. In addition, there exists a large group of mental health professionals who were trained long before issues of culture were ever discussed as a serious topic (Baruth and Manning 1999; Bernal and Castro 1994; Lee and Ramirez 2000).

Data suggest that many psychotherapists do not perceive themselves to be competent enough to work with culturally different clients, even though many of them have received some form of multicultural training at the graduate and postgraduate levels (Allison et al. 1996). Often, multicultural perspectives are relegated to optional courses within graduate curricula or are covered during one session (many times at the end of the semester) in graduate seminars in a disjointed manner, making it difficult for students to integrate the material presented with other required topics such as psychopathology, assessment, and practica. Many scholars and researchers have additionally pointed to the underrepresentation of culturally diverse faculty in graduate training programs as a predictor of the lack of minority courses offered, the minimal amount of culturally diverse research produced by the program, and the limited number of culturally diverse students recruited, retained, and graduated from the program (Bernal and Castro 1994; Hall and Barongan 1997).

If therapists lack multicultural competence in time-unlimited therapies, they can hardly be expected to be able to integrate culturally informed assessments and interventions into their short-term work. In the manualization of many brief therapies, little, if any, attention has been paid to multicultural competence, reinforcing the impression that cultural factors are not central to the helping process. Indeed, the entire notion of manualization runs counter to the notion that therapy should be tailored to the varied needs, values, and worldviews of patients.

Ultimately, it is the responsibility of therapists to assess their own comfort level and self-perceived competence in working with diverse populations. An accurate self-appraisal will generally lead to the conclusion that we are fundamentally unprepared to provide adequate services to individuals who are culturally different than we are. This recognition does not make us "bad" or incompetent; it just means that we are aware of our limitations and have some work to do. In some cases, it means that our most responsible course of action is to refer the patient. This is particularly true in the case of linguistic differences. In other cases, it may mean that we need to secure additional training in the form of self-study, attending workshops and seminars, and consultation with other professionals more knowledgeable in the particular culture. Perhaps the best type of additional training is seeking supervision from a colleague who is recognized to be expert in the area. This training is suggested for all clinicians, not just those from the majority culture. Sometimes minority culture practitioners assume that they are competent to work with minority populations because they themselves are from an underrepresented group. Minority status, in and of itself, is not an indication of multicultural competence.

Conclusion

We live in an increasingly diverse society that demands appropriate mental health services for all of its constituents. The integration of multicultural perspectives into psychotherapy (and assessment) may seem daunting and at times overwhelming, especially in short-term therapies. As we all know, it is easier to maintain the status quo than it is to question our abilities and perhaps change our practices. However, we believe that the inclusion of cultural perspectives into each of the psychotherapeutic approaches discussed in the previous chapters of this book will improve the effectiveness of these approaches with culturally different clients.

Just as contemporary research has focused on identifying common elements across psychotherapies that facilitate clinical change, integrating multicultural competencies into training and practice can contribute to increasing effective mental health service delivery among culturally different clients. The continued failure to do so can only portend the development of an even wider chasm between psychotherapy and multicultural populations in the United States and provide a disservice to the very people who place their care in our trust.

References

Allison KW, Echemendía RJ, Crawford I, et al: Predicting cultural competence: implications for practice and training. Prof Psychol Res Pr 27:386–393, 1996

American Psychiatric Association: Diagnostic and Statistical Manual of Mental Disorders, 2nd Edition. Washington, DC, American Psychiatric Association, 1968

American Psychiatric Association: Diagnostic and Statistical Manual of Mental Disorders, 3rd Edition. Washington, DC, American Psychiatric Association, 1980

American Psychological Association: Guidelines for providers of psychological services to ethnic, linguistic, and culturally diverse populations. Am Psychol 48:45–48, 1993

Atkinson DR, Morten G, Sue DW: Counseling American Minorities, 5th Edition. Boston, MA, McGraw-Hill, 1998

Baruth LG, Manning ML: Multicultural Counseling and Psychotherapy: A Lifespan Perspective, 2nd Edition. Upper Saddle River, NJ, Merrill, 1999

Bernal ME, Castro FG: Are clinical psychologists prepared for service and research with ethnic minorities? Report of a decade of progress. Am Psychol 49:797–805, 1994

Cross WE: Shades of Black: Diversity in African-American Identity. Philadelphia, PA, Temple University Press, 1991

Cuéllar I: Cross-cultural clinical psychological assessment of Hispanic Americans. J Pers Assess 70:71–86, 1998

Cuéllar I, Paniagua FA (eds): Handbook of Multicultural Mental Health. San Diego, CA, Academic Press, 2000

Fontes LA: Sexual Abuse in Nine North American Cultures: Treatment and Prevention. Thousand Oaks, CA, Sage, 1995

Gopaul-McNichol S, Brice-Baker J: Cross-Cultural Practice: Assessment, Treatment, and Training. New York, Wiley, 1998

Hall GCN, Barongan C: Prevention of sexual aggression: sociocultural risk and protective factors. Am Psychol 52:5–14, 1997

Harris J, Echemendía R, Ardila A, et al: Cross cultural competencies and neuropsychological assessment, in Handbook of Psychoeducational Assessment. Edited by Andrews J, Janzen H, Saklofske D. San Diego, CA, Academic Press, 2001, pp 391–414

Lee RM, Ramirez M: The history, current status, and future of multicultural psychotherapy, in Handbook of Multicultural Mental Health. Edited by Cuéllar I, Paniagua FA. San Diego, CA, Academic Press, 2000, pp 279–309

Negy C: Limitations of the multicultural approach to psychotherapy with diverse clients, in Handbook of Multicultural Mental Health. Edited by Cuéllar I, Paniagua FA. San Diego, CA, Academic Press, 2000, pp 439–453

Patterson CH: Multicultural counseling: from diversity to universality. J Couns Dev 74:227–231, 1996

Ponterotto JG: Handbook of Multicultural Counseling, 2nd Edition. Thousand Oaks, CA, Sage, 2001

Spence JT, Helmreich RL: Masculinity and Femininity: Their Psychological Dimensions, Correlates, and Antecedents. Austin, University of Texas Press, 1978

Steenbarger BN: A multicontextual model of counseling: bridging brevity and diversity. J Couns Dev 72:8–15, 1993

Sue DW, Sue D: Counseling the Culturally Different: Theory and Practice, 3rd Edition. New York, Wiley, 1999

Szasz TS, Reiman J, Chambliss WJ: Constructing difference: social deviance, in Sociology: Exploring the Architecture of Everyday Life. Edited by Newman DM. Thousand Oaks, CA, Pine Forge Press/Sage, 1995, pp 121–150

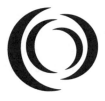

10

Combining Brief Psychotherapy and Medications

Mantosh J. Dewan, M.D.

For many patients with a variety of disorders, brief psychotherapy by itself is very effective. However, for some patients, the judicious use of medications in addition to brief therapy allows for—or accelerates—change. Furthermore, several excellent studies that have compared psychotherapy alone and medications alone with the combination of psychotherapy and medication have reported two important findings: 1) the combination is better than either treatment alone, and 2) biological symptoms (e.g., sleep disturbance, agitation) generally respond better to medications, whereas psychological and interpersonal deficits are more effectively treated with psychotherapy (reviewed in Barlow et al. 2000; Dewan and Pies 2001; Keller et al. 2000). Therefore, therapists need to constantly update their biopsychosocial understandings of their patients and repeatedly evaluate whether their patients would be best treated by psychotherapy or medications or a combination of both.

In this chapter, I present guidelines for the use of medications and then address the psychological effects on the therapist and patient of adding medications to brief psychotherapy. Psychotherapy by itself is a complex procedure that requires great skill to perform competently and has the potential for both benefit and harm. Adding another modality (medication) and another partner (a prescribing physician) requires an even greater sensitivity and skill on the part of clinicians. I recommend steps to foster effective collaboration among the treatment triad—the patient, the therapist, and the prescribing physician—so that change can proceed both efficiently and forcefully.

Evaluating the Need for Medication

During the initial evaluation, the brief therapist may decide that medications could be helpful. Severe symptoms (e.g., panic attacks) may prevent a willing patient from actively engaging in brief behavior therapy. Medication could quickly relieve these crippling panic symptoms and allow for psychotherapy to proceed. Similarly, patients exhausted and drained from days of not having slept, eaten, or taken a break from struggling with the consequences of acute trauma may benefit from a few days of medications to help them sleep before they can actively participate in brief therapy.

During the course of brief therapy, dealing directly with their trauma or fears may exacerbate patients' symptoms and make them unable to function in therapy and/or in their lives. These patients may benefit from short-term, targeted medications to treat their disabling anxiety (e.g., benzodiazepines) or even the micropsychotic episodes of borderline personality disorders (e.g., low-dose antipsychotics). Medication should be given only if patients' symptoms prevent them from being active in psychotherapy at that moment. After medication makes symptoms (e.g., sleep medications for a person with an acute grief reaction, short-term use of benzodiazepines for a patient experiencing panic attacks) more manageable, patients often return to the active focus of brief psychotherapy.

At the end of brief therapy, nonresponders and patients with significant residual symptoms may benefit from a trial of medications. This is supported by a small study of depressed patients who were unaffected by cognitive therapy but then responded to an antidepressant. The reverse also has been shown to be true: after a trial of antidepressants was ineffective, brief therapy was helpful in treating residual symptoms and nonresponders. Furthermore, even after medications have been effective, adding specific brief therapies may help prevent relapse, such as cognitive-behavioral therapy for patients with depression and exposure and response prevention for obsessive-compulsive disorder (reviewed in Dewan and Pies 2001).

Medications also should be considered when the patient expresses a strong preference for them. It is appropriate to educate them on their options and to point out (if this pertains) that for many conditions, brief psychotherapy alone is as effective as medication, generally has fewer side effects, and can have a shorter treatment course (e.g., 10 sessions of interpersonal psychotherapy for depression compared with a yearlong course of antidepressant medications). In some disorders, brief psychotherapy also is more effective than medications in preventing relapse (e.g., when behavior therapy for obsessive-compulsive disorder is stopped, significantly fewer relapses occur than when effective medications such as the serotonin reuptake inhibitors are discontinued).

Psychological Meaning of Medications

The old proverb "A cigar is not *just* a cigar" can be rephrased as "A pill is not *just* a pill." Each patient and therapist brings his or her own unique and personal attitudes toward medications. Therefore, therapists must carefully assess their own reasons for considering medications and also look for reactions—both obvious and covert—and the psychological meaning that these medications have for each particular patient.

Some patients derive a psychological benefit from being given medications, because they consider it a caring, nurturing act that feeds their dependency needs or validates their suffering as genuine. Other patients may see the prescription of medications as an imposition of external control or as a statement by the therapist that they are not strong enough to solve their problems by themselves. These feelings may contribute to noncompliance with both medications and brief therapy. I have also seen patients who are desperately denying the severity of their symptomatology and dysfunction. Offering them medications means that they have to confront their worst nightmare and acknowledge that they are "very sick," perhaps even psychotic (Dewan 1992).

Not offering medications is also interpreted in different ways. Some patients view it in a positive way because they believe that the therapist "must be interested in me as a person and not just in my symptoms" or that the therapist thinks that "I am competent enough to do it by myself." Angry and dependent patients, however, may regard it in a negative way because the therapist is believed to be withholding support or prolonging their agony. This is particularly potent because our culture vigorously promotes the false idea that a pill can fix everything, with patients frequently asking for a specific (but sometimes unrelated) drug because "my friend takes it, and she is doing well." Other patients feel that they are not being taken seriously or are not considered sick enough or even that the therapist thinks that they are faking their symptoms.

Some patients so overvalue their medication that they will carry around the unfilled prescription as a soothing—and often very effective!—good-luck charm or transitional object.

Psychotic patients, in particular, also may have an idiosyncratic association to the name of a medication. One of my patients was vehemently opposed to taking Stelazine (trifluoperazine) ("I hate it! It reminds me of my sister Stella.") but graciously agreed to take an equivalent drug, Mellaril (thioridazine), saying, "That's fine. It will make me mellow, right, Doc?" (Dewan 1992).

Therapists, like patients, also have strong biases and reactions toward the use of medications. Some therapists are absolutely opposed to certain medication groups, most commonly the benzodiazepines, because they believe that they are addicting, and they will deprive patients of them even when they could be enormously helpful and prescribed safely. The therapist's unrecognized feelings (countertransference), be they fear, hate, or sexual attraction toward a particular patient, may unfairly dictate the addition of medication as a way of distancing, controlling, or even punishing the patient.

Although these distortions may not be overtly discussed in brief therapy, therapists must be aware of the possibilities because they sometimes serve as a powerful distraction from the agreed-on therapeutic focus.

Fostering Collaboration Within the Clinical Triad: Patient, Nonphysician Therapist, and Prescribing Physician

Setting the Stage

Although psychiatrists can provide both therapy and medications themselves, most brief therapy is done by nonphysician therapists. Because medications are frequently combined with therapy, collaborative treatment is common. Collaboration between disciplines has many advantages for the patient and the collaborators. The patient receives greater amounts of time and expertise, which may lead to better adherence to medications and a more active participation in brief therapy. Collaboration provides an invaluable opportunity for mutual professional and emotional support on an ongoing basis but especially at times when the patient is in crisis.

It is essential that the therapist and the psychiatrist build a mutually trusting and respectful relationship, one that clearly recognizes the special and differing skills that each partner brings to the collaboration (Balon 2001). Furthermore, the therapist and psychiatrist must clarify the important elements of their practice: clinical orientation, who will provide what part of the treatment, how to contact each other after hours and during vacation coverage (the therapist and psychiatrist should not cover each other; each should provide someone from his or her own discipline), how emergencies will be handled, and confidentiality.

The patient needs to know that all information will be shared between the collaborating partners and should sign appropriate releases at the outset. There is no place for "secrets." For example, the patient says to the therapist, "Don't tell the doctor, but I have stopped taking his horrible medication, even though I tell him that I am taking it," or to the psychiatrist, "I do not feel like my therapist listens to me, so I don't tell her about cutting myself." If the patient shares something "in confidence," warning bells should go off (Meyer and Simon 1999). Given this scenario, it is common and even advisable for a therapist and a psychiatrist to get to know the backgrounds and practices of, learn to respect, and then cross-refer to each other.

Making the Referral

It is important that the therapist set the stage appropriately with the patient about the referral for medication consultation. The therapist should summarize the need for medications by describing to the patient the troublesome clinical symptoms that are to be targeted, the research data that suggest medications are likely to be helpful, and the fact that medication is an added resource to improve outcome. Unless the patient is psychotic, I present the medication consultation as a useful adjunct to the more important work being done, which is the brief therapy. Patients need to be told explicitly that the consultation may or may not result in medication being prescribed.

It is important that the referral be for an open-ended consultation and not for a specific medication. "If you agree, we will ask Dr. D to consult with us on whether medications may be helpful to you at this time" is more appropriate than "I think you should be taking Prozac. I will refer you to Dr. D." The therapist may in fact be correct that the patient needs an antidepressant and may indeed have a strong preference for a particular one, but sharing this with the patient is inappropriate and almost always antagonizes the prescribing physician. This recommendation may, however, be conveyed directly to the physician.

It is best when therapists obtain a consultation proactively rather than when they feel they are "stuck," at a therapeutic impasse, or when they have discovered the patient to be at high risk for suicide or homicide and want to "pass on the risk." Sometimes a managed care company pressures a therapist to get a medication consultation if it judges that the patient is not improving quickly enough. When the psychiatrist agrees with the therapist and decides to recommend medications, it is important to again explain the reasons to the patient and then to discuss the available options. Given that patients have very personal reactions to medications, the specific medication is best chosen as a collaborative venture to improve adherence. How to take the medication, expected improvement, and potential side effects are clearly described and perhaps even written down so that both the patient and the therapist are aware of them. The schedule for follow-up appointments is also clearly spelled out (Himle 2001).

After the first or second appointment, the psychiatrist and therapist need to communicate directly, share their impressions, and agree on a treatment plan. The psychiatrist is expected to support the psychosocial treatment plan and refrain from recommending changes in it to the patient (e.g., "I think that solution-focused therapy would be more effective than the behavior therapy you are receiving."). If the psychiatrist thinks that a change is needed, he or she may recommend this only to the therapist. Furthermore, the consulting psychiatrist must not be drawn into discussing psychotherapeutic issues with the patient. Likewise, therapists are expected to fully support the medication regimen and are an important ally in improving adherence. If the therapist disagrees with or wants to change medications, this discussion should take place directly with the physician and not indirectly through the patient. Similarly, specific questions from the patient about medications should be referred back to the prescribing physician (Himle 2001).

It takes a great deal of effort to keep the clinical triad "on the same page." Interdisciplinary tensions, honest differences in clinical approach, and a lack of time to keep regularly in touch all potentially stress the therapist–psychiatrist relationship. Some patients with a penchant for splitting may quickly aggravate the situation. The functional triad often deteriorates into two parallel dyads. Besides the obvious (i.e., the therapist and psychiatrist must invest in an ongoing relationship), we have found that doing the initial medication evaluation as a triad (i.e., having the therapist present) allows for all parties to evaluate the symptoms, agree on a treatment plan, and assign roles in an open manner, thereby minimizing distortions and fostering a collaboration that allows for maintaining the focus on therapeutic goals.

Conclusion

Therapists who provide long-term therapy will inevitably have some patients in combined treatment. Even therapists who primarily do brief therapy will have some patients who are taking medication. Many patients will be receiving both treatments from the start (e.g., a psychotically depressed patient taking an antipsychotic and/or antidepressant plus undergoing brief cognitive or interpersonal therapy). Some patients will start in brief therapy alone and may need medication added (e.g., a benzodiazepine being added to brief behavior therapy to control panic attacks) during the course or at the end of therapy for residual symptoms. Others will benefit from brief therapy after a course of medications. For instance, some patients with obsessive-compulsive disorder are initially unable to tolerate the treatment of choice, exposure and response prevention behavior therapy. Medications are used to bring symptom relief before the addition of exposure and response prevention therapy, which usually is then better tolerated. It is heartening that several brief therapies and medications are available to bring relief to our patients. It is essential that therapists and psychiatrists know the biopsychosocial aspects of their patients well, recognize the powerful treatment options that are available, and tailor their treatments (singly and in combination, either simultaneously or sequentially) to the patient's needs according to the available clinical and research evidence rather than maintain an old-fashioned adherence to ideology.

When combining brief therapy and medication, therapists must be aware that the simple dyadic relationship (therapist–patient) of psychotherapy alone has been converted into two complex, overlapping triadic relationships—therapist–patient–medication and therapist–patient–prescribing psychiatrist—each with powerful psychological dynamics. A thoughtful and often energetic engagement is required by all partners to avoid the many potential pitfalls and to benefit from the rich promise of medications and collaborative care.

References

Balon R: Positive and negative aspects of split treatment. Psychiatric Annals 31:598–603, 2001

Barlow D, Gorman J, Shear K, et al: Cognitive-behavioral therapy, imipramine, or their combination for panic disorder. JAMA 283:2529–2536, 2000

Dewan M: Adding medications to ongoing psychotherapy: indications and pitfalls. Am J Psychother 66:102–110, 1992

Dewan MJ, Pies RW (eds): The Difficult-to-Treat Psychiatric Patient. Washington, DC, American Psychiatric Publishing, 2001

Himle J: Medication consultation: the nonphysician clinician's perspective. Psychiatric Annals 31:623–628, 2001

Keller M, McCullough J, Klein D, et al: A comparison of nefazodone, the cognitive behavioral analysis system of psychotherapy, and their combination for the treatment of chronic depression. N Engl J Med 342:1462–1470, 2000

Meyer D, Simon R: Split treatment: clarity between psychiatrists and psychotherapists, part 2. Psychiatric Annals 29:327–332, 1999

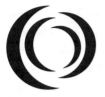

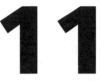

Evaluating Competence in Brief Psychotherapy

John Manring, M.D.
Bernard Beitman, M.D.
Mantosh J. Dewan, M.D.

A trainee reads this book, observes experts present the art and science of their craft, uses each of the six specific brief therapies in work with a few patients, and is carefully supervised. Is the trainee now demonstrably competent in brief psychotherapy?

As part of a broader movement in medicine to use outcome-based and evidence-based treatments, there is now increasing pressure from the public (via government), health insurers, and certification agencies to show that trainees actually learn what training programs claim they are teaching them. But how does one dependably test competence in something as complex and varied as psychotherapy? We have much yet to learn about which aspects of these psychotherapies are essential for them to be effective, which are sufficient, and which go beyond what is required to facilitate therapeutic change in a patient. As a result, we cannot define what the minimum is that one must *do* to have a successful outcome. Thus, we are left with two problems: what to measure and how to measure it. In this chapter, we present some basic building blocks in these two areas that may allow programs to construct their own competence assessments.

What to Measure: Enumerating Skills Needed for Competence in Psychotherapy

Lacking research data and consensus, the field has turned to experts to help define those skills believed to be important for effective brief therapy (e.g., the American Association of Directors of Psychiatric Residency Training [AADPRT] Psychotherapy Task Force, the Association of Directors of Psychology Training Clinics [ADPTC] Practicum Competencies Workgroup). In Chapter 12 (see Tables 12–1 through 12–3), Steenbarger et al. present a list of skills deemed common to all schools of brief therapy and match them to the three phases of therapy. Another set of *general* psychotherapy skills, based on the work of the AADPRT group[1] and Beitman and Yue (1999), which are deemed necessary but *not* sufficient, include abilities to manage boundaries, to develop a therapeutic alliance, to listen, to handle emotions and be understanding, to use supervision, to deal with obstacles to therapy, and to intervene therapeutically.

Some believe that the more specifically we can define these skills (e.g., the ability to begin and end a session on time as a specific task within the global skill "to manage boundaries"), the more likely psychotherapy will be effectively taught and learned. For this reason, several groups have distilled general psychotherapy skills into their smallest identifiable units, the acquisition of which will lead to competent performance of psychotherapy (Bienenfeld et al. 2000). Three examples are illustrative:

- *Boundaries*—The ability to 1) establish and maintain a treatment frame (e.g., setting schedules and sticking to times, dealing with outside agencies and relationships), 2) establish and maintain a professional relationship, 3) protect patient privacy and confidentiality, and 4) appropriately handle financial arrangements with the patient

---

[1]AADPRT Psychotherapy Task Force: David Goldberg, Ron Reider, Ron Krasner, and Lisa Mellman. Further refined by Carol Bernstein and New York University faculty and Hinda Dubin and University of Maryland faculty.

- *Therapeutic alliance*—The ability to 1) establish rapport and a therapeutic alliance with the patient, 2) enable the patient to actively participate in the treatment, 3) recognize and repair disturbances in the alliance, and 4) establish a treatment focus
- *Techniques of intervention*—The ability to 1) maintain focus in treatment; 2) confront a patient's statement, affect, or behavior and assess his or her response; and 3) assess readiness for and manage termination of treatment

To convert the previously mentioned *necessary* skills into skills *sufficient* for effective *generic* brief therapy, sets of additional skills have been prescribed by several groups. One, by Steenbarger et al., is presented in Chapter 12 (Tables 12–1 through 12–3); another, by Beitman and Yue (1999), requires

- *Verbal interventions*—The ability to use a broad array of verbal interventions, including providing hope, reassurance, information and guidance, reflection, interpretation, and confrontation; focus the patient; promote the patient's identification of feelings, thoughts, and behavior patterns; and encourage and reinforce change
- *Identifying patterns*—The ability to use inductive reasoning to generalize from specific pieces of information to patterns of behavior, feelings, or thoughts that fit the patient; are viewed by both the patient and the therapist as needing change; and, once changed, lead to the desired outcome
- *Strategies for change*—The ability to 1) recognize three *stages* of change—relinquishing dysfunctional patterns, initiating functional patterns, and maintaining functional patterns; 2) identify the three *orders* of change—helping a patient do something different, helping a patient alter a pattern in a way that generalizes to new situations, and teaching the patient to change patterns without the help of a therapist; 3) identify the five domains of patient functioning—emotion, cognition, behavior, interpersonal, and system; and 4) use a sufficient breadth of techniques in each domain to help patients change

Additional skill sets will be required for the specific brief therapies. For instance, the AADPRT group (L. Mellman and E. Beresin, co-chairs, AADPRT Psychotherapy Task Force [AADPRT-list@aadprt.org]; July 3, 2000) suggested the following abilities for brief cognitive-behavioral therapy:

1. State the cognitive model.
2. Socialize the patient into the cognitive model.

3. Use structured cognitive model activities (mood check, bridging to prior session, agenda setting, homework review, capsule summaries, and patient feedback).
4. Identify and elicit automatic thoughts.
5. State and employ knowledge of cognitive triad of depression.
6. Use dysfunctional thought records as a tool in therapy.
7. Identify common cognitive errors in thinking.
8. Use activity scheduling as a tool in therapy.
9. Use behavioral techniques as a tool in therapy.
10. Plan booster, follow-up and self-help sessions appropriately with patients when terminating active therapy.

Listing specific skills sufficient for effective brief therapy is an important start toward learning these skills; to certify competence, we still must decide which skills are essential, whether all skills are necessary, or whether some critical mass or percentage of the skills is required for competence. Unfortunately, these questions remain to be answered by empirical research.

How to Measure It: Tools to Assess Competence

Competent is defined as "suitable, sufficient, or adequate" (*Webster's 20th Century Unabridged Dictionary*, 2nd Edition). It may be helpful to think about competence on a continuum of increasing skill as described in the Dreyfuss model of skill acquisition (Figure 11–1).

Significantly, competent is a skill level *midway* between novice and expert. The implication, therefore, is that a trainee may not need to master all the skills of psychotherapy to be considered competent.

Once we agree on the list of skills necessary for competence in psychotherapy, how do we assess adequacy or competence in each of these skills? The Accreditation Council for Graduate Medical Education (ACGME—the parent certifying body for all medical specialties) constructed a "toolbox" of 13 "best methods" for evaluating competence in all aspects of medical education (ACGME Outcomes Project 2000). In the following subsections, we list seven methods most applicable to the brief psychotherapies.

Written Examination

The familiar printed or computer-based multiple-choice questionnaire examination is designed not only to sample easy-to-recollect facts and knowledge but also to evaluate a candidate's understanding of the sub-

	Novice	→	Beginner	→	Competent	→	Proficient	→	Expert
Learning issues	Isolated facts, some choices		Some synthesis, self-control		Independence, identity		Professional norms, patient centered		Internalized
Learning methods	Lectures, laboratories, faculty control		Seminars, laboratories, supervised work		Realistic work setting		Specialized training, socialization		Self-managed
Evaluation method	Tests		Simulations		Real evaluations, portfolios		Work-related markers		Self-assessment, internalized standards

Figure 11–1. Competence on a continuum of increasing skill as described in the Dreyfuss model of skill acquisition.

ject. In a computer adaptive test, fewer test questions are needed because statistical rules are programmed into the computer to quickly measure the examinee's ability, and the test is stopped when the candidate has clearly proven his or her ability. Comparing test scores on in-training examinations with national norms can identify strengths and limitations of individual trainees to help them improve. Comparing test results aggregated for trainees in each year of a program can be helpful to identify training experiences that might be improved. Multiple-choice questionnaire examinations are universally used for in-training examinations and for initial certification. Although the multiple-choice questionnaire is useful for testing knowledge, it cannot evaluate subtle interactions and cannot be the sole device used to assess competence in psychotherapy.

Chart-Stimulated Recall Oral Examination

A chart-stimulated recall examination uses the trainee's case record, "process notes," or tapes as the basis of a standardized oral examination of the care provided, probing for reasons behind the diagnoses, interpretations of clinical findings, and treatment plans. Examiners rate the trainee with a well-established protocol and scoring procedure. Reliability ranges from 0.65 to 0.88. For instance, a trainee's videotapes from several stages of treatment (e.g., initial interview, selection of a focus, use of strategies for change, termination) could provide an accurate record of a trainee's skills and decision making. Trained examiners would follow a standard protocol to orally examine a single case or a "portfolio" of the trainee's work (discussed in "Portfolios" later in this chapter). Drawbacks can arise in the expense of equipment, acquiring informed consent, and examining a sufficient number of stages of therapy in an adequate range of patients in the various schools of therapies. No data are available on chart-stimulated recall and psychotherapy; however, this is a promising technique for both evaluation and teaching, different versions of which are currently operational at McMaster University (Hamilton, Ontario, Canada).

Checklist Evaluation

Checklist evaluation consists of using a list of essential or desired specific behaviors, activities, or steps that make up a more complex skill. Research supports the usefulness and reliability (0.7–0.8) of checklists for evaluation of patient care skills (e.g., history taking) and for interpersonal and communication skills when directly observed by a trained rater. Checklists are developed by expert consensus. Criteria for evaluating performance benefit from descriptive "anchor points." Earlier in this chapter and in Chapter 12, we present several lists of skills believed to be essential for brief therapy. Some simple tasks lend themselves to checklists, but many of them (e.g., ability to establish rapport or a therapeutic alliance) represent complex abilities that cannot be broken down into their component skills. Therefore, their evaluation by checklists may not be valid, and we are left in the uncomfortable position of saying that we cannot define competence precisely but that "we recognize it when we see it." If carefully constructed and tested for validity and reliability, checklists could be effective tools for evaluating actual or recorded trainee therapy sessions (see "Portfolios" later in this chapter).

Global Rating of Live or Recorded Performance

Global rating forms are distinguished from other rating forms in that 1) a rater judges general categories of ability (e.g., interpersonal and communication skills) instead of specific skills, tasks, or behaviors; and 2) the ratings are completed retrospectively based on general impressions collected over time (e.g., end of a clinical rotation) and derived from multiple sources of information (e.g., direct observations or interactions; input from other faculty, trainees, or patients; review of work products or written materials). Rating scales are numeric but presented as qualitative indicators (e.g., outstanding=1, good=2, fair=3, poor=4). Written comments allow evaluators to explain their ratings. Global ratings of patient interviews directly observed by trained examiners are currently used in the oral examination portion of the American Board of Psychiatry and Neurology certification process and in many training programs.

With global ratings, scores can be highly subjective and biased with untrained raters. However, global rating forms can be easily constructed and can be completed quickly. Reliability and validity improve when standards are created and "anchors" (i.e., examples of behaviors or attitudes) for each point on the scale are provided.

Portfolios

A portfolio is a collection of products prepared by the trainee that provides evidence of learning and achievement related to training goals. It typically contains written documents (e.g., logs and transcripts) but can include video or audio recordings. It can include statements about what has been learned, its application, and remaining learning needs and how they can be met. In graduate psychotherapy training, a portfolio might include a log of diagnoses treated, a log of therapies used, a summary of the research literature reviewed when selecting a treatment option, a quality improvement project, descriptions of ethical dilemmas faced and how they were handled, or a recording or transcript of interactions with patients. The contents of a portfolio do not have to be standardized, because the purpose is to show individual learning gains relative to individual goals. A portfolio is also one of the best tools for combining teaching with assessment of continuity-of-care concerns that are the essence of psychotherapy. Developing protocols for assessing such portfolios would be crucial to the reliability of such assessments.

360-Degree Evaluation Instrument

The 360-degree evaluation instrument is a questionnaire completed by multiple people in a trainee's sphere of influence (e.g., superiors, peers, subordinates, patients, and families). Used in business, military, and education settings, this method is an appealing one for collecting reliable, primary outcome data. However, it is difficult to design a single questionnaire for rating a trainee's brief therapy skills that is appropriate for use by supervisors, co-trainees, clinic staff, patients, and families, because each is looking for something different from the trainee and is likely to use and understand language differently. Also daunting is the administrative complexity of distributing and collecting the forms and quantifying the results meaningfully. However, with sufficient resources, the 360-degree evaluation instrument has the potential to become a powerful tool.

Simulations and Models

A wide array of simulations used for assessment of clinical performance closely imitate reality and allow examinees to reason through a clinical problem, make life-threatening errors without hurting a real patient, and obtain instant feedback so that they can correct a mistake in action. Simulations can be used to rate performances on clinical problems that are difficult to evaluate effectively in other circumstances. Simulation formats have been developed as paper-and-pencil branching problems (patient management problems), computerized versions of patient management problems called *clinical case simulations*, role-playing situations (e.g., standardized patients), clinical team simulations, and combinations of all formats. Experts set the scoring rules.

To build a simulation, clinical experts craft scenarios from real patient cases to focus on specific skills. Technical experts then create scripts for standardized patients or computer-based simulations and add, when feasible, automated scoring rules. Simulations are expensive to create. None are currently available for assessing the nuances of psychotherapy. However, simple clinical vignettes to assess the recognition and handling of psychotherapeutic phenomena have been incorporated into the Columbia Psychodynamic Psychotherapy Skills Test (a multiple-choice examination). We expect that the rich literature on simulation and gaming (Meyers et al. 1999; Satish et al. 2001) will power the development of sophisticated and useful computerized simulations of the more subtle aspects of therapy in the future.

Evaluating Competence in Brief Therapy Today

Brief psychotherapy is a complex interplay of interpersonal skills and therapeutic techniques played out during 2–20 sessions over weeks to a year. No obvious method is available to adequately evaluate the art and science of an ongoing relationship. How, then, can we best use the ACGME toolbox and the list of skills developed by experts to certify competence?

A review of several models that already exist may be helpful. At McMaster University in Canada, they teach seven brief therapies using manuals (except for psychodynamic therapy) to increase fidelity. Audio- or videotaped sessions are assessed in weekly supervision. For supportive, cognitive-behavioral, interpersonal, and family therapy, trainees present recordings of early and late sessions for each specific therapy, which are evaluated with standardized scales for rating the therapeutic relationship (e.g., the Working Alliance Inventory and the Truax Empathy Scale) and the technical competence of the therapist (e.g., the Cognitive Therapy Scale and the Therapist Strategy Rating Form for interpersonal therapy, Weerasekera 1997, 2003).

Beitman and Yue (1999) took a very different approach at the University of Missouri. From their detailed list of skills considered important for competent psychotherapy, they culled the essential ones to construct a portfolio (see below). All skills are not tested, yet a trainee completing the portfolio requirements satisfactorily will likely be at least competent in the brief therapies and will, of necessity, have learned a great deal in the process.

Another, more comprehensive approach may include

- *Periodic examinations* at the end of a module, quarterly, or yearly. Knowledge is tested by giving multiple-choice questionnaire examinations with clinical vignettes (e.g., Columbia Psychodynamic Competency Psychotherapy Test [formerly called Columbia Psychodynamic Psychotherapy Skills Test]). Clinical skills can be tested cross-sectionally by administering an oral examination based on tapes, live patient interviews, or simulations, which are used to probe reasons behind formulations and treatment plans. Trained examiners score the examination according to a standardized protocol.

- *Weekly supervision*, a powerful tool for teaching and evaluating therapy because it is a longitudinal process. Supervisors can improve the validity of their evaluations by using "anchored" global ratings to periodically assess knowledge and clinical skills. Trainees can be rated on both a list of key skills common to all therapies and skills specific to a therapy being practiced (e.g., behavioral or solution focused).
- *Portfolios*, which create a permanent record of requirements met (e.g., a "minimum clinical expectation" of having treated three patients with at least two specific brief therapies) and the objective demonstration (e.g., via tapes) of specific skills. Examples of portfolios assembled over long periods of training and used at the University of Missouri at Columbia include

1. A Counseling Self-Estimate Inventory, a 37-item Likert-scaled questionnaire about the trainee's attitudes and skills, every 3 months
2. Both a trainee and a patient version of the Working Alliance Inventory, a 12-item rating scale to assess the state of the therapeutic alliance
3. Two analyses of psychotherapy sessions in which the trainee categorizes each intervention as to mode of response as well as his or her own intention; these analyses are then compared with later sessions for the variety of interventions used
4. A description of five boundary violations with specific cases based on an Exploitation Index, another Likert-scaled questionnaire of 32 thoughts, feelings, or behaviors that may lead to boundary violations
5. A vignette from the trainee's own cases of how a stressor became the focus of brief therapy, and a vignette of psychodynamic as well as cognitive-behavioral patterns evident in the same case
6. Examples from the trainee's own practice of transference, resistance, and countertransference
7. Copies of two dysfunctional thought records from the trainee's own patients and two examples illustrating cognitive distortion, to show use of cognitive therapy
8. Two brief descriptions of the relationship between past experiences and current difficulties, to show understanding of psychodynamics
9. Two examples of finding a focus with two patients in brief therapy
10. Global Evaluations of Trainee Change (a single-item rating scale from "very poor" to "excellent") by supervisors every 3 or 6 months

11. Two vignettes in which the supervisor stops the tape or transcript and the trainee provides an empathic summary of what the patient has just said, to assess ability for supportive psychotherapy

The portfolio can be strengthened by the addition of two 360-degree evaluations (or at least the subjective and objective rating of patient outcome). This could help show that a trainee's competence correlates with good patient outcome. The reliability of portfolios would be enhanced by training raters in the application of rating criteria to each aspect of the portfolio to ensure consistent evaluation across portfolios.

Finally, as controlled trials inform us about which psychotherapies are effective for which problems and the behaviors and techniques specific to those psychotherapies, we will become more specific about what we expect from a competent trainee. We are optimistic that we will also be able to construct sophisticated computer models of the psychotherapeutic situations that call on those essential skills. Until then, we will likely be best served by a broad-based portfolio with multiple-choice questionnaire examinations, global ratings of ongoing supervision, and recorded samples that show specific technical skills (especially helpful when anchored by successful patient outcomes) and by tolerating the ambiguity (we hope for only a bit longer) that has been an integral part of our profession from its inception. Fortunately, despite all the distracting "noise" in the system, research consistently shows that patients do benefit from brief therapy, even when provided by trainees.

References

ACGME Outcomes Project: Toolbox of Assessment Methods, Version 1.1. September 2000

Beitman BD, Yue D: Learning Psychotherapy. New York, WW Norton, 1999

Bienenfeld D, Klykylo W, Knapp V: Process and product: development of competency-based measures for psychiatry residency. Acad Psychiatry 24:2, 2000

Meyers H, Dorsey K, Benz E: DxR Patient Simulation Software. Carbondale, IL, DxR Development Group, Copyright 1992–1999

Satish U, Streufert S, Barach P: Assessing and improving medical competency: using strategic management simulations; and improving medical care: the use of simulation technology. Simulation and Gaming 32:156–174, 2001

Weerasekera P: Postgraduate psychotherapy training. Acad Psychiatry 21:122–132, 1997

Weerasekera P: Competency-based psychotherapy training: can we get there? Annual meeting, American Association of Directors of Psychiatric Residency Training, San Juan, Puerto Rico, March 2003, p 24

Part III

Overview and Synthesis

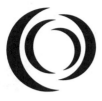

12

Doing Therapy, Briefly

Overview and Synthesis

Brett N. Steenbarger, Ph.D.
Roger P. Greenberg, Ph.D.
Mantosh J. Dewan, M.D.

In the preceding chapters of this book, readers have encountered six models of brief therapy that have been successfully incorporated into training efforts in the mental health professions. In cognitive therapy, behavior therapy, solution-focused brief therapy, brief interpersonal therapy, time-limited dynamic therapy, and cognitive-behavioral couple therapy, we can observe the broad scope of the art and science of short-term intervention. As we suggested in Chapters 1 and 8, significant overlaps are found among these models. The brief therapies are not fundamentally different from time-unlimited therapies; rather, their uniqueness stems from their efforts to accelerate change processes through careful patient selection, maintenance of a well-defined therapeutic focus, and a high level of involvement and activity on the parts of therapists and patients.

This concluding chapter draws on the six preceding models to derive a set of core competencies underlying brief therapeutic practice. It is hoped that this effort can inform efforts in the mental health professions to assess both therapist skill and the outcomes of training efforts, issues highlighted in Manring et al., Chapter 11, in this book. Although each specific model of brief work necessarily uses these competencies differently, in this chapter, we propose that the following three skill sets form the backbone of what it means to be a competent practitioner of brief therapy.

Skill Set One: Relationship Skills

As Greenberg emphasized in Chapter 8, the alliance between therapist and patient is a hallmark of effective therapy in all examined therapies. *The brief therapist must have the same core relationship skills that are essential to all forms of counseling and therapy but—given time limitations—must be particularly active in fostering and maintaining the positive working alliance.*

The various chapter authors note that their approaches to change hinge on the formation of a successful working alliance between therapist and client. Indeed, as Stuart, Chapter 5, and Levenson, Chapter 6, noted, brief work becomes very difficult, if not impossible, when patients lack an interpersonal history and attachment styles conducive to the ready formation of an alliance. A term used by many of the authors is *collaborative;* the short-term therapist actively involves patients in all phases of planning and implementing the treatment. In Chapter 7, Baucom and colleagues, for example, noted that it would be overwhelming for therapists and clients to tackle all facets of a couple's life. Therapists work collaboratively with couples to identify the facets most central to their presenting complaints and establish these as targets for change. Once achieved, these focal changes can spill over to other areas of life for individuals and couples, as stresses are lowered and methods for dealing with problems are learned.

In cognitive and behavior therapies, the alliance is furthered by efforts at psychoeducation: educating clients about the origins of problems, the rationale for therapy, and the methods used. Stuart's description of the short-term therapist as a "benevolent expert" captures the dual roles of support agent and change agent in brief work. Thus, in solution-focused brief therapy, for example, goal setting is accomplished in a highly interactive, collaborative mode, cementing the alliance even while framing the instrumental ends of treatment.

This active alliance building includes the core therapeutic elements of warmth, genuineness, and empathy found among all successful helping interventions. Brief work goes beyond these elements, however, in fostering an active sense of involvement among clients, a tangible sense of teamwork that pervades each phase of the helping process. Brief therapy done well is not done *to* a patient but *with* that patient. It is truly, in the tradition of cognitive therapy, "collaborative empiricism," in which the participants share responsibility for examining and modifying patterns of thought, feeling, and behavior. To accomplish this, the brief therapist must be able to foster an environment conducive to such endeavors. As Baucom et al. (Chapter 7) observed in brief couple work, the short-term therapist must be a facilitator, creating a sense of safety that permits the exploration of difficult issues.

Students in the mental health professions often learn their craft in a mode in which time is not an explicit dimension of treatment planning. This confers both advantages and disadvantages. On the positive side, learning therapy without time pressures allows one to cultivate basic relationship skills—in essence, learning to crawl before walking or running. On the negative side, the absence of time constraints tends to remove an element of urgency from therapists, allowing them to rest on their warm, caring laurels rather than actively pursuing a collaborative stance. Table 12–1 proposes several markers of competent collaborative behavior across the brief therapies. These can be modeled and assessed in training, even in settings where much of the work may not be limited by time. This table and Tables 12–2 and 12–3 organize the markers by the proposed stages of change in brief work outlined in Chapter 1. The resulting matrix may be particularly helpful for readers' self-assessments, providing a broad heuristic of "to do" tasks in brief work.

In Chapter 9, Echemendía and Núñez raised cultural awareness as an important dimension of brief work, given the diverse expectations that clients bring to therapy. Collaboration proceeds differently when English is the second language of a client or when clients come to therapy with significant concerns over the ability to trust a therapist who is of a different gender, race, or nationality. Once again, the active, collaborative stance of short-term work transcends a mere avoidance of racial or cultural stereotypes or broad and bland efforts to convey "respect." Rather, patients are treated as informants who educate therapists in their distinctive values, traditions, and beliefs. Blindly applying a cognitive-behavioral model of assertiveness training to a client whose cultural background emphasizes deference to one's elders, for example, can court only unfavorable outcomes. The competent brief therapist who notes conflicts in this client's home must be educated in the ways such domestic difficulties *are*

Table 12–1. Markers for relationship skills among brief therapists

Engagement phase

✓ The therapist shows warmth, genuineness, and empathy toward clients in the process of eliciting background information.

✓ The therapist actively engages clients in educative efforts that describe how problem patterns are formed and how they are addressed in therapy, responding helpfully to client questions and concerns.

✓ The therapist is actively educated by clients, eliciting an understanding of how the unique educational, socioeconomic, cultural, racial, and gender backgrounds of clients help to shape their experience.

✓ The therapist actively seeks the involvement of clients in framing the means and ends of therapy, making sure that there is a shared understanding of the responsibilities and expectations for both parties.

Discrepancy phase

✓ The therapist actively delivers and solicits feedback during the course of therapy, ensuring that change efforts move at a pace appropriate to each client.

✓ The therapist avoids complicated and negative transference reactions and resistances rather than focusing on them.

Consolidation phase

✓ The therapist maintains a collaborative stance even at the end of treatment, opening the door for intermittent visits and ongoing assistance as needed and desired.

successfully resolved in the client's culture. Ensuring that clients are co-contributors to therapeutic means and ends is an important way in which the cultural congruence of helping efforts can be sustained.

An examination of the six clinical chapters finds broad acceptance of the idea that brief therapy does not treat all problems or all facets of personality. It is accepted that short-term intervention starts a change process, without necessarily completing it, that "cure" is not the goal of therapy. The collaboration that marks the conduct of short-term work also permeates its completion, as therapists replace the notion of "termination" with the idea of intermittent visits. Stuart (Chapter 5) and Levenson (Chapter 6), for example, noted the value of intermittent therapy in brief interpersonal therapy and time-limited dynamic therapy, drawing on the analogy between brief therapy and family practice. The goal, Hembree and colleagues noted in Chapter 3, is to make the patient an expert in his or her own treatment. In Chapter 2, Beck and Bieling described this as teaching patients to become their own therapists. A key task of the therapist, Baucom and associates observed in Chapter 7, is to help couples become better observers and evaluators of their own patterns. By making the therapist available for "booster" sessions, short-term treatments maintain a collaborative stance even after regularly scheduled meetings have ended. Stuart's notion of dividing therapy into two phases, acute and maintenance, makes sense in this regard, with the maintenance phase extending indefinitely to accommodate future needs.

Finally, the notion of collaboration also highlights what brief therapists do *not* do. Whereas longer-term practitioners may involve themselves in lengthy analyses of resistances and transference reactions, brief therapists are apt to view such forays as counterproductive. In Chapter 4, Steenbarger noted, for example, that solution-focused brief therapists take pains to define goals in user-friendly ways, so as to ensure client participation in tasks and exercises. Similarly, in Chapter 5, Stuart observed that brief interpersonal therapists assiduously avoid the development of transference responses that would detract from the primary therapeutic focus. Even in time-limited dynamic psychotherapy, in which transference is actively used, the emphasis is not on an analysis of the transference but on the provision of new relationship experiences in the here and now. In Chapter 6, Levenson cited research from Strupp and colleagues that found suboptimal therapeutic outcomes in therapies that feature transference interpretation. Such an emphasis may unwittingly contribute to a divide between therapist and client, rupturing the teamwork essential to successful short-term work. In Chapter 8, Greenberg echoed the research-supported notion of noxious effects stemming from an overemphasis on transference interpretations.

Skill Set Two: Instrumental Skills

The active goal orientation of brief therapy was a universal theme sounded by the chapter authors. *The brief therapist must be task focused, actively gathering information that aids in determining the appropriateness of short-term work and in selecting and maintaining a proper therapeutic focus.*

As we noted in Chapter 1, brief therapy is not appropriate for all clients or presenting concerns. Chronic and severe problems, particularly those that are accompanied by disruptions in the ability to form relationships, tend to require sustained intervention and support. In such cases, brief treatments may be useful but will be conducted in sequential fashion to achieve long-term ends, as in the dialectical behavior therapy of Linehan (1993). Levenson, in Chapter 6 on time-limited dynamic psychotherapy, identified several factors that guide the application of her brief work. She stressed that patients must be in a state of emotional discomfort, must be able to engage the therapist in an examination of relationship patterns, and must be capable of forming meaningful relationships. In a similar vein, Stuart, in Chapter 5, noted that brief interpersonal therapy is difficult in patients with Axis II disorders because these disorders often reflect difficulties in forming and maintaining relationships that necessarily interfere with the creation of a ready therapeutic alliance.

Another indication for brief therapy noted by Stuart is client motivation. This is intimately linked to the issue of client distress because individuals in a state of discomfort are most likely to possess the motivation to actively sustain change efforts. Some of the brief models discussed in the preceding chapters, including behavior therapy, cognitive therapy, and solution-focused brief therapy, make considerable use of homework assignments as part of the helping process. This requires a meaningful degree of client motivation. Indeed, Hembree and colleagues (Chapter 3) cited evidence that suggests a linkage between homework completion and positive outcomes in behavior therapy. The brief therapist's assessment of client suitability for short-term work, therefore, should include a frank discussion with the patient as to whether between-session efforts at change will be feasible. If the client is ambivalent about change, or if he or she is so emotionally overwhelmed that homework completion is not possible, then brevity is unlikely to be achieved in treatment. Similarly, if the client lacks a support system that encourages the completion of homework and the ends of treatment—or if such a lack leads the client to seek ongoing support rather than change efforts from the therapist— therapy is unlikely to be completed in a brief duration.

Table 12–2 proposes that an important marker of competence in brief work is a thorough assessment as to these indications and contraindications for brevity. In Chapter 1, we suggested six factors that can form the basis for such an assessment, forming the acronym *DISCUS*: Duration of the presenting problem, Interpersonal history of the client, Severity of the presenting problem, Complexity of the problems that are presented, degree of Understanding and motivation possessed by the client, and degree of Social support enjoyed by the client. Certainly, other formulations of inclusion and exclusion are possible. What is important is that clients who need more extensive intervention be promptly routed to the most promising forms of assistance. In Chapter 10, Dewan cited evidence that indicates superior therapeutic outcomes for particular problems when psychopharmacological interventions (medications) are blended with psychosocial ones (psychotherapy). This can be helpful in working with clients who have had recent traumatic stresses or acute levels of distress associated with panic disorder. The use of a medication to control overwhelming anxiety often makes it possible for a client to focus on the aims of short-term work. The same DISCUS criteria that are useful in

---

Table 12–2. Markers for instrumental skills among brief therapists

Engagement phase

✓ The therapist conducts a thorough assessment of the factors associated with indications and contraindications for brief therapy, making proper referrals and/or treatment planning decisions with clients who would benefit more from other extended forms of treatment.

✓ The therapist conducts a focused and structured assessment of client concerns to help formulate potential goals for short-term therapy.

✓ The therapist ensures that goals are stated in a clear and concrete manner, so that they are unambiguously understood and endorsed by all parties to the helping process.

Discrepancy and consolidation phases

✓ The therapist facilitates activities during each session to ensure that the goal orientation is sustained, including redirection when sessions lose their focus, summaries of session progress, and assignment of tasks and exercises.

✓ The therapist enters each session with a mutually understood and flexible "game plan" derived from the client's goals and ensures that this plan is either implemented as intended or modified as needed.

---

framing contraindications for brief work can be of value in determining when consideration should be given to pharmacological therapies.

The second function of a careful assessment is the determination of a concrete focus for treatment. If there was one theme that was sounded unanimously among the chapter authors, it was the importance of establishing and maintaining a focus to keep therapy time-effective. Very often, this focus is established through a structured evaluation that ensures that all relevant aspects of client experience are addressed. In Chapter 2 on cognitive therapy, Beck and Bieling stated that the evaluation is conveyed through a cognitive conceptualization diagram that outlines automatic thought patterns, their origins, and their consequences. Levenson (Chapter 6) described the formulation of cyclical maladaptive patterns in providing a blueprint for time-limited dynamic psychotherapy; Stuart (Chapter 5) used an interpersonal inventory to assess relationship needs in brief interpersonal work; and Steenbarger (Chapter 4) described how formula first-session tasks are used to provide an initial assessment of client goals.

These structured assessment methods provide a high degree of focus for client evaluations. The idea is to engage in a rapid pattern search (Beitman and Yue 1999) to aid in the formulation of mutual goals that can quickly proceed to an action phase of treatment. Such methods, being standardized, also ensure that new therapists cover the most important areas for assessment within their particular modality, a training goal consistent with mandates for ensuring therapist competence noted by

Manring and colleagues in Chapter 11. Here, again, the analogy with family medicine seems apt. For established patients who do not have significant illness, a family physician is unlikely to conduct an entire history and physical, or even an exhaustive review of systems. Rather, the assessment will lightly touch on the various systems but focus on the areas of particular patient complaint. A similar assessment, highlighting the particular areas of client concern, guides the brief therapist once clients have been screened to determine the appropriateness of short-term work. This tailored assessment facilitates an efficient movement from assessment to goal formation to intervention.

Finally, a related marker of competence for the brief therapist is the formulation of goals in highly concrete terms. This helps ensure that client and therapist share an understanding of the ends of treatment—a factor important to the alliance—but also allows therapy to proceed time-effectively by keeping sessions "on task." Indeed, many of the brief therapies are highly structured to ensure such a goal orientation. In Chapter 3, Hembree et al. noted that relatively little talking and much doing occur in behavior therapy, with the doing structured by methods such as the creation of anxiety hierarchies for use in desensitization. Beck and Bieling (Chapter 2) similarly spoke of using graded tasks and therapist summaries in cognitive therapy to maintain a concrete goal orientation. Baucom et al. (Chapter 7) described the targeting of focal relational patterns, with interventions aimed at guided behavior change and skills development. Goals are also stated concretely and behaviorally in solution-focused brief therapy, with the assignment of specific tasks to maintain the focus between sessions. Indeed, Steenbarger (Chapter 4) noted that solution-focused work is so structured that it can be captured in a flow diagram, a characteristic also shared by many manualized therapies, including behavioral, interpersonal, and cognitive modalities. In no small measure, brief therapy is able to achieve brevity thanks to its circumscribed focus and concrete goal orientation. This leaves less room for lengthy digressions, explorations, and discussions that can dilute change efforts in time-unlimited treatments.

Although this structured approach has clear advantages, important caveats exist. One of these, noted in the work of Prochaska et al. (1994), is that not all clients are ready for active change. They come to therapy in a state of relative ambivalence, unsure of whether they want or need to make the efforts to alter long-standing patterns. Clients also may enter therapy too emotionally overwhelmed to undertake the ongoing commitment needed to define and work on therapeutic goals. Another caveat, highlighted by Echemendía and Núñez in Chapter 9, is that clients may come to therapy with needs different from those of their therapists, particularly needs shaped by their gender or culture. A client who pursues therapy for support and understanding may be frustrated by treatments that consist of highly instrumental tasks and exercises. Standardized assessments may be so focused that they fail to evaluate the very personal and sociocultural factors that help define a person's individuality.

What this means is that the competent brief therapist walks a continual tightrope. On the one hand, therapy must actively build and maintain an alliance. The therapist's work is thus highly collaborative and user-friendly. On the other hand, the therapist must be especially task focused, both in assessment and in intervention. To be sure, brief therapy is not unique in blending these expressive and instrumental demands. Teachers and parents, to name but two common examples, often must provide directive guidance even as they maintain strong affective and collaborative bonds. The element of time constraint in brief work, however, lends a particular note of challenge. The competent brief therapist must be caring and collaborative in a goal-oriented manner, continuously maintaining a mutually forged game plan for change.

Skill Set Three: Change-Agency Skills

In brief therapy, the ideal of the therapist-as-blank-screen is replaced by the notion that therapists serve as active change agents. *The brief therapist must possess a range of skills that evoke patterns of client thought, feeling, and behavior in the here and now, providing opportunities for an understanding and reworking of these patterns.*

A common theme among the chapter authors is that change efforts are accelerated and enhanced by the creation of active learning experiences both in and out of session. Levenson's (Chapter 6) quotation from Fromm-Reichmann, indicating that what patients need are experiences rather than explanations, goes to the heart of the matter. In no small measure, the differing forms of brief therapy appear to be "technologies" for generating novel learning experiences for clients. An important marker for competence in brief therapy, as Table 12–3 suggests, is the ability to transcend mere talking about problems by creating opportunities to actually experience and rework these.

Trauma provides an illustrative, if painful, example of the power of emotional learning, as vivid experiences shatter long-standing behavior patterns and even personality characteristics. The "corrective emotional experiences" identified by Alexander and French (1946) are, in a sense, *positive traumas*, bypassing normal critical, conscious awareness and exercising a relatively direct emotional imprinting. It is noteworthy that the

---

Table 12–3.   Markers for change-agency skills among brief
therapists

Engagement phase

✓   The therapist elicits existing problem patterns, including their
accompanying thoughts, feelings, and behaviors, through sensitive inquiry,
imagery, and experiential methods.

Discrepancy phase

✓   The therapist takes active measures to ensure that the affective intensity of
sessions is neither so low that it fails to facilitate experiential learning nor so
high that it overwhelms patients and frustrates efforts at change.

✓   The therapist is intimately familiar with one or more therapeutic modalities
and the techniques used within these to evoke and rework problem patterns
and generate experiences of mastery.

✓   The therapist is flexible within his or her repertoire of therapeutic modalities
so that if one set of methods does not successfully evoke or rework old
patterns, then other methods can be readily employed.

Discrepancy and consolidation phases

✓   The therapist paces change efforts to provide support and structure and to
encourage client autonomy, with the primary locus of change efforts
gradually shifting from therapist-initiation to client-initiation.

✓   The therapist provides multiple contexts for rehearsing changes in client
patterns, so as to promote an internalization of new skills, insights, and
experiences.

---

primary mode of change in all of the brief modalities presented in this
volume is experiential; none primarily emphasizes dialogue and insight.
These, Hembree and colleagues (Chapter 3) noted, are *doing* approaches
to therapy and require the therapist to be far more active and directive
than is normally the case in time-unlimited treatment.

The provision of these powerful learning experiences has two facets.
The first is the evocation of current client patterns, accompanied by their
full range of emotion. In behavior therapy, for example, interoceptive exposure is used to evoke the very sensations of anxiety that have proven
troublesome. Cognitive therapy conducts collaborative behavioral experiments to allow patients to directly face their fears. In time-limited dynamic psychotherapy, client problems are evoked within the context of
the therapeutic interactions, as therapists willingly enter into their clients' cyclical maladaptive patterns. Tasks assigned in brief interpersonal
and solution-focused brief therapies invariably involve facing situations
that had proven challenging in the past. Cognitive therapists note that a
schema, to be modified, first must be activated. This appears to be a tru-
ism across the range of short-term modalities.

An important implication of this experiential component of brief work is that short-term interventions generally raise clients' levels of anxiety and discomfort before offering relief and resolution. Indeed, Hembree et al. (Chapter 3) noted that in their behavioral work, the duration of exposure is an important element in its success. Their sessions often extend well beyond the traditional therapeutic hour to facilitate this immersion. "The more the patient is affectively involved in therapy, the more likely he or she will be motivated to change behavior or communication style," Stuart (Chapter 5) noted of brief interpersonal therapy. The competent brief therapist must titrate this affective involvement, ensuring that therapy is "hot" enough to touch long-standing emotional and behavioral tendencies but not so heated that it threatens to traumatize or retraumatize patients. Maintaining the positive therapeutic alliance even during the heightening of discomfort is a vital marker of skill in brief work, reflecting an ongoing sensitivity to the experience of clients and the pacing of change efforts.

This makes particular sense if we view short-term therapy as a process of emotional learning. Like most learning processes, therapy will bog down if the tasks are too simple and insufficiently challenging. Conversely, if learning tasks are too challenging, the result is likely to be frustration and a sense of discouragement and failure. Bandura (1977) proposed that therapy provides experiences of mastery for clients by providing experiences that are challenging but within their reach. The most valuable aspect of successful brief therapy may be its ability to provide opportunities for individuals to directly face their problems and exercise a degree of mastery over these. This fits very well with research cited by Steenbarger, in which success in solution-focused work was associated with a client shift toward an internal locus of control. It also supports the use of guided discovery in the cognitive-behavioral couple therapy of Baucom and colleagues (Chapter 7), which "creates experiences for a couple so that one or both people may start to question their thinking and develop a different perspective on the partner and/or relationship." The challenge of the brief therapist is to facilitate sufficient activation of client patterns so that experiences of mastery can result but not so much activation that helplessness is unwittingly reinforced.

Such mastery building is an example of the second facet of providing powerful learning experiences: the introduction of novelty during these periods of emotional activation. As Levenson noted in Chapter 6 on time-limited dynamic psychotherapy, this novelty includes the provision of new understandings and new experiences. It is not enough to simply activate old problem patterns; this, by itself, would only replicate what is already occurring in the client's life. Rather, once these behaviors and their associated thoughts and feelings are stimulated, the short-term therapist must encourage the enactment of new, constructive actions to provide the requisite experience of mastery. This, as Table 12–3 notes, requires that competent brief therapists possess a sizable toolbox of methods designed to generate successful novel experiences.

The toolbox for cognitive therapists includes the use of graded tasks, activity monitoring, behavioral experiments, and coping cards. In solution-focused work, the therapist elicits novelty first by searching for exceptions within the client's own behavioral repertoire. If this fails, the therapist elicits hypothetical solutions by encouraging clients to use their imagination or draw on their observations of others. The toolbox for behavior therapy includes imaginal as well as in vivo exposure methods, with in-session efforts augmented by homework. Cognitive-behavioral couple therapy embraces a wide collection of tools for change, including those drawn from behavior, cognitive, dialectical behavior, and emotion-focused therapies. Use of interpersonal situations inside and outside of therapy to rehearse new communication patterns and solve problems is a central element in aiding clients to master grief reactions, interpersonal disputes, role transitions, and social sensitivity in brief interpersonal therapy. The ability to quickly use such toolboxes when old problem patterns have been activated requires an intimacy with the various models of short-term work that can be obtained only via intensive, dedicated training.

Echoing Greenberg in Chapter 8, whether a short-term therapist adheres to one approach or another may be less crucial to outcome than the ability to work consistently within *some* approach. Few, if any, data suggest that one particular modality of short-term work is consistently more efficacious than another across the broad range of patients and disorders. Without the guidance of a particular method, however, therapy may be fatally wounded. The presence of a specific method provides a treatment rationale and expectations for improvement that elicit the cooperation of clients and their commitment to the alliance. It also provides a ready-made toolbox for therapists—especially beginning ones—in the form of specific techniques that sustain a treatment focus, enhance client experiencing, and provide for the novel reworking of old patterns.

Although it is certainly possible for therapists to mix and match techniques from different therapies for a given client, this also runs the risk of devolving into incoherence. Conducting treatment behaviorally for anxiety one session, emphasizing insight and reworking of relational patterns the next meeting, and still later targeting dysfunctional cognitions suggests a lack of focus that almost certainly will prove confusing for clients. It is difficult to imagine that such "seat of the pants" treatment can provide the purposeful reworking of focal client patterns that is the hallmark of successful brief therapy. Integration, in the sense of mixing methods from various modalities, generally requires the cultivation of experience and expertise in each of these schools and an overarching *rationale* for the combination. Such eclecticism is a reasoned integration of modalities, not a substitute for them.

Finally, an important element in the practice of brief therapy is the ability to foster the generalization of changes once these have commenced. The successful brief therapist creates a variety of contexts for the enactment of new patterns so that these can be readily internalized. Some of these contexts are constructed within sessions, through means such as anxiety hierarchies and repeated behavioral experiments. Others are structured as out-of-session homework assignments and tasks. In brief interpersonal therapy and time-limited dynamic psychotherapy, for example, clients are encouraged to try out new interactional patterns in their social relationships as a means of cementing them. Change efforts may begin in the therapy office, but they quickly move beyond the four walls to tackle real-life situations. This contributes to the sense of mastery noted earlier and helps ensure that initial changes truly become part of the client's repertoire. The need to generalize change is similar to what Freud described as the "working through" process. Freud, however, relied on events and repeated patterns unfolding naturally in the client's life, whereas brief therapists seem to speed the process through actively prescribed tasks and techniques.

One way that short-term therapists facilitate this consolidation of emotional learning is by structuring sessions in an intermittent fashion once initial changes have taken root. Stuart's (Chapter 5) aforementioned division of brief interpersonal therapy into acute treatment and mainte nance phases is particularly noteworthy in this regard. None of the short-term methods outlined in this text emphasize the notion of "cure," followed by a complete "termination" of sessions. Rather, the family practice model noted by Stuart is the norm, with later sessions scheduled intermittently to allow for sufficient opportunity to apply insights, skills, and experiences generated within sessions. The pacing of change efforts is thus an important skill for the brief therapist. These efforts may begin on an intensive basis during the acute treatment phase of therapy and shift to intermittent visits during the maintenance phase. This change in pacing is accompanied by a movement in the relative locus of change efforts. Early in treatment, the therapist is particularly active in gathering information, structuring initial topics for inquiry, and proposing between-session exercises. As changes begin, clients naturally assume more of the responsibility for generalizing their gains by applying what they have learned from therapy. The goal of the work, as noted by Beck and Bieling in Chapter 2, is to teach patients to become their own therapists. A marker of competence among brief therapists is the ability to both take control and relinquish it, encouraging client autonomy while providing the support and structure needed for experiences of mastery. This blending of the directive/nondirective and supportive/challenging elements of treatment forms a great deal of the art of short-term work.

Conclusion

The goal of this book has been to give readers a taste of different brief therapies and their underlying strengths and similarities. Although reading a text cannot be expected to provide expertise in itself, it can start the process of applying new approaches and learning from this application. Ultimately, nothing substitutes for the observation and mentorship of experienced professionals. Learning short-term work is not unlike therapy itself: best learned by doing. Via workshops, tapes, and direct supervision, readers can examine their own patterns of practice and acquire new ways of assisting others.

In this chapter, we have outlined some of the specific elements that are associated with the skillful practice of brief therapy. Other formulations of therapist competence are possible and indeed have been proposed (see, for example, Beitman and Yue 1999). We hope that readers and researchers will refine and investigate these criteria, contributing to our understanding of how therapists can serve as effective and efficient change agents. Such a refinement promises much, anchoring training efforts in graduate and residency programs and enhancing our understanding of how therapist skills are best transmitted and developed. We are unlikely to ever completely unravel the artistry and science of brief therapy. To the extent that we can model the best therapists, therapies, and teachers, however, we may gain a measure of understanding that will enrich the lives of patients and therapists alike.

References

Alexander F, French TM: Psychoanalytic Therapy: Principles and Applications. New York, Ronald Press, 1946

Bandura A: Self-efficacy: toward a unifying theory of behavioral change. Psychol Rev 2:191–215, 1977

Beitman BD, Yue D: Learning Psychotherapy. New York, WW Norton, 1999

Linehan MM: Skills Training Manual for Treating Borderline Personality Disorder. New York, Guilford, 1993

Prochaska JO, Norcross JC, DiClemente CC: Changing for Good. New York, Avon, 1994

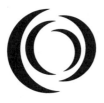

Index

*Page numbers printed in **boldface** type refer to tables or figures.*